Hormone Replacement Therapy *and* The Brain

The Current Status of Research and Practice

CONTROVERSIAL ISSUES IN CLIMACTERIC MEDICINE SERIES

Hormone Replacement Therapy *and* The Brain

The Current Status of Research and Practice

Edited by
A. R. Genazzani
Past President of the International Menopause Society
and
Chairman of the Division of Obstetrics and Gynecology
University of Pisa, Italy

Published under the auspices of
the International Menopause Society

The Parthenon Publishing Group
International Publishers in Medicine, Science & Technology

A CRC PRESS COMPANY
BOCA RATON LONDON NEW YORK WASHINGTON, D.C.

Library of Congress Cataloging-in-Publication Data

Data available on application

British Library Cataloguing in Publication Data
Hormone replacement therapy and the brain
1. Menopause - Hormone therapy. 2. Estrogen - Physiological effect 3. Dementia - Hormone therapy
I. Genazzani, Andrea
618.1′75′061

ISBN 1-84214-168-6
ISSN 1474-3930

Published in the USA by
The Parthenon Publishing Group Inc.
345 Park Avenue South
10th Floor
New York, NY 10010, USA

Published in the UK and Europe by
The Parthenon Publishing Group Limited
23–25 Blades Court, Deodar Road
London SW15 2NU, UK

Typeset by AMA DataSet, Preston, UK

Printed and bound by Butler & Tanner Ltd, Frome and London

Contents

Section VI: Hormone replacement therapy: effects on mood and behavior

Section VII: Menopause, hormone replacement therapy and psychiatric diseases

Section VIII: Cognition, memory, menopause and aging

Section IX: Hormone replacement therapy and neurological disorders

Section X: Selective aspects of specific therapies

List of principal contributors

J. M. Alt
Solvay Pharmaceuticals
Hans-Böckler-Allee 20
30173 Hannover
Germany

J. Angst
University of Zurich Psychiatric Hospital
Lenggstrasse 31
PO Box 68
8029 Zurich
Switzerland

T. Bäckström
Umea Neurosteroid Research Center
Department of Clinical Sciences, Obstetrics and Gynecology
Norrland University Hospital
Umea 90185
Sweden

S. L. Berga
Department of Obstetrics, Gynecology and Reproductive Sciences
University of Pittsburgh School of Medicine
300 Halket Street
Pittsburgh
PA 15213
USA

E. O. Bixler
Sleep Research and Treatment Center
Penn State University College of Medicine
500 University Drive
Hersey
PA 17033
USA

R. D. Brinton
Molecular Pharmacology and Toxicology
University of Southern California
Pharmaceutical Sciences Center
1985 Zonal Avenue PSC 502
Los Angeles
CA 90089
USA

H. U. Bryant
Department of Gene Regulation and Bone
d/c 0424
Lilly Corporate Center
Indianapolis
IN 46285
USA

V. P. Eymer
Mason, Ohio, USA
c/o A. Moufarege
Hormonal Development
Procter & Gamble Pharmaceuticals
Rusham Park
Whitehall Lane
Egham
Surrey TW20 9NW
UK

R. R. Freedman
Obstetrics, Gynecology, Psychiatry and Behavioral Neurosciences
Wayne State University SOM
C.S. Mott Center
275 E. Hancock Avenue
Detroit
MI 48201
USA

L. M. Garcia-Segura
Instituto Cajal
CSIC
Av. Dr. Arce 37
28002 Madrid
Spain

A. R. Genazzani
Department of Obstetrics and Gynecology
University of Pisa
Via Roma 35
56100 Pisa
Italy

P. W. Gold
Clinical Neuroendocrinology Branch
National Institute of Mental Health
Building 10, Room 2D-46
10 Center Drive (MSC 1284)
Bethesda
MD 20892-1284
USA

R. Guennoun
INSERM U488
80, rue du Général Leclerc
94276 Bicêtre
France

U. Halbreich
School of Medicine and Biomedical Sciences
SUNY at Buffalo, Haynes C, Suite 1
3435 Main Street, Building 5
Buffalo
NY 14214-3016
USA

V. W. Henderson
Reynolds Center on Aging
University of Arkansas for Medical Sciences
4301 W. Markham Street, #810
Little Rock
AR 72205
USA

H. Honjo
Department of Obstetrics and Gynecology
Kyoto Prefectural University of Medicine
465 Kajii-cho, Kawaramachi-Hirokoji
Kamigyo-ku
Kyoto 602-8566
Japan

P. M. Maki
Departments of Psychiatry and Psychology
Center for Cognitive Medicine
Neuropsychiatric Institute, Room 130G
University of Illinois at Chicago
912 S Wood St. MC913
Chicago
IL 60612
USA

E. Martignoni
Department of Medical Sciences
University of Piemonte Orientale
Via Solaroli 17
28100 Novara
Italy

M. Mauri
Department of Psychiatry, Neurobiology, Pharmacology and Biotechnologies
Psychiatric Section
University of Pisa
Pisa
Italy

R. C. Melcangi
Department of Endocrinology and Center of Excellence for Neurodegenerative Disorders
Via Balzaretti 9
Milan 20133
Italy

F. Naftolin
Department of Obstetrics and Gynecology
Yale University
333 Cedar Street, FMB 335
New Haven
CT 8063
USA

R. E. Nappi
Department of Obstetrics and Gynecology
IRCCS Policlinico S. Matteo
University of Pavia
Piazzale Golgi 2
27100 Pavia
Italy

A. Riecher-Rössler
Psychiatrische Universitatspoliklinik
Kantonsspital Basel
Petersgraben 4
4031 Basel
Switzerland

E. Sanna
Department of Experimental Biology
Section of Neuroscience and Center of Excellence for the Neurobiology of Dependence
University of Cagliari
090123 Cagliari
Italy

P. J. Schmidt
NIMH, Building 10
Room 3N238
10 Center Drive MDC 1276
Bethesda
MD 20892-1276
USA

E. R. Simpson
Prince Henry's Institute of Medical Research
Monash Medical Centre
PO Box 6125
Clayton
Victoria 3168
Australia

J. Studd
Department of Gynaecology
Chelsea and Westminster Hospital
369 Fulham Road
London SW10 9NH
UK

D. F. Swaab
Netherlands Institute for Brain Research
Meibergdreef 33
1105 AZ Amsterdam ZO
The Netherlands

E. Syková
Institute of Experimental Medicine AS CR
Videnska 1083
14220 Prague 4
Czech Republic

K. Yaffe
Department of Psychiatry, Neurology, Epidemiology and Biostatistics
University of California, San Francisco
Box 111G, 4150 Clement Street
San Francisco
CA 94121
USA

Introduction

The fact that the brain is a major target for sex steroid hormones has been known for many years, but a great amount of research has recently been carried out to clarify the different roles of estrogens, progesterone and androgens, both in basic experiments and in clinical studies.

The present book, the third volume in the Series on Controversial Issues in Climacteric Medicine, published under the auspices of the International Menopause Society, contains the presentations made at a Workshop held in Pisa, March 15-18, 2003, on 'HRT in Climacteric and Aging Brain'.

The brain cells, the aging process and the impact of aging on integrated brain functions are discussed in the introductory part of the book, in which the cells, mitochondrial function, the immune system, the brain aromatase and neurotransmitter systems are analyzed for their part in the aging process of neurons and glia cells.

As the volume analyzes the changes occurring through the climacteric transition and aging, estrogens, the effects of progesterone and androgens on different brain cells and different areas are covered in the section on the neurobiology of steroids and their receptors. Menopausal hot flushes and sleep disturbances are discussed as central symptoms of menopause, as well as the relationship between sex hormones and headaches in females and the impact of androgen deficiency syndrome on female sexuality.

The chapter on gender differences in affective disorders introduces a more analytic section on the effects of hormone replacement therapy on mood and behavior, in which estrogens, progesterone and androgens are discussed separately. The impact of the menopause on psychiatric diseases such as depression, anxiety, panic disorders and schizophrenia is extensively analyzed and discussed, as are the protective mechanisms of estrogens on cognition and memory.

The biological basis of menopause as a risk factor in dementing illness and the neuroendocrine aspects of aging and the effects of hormone replacement therapy provide the basis for analyzing the role of hormone replacement therapy as preventive therapy for Parkinson's disease and its significance in Alzheimer's disease.

The last section of the book examines specific aspects of selected therapies where the central effects of estrogens, androgens and SERMS are analyzed and discussed for their clinical activities in menopausal women and aging individuals.

For scientists, clinicians and students, this book provides extensive and valuable information and represents the state of the art of hormone replacement therapy in the climacteric and aging brain.

We wish to thank all the scientists and clinicians who have contributed in any way to the publication of this book.

Andrea R. Genazzani
Past President of the IMS

Glia and extracellular space in the aging brain

1

E. Syková

Aging, Alzheimer's disease and many degenerative diseases are accompanied by serious cognitive deficits, particularly impaired learning and memory loss. This decline in old age is a consequence of changes in brain anatomy, morphology and volume and functional deficits. Nervous tissue, particularly in the hippocampus and cortex, is subject to various degenerative processes including a decreased number and efficacy of synapses, a decrease in transmitter release, neuronal loss, astrogliosis, changes in astrocytic morphology, demyelination, deposits of β-amyloid and changes in extracellular matrix proteins[1–4]. These and other changes affect not only the efficacy of signal transmission at synapses, but also the functioning of glia and extrasynaptic ('volume') transmission mediated by the diffusion of transmitters as well as other substances through the volume of the extracellular space (ECS)[5-10]. This mode of communication without synapses provides a mechanism of long-range information processing in functions such as vigilance, sleep, chronic pain, hunger, depression, long-term potentiation (LTP), long-term depression (LTD), memory formation and other plastic changes in the central nervous system (CNS)[7,11,12].

Neurons interact both via synapses and by the diffusion of ions and neurotransmitters in the ECS. Since glial cells do not have synapses, their communication with neurons is mediated only by the diffusion of ions and neuroactive substances in the ECS. Neurons and glia release ions, transmitters and various other neuroactive substances into the ECS. Substances released non-synaptically diffuse through the ECS and bind to extrasynaptic, usually high-affinity, binding sites located on neurons, axons and glial cells.

Diffusion in the ECS is critically dependent on the structure and physicochemical properties of the ECS: the nerve cell microenvironment. These properties vary, however, around each cell and in different brain regions. Certain synapses ('private synapses') or even whole neurons are clearly tightly ensheathed by glial processes and by the extracellular matrix, so-called perineuronal nets[13]; others are left more 'naked'. These 'open' synapses are more easily reached by molecules diffusing in the ECS. On the other hand, many mediators, including glutamate and γ-aminobutyric acid (GABA), bind to high-affinity binding sites located at non-synaptic parts of the membranes of neurons and glia. Mediators that escape from the synaptic clefts at an activated synapse, particularly following repetitive stimulation, diffuse in the ECS and can cross-react with receptors in nearby synapses. This phenomenon, called 'cross-talk' between synapses caused by the 'spillover' of a transmitter (e.g. glutamate, GABA, glycine), has been proposed to account for LTP and LTD in the rat hippocampus[14,15]. This cross-talk between synapses, and the efficacy and directionality of volume transmission, could be critically dependent on the diffusion properties of the ECS.

There is increasing evidence that changes in neuron–glia interactions, for example glial coverage and/or the retraction of glial processes from synapses, occur during physiological and pathological functional changes in many brain regions. The glial environment of neurons is likely to be a key factor in the regulation of intersynaptic communication mediated by glutamate. For instance, most synaptically released glutamate is taken up by high-affinity transporters such as GLT-1 and GLAST, which are located on surrounding astrocytes[16]. Moreover, glial cells represent a diffusion barrier in the ECS, hindering the movement of neuroactive substances within the tissue[8,10,17].

Long-term changes in the physical and chemical parameters of the ECS accompany many physiological and pathological states, including CNS trauma and aging. The 'acute' or relatively fast changes in the size of the intercellular channels are apparently a consequence of cellular (particularly glial) swelling. Abrupt ECS volume decrease may cause 'molecular crowding', which can lead to an acute increase in tortuosity. Long-term changes in diffusion would require changes in ECS composition, either permanent changes in the size of the intercellular channels, changes in extracellular matrix molecules or changes in the number and thickness of cellular (glial) processes. Available data suggest that in some pathophysiological states, the extracellular space volume fraction (α) and tortuosity factor (λ) behave as independent variables. A persistent increase in λ (without a decrease in ECS volume) was found during astrogliosis[17,18] and in myelinated tissue[19], suggesting that glial cells can form diffusion barriers, make the nervous tissue less permissive and play an important role in signal transmission, tissue regeneration and pathological states. This observation has important implications for our understanding of the function of glial cells. The extracellular matrix apparently also contributes to diffusion barriers and to diffusional anisotropy, since its loss, such as during aging, correlates with a tortuosity decrease and a loss of anisotropy[3,4].

DIFFUSION PARAMETERS OF THE EXTRACELLULAR SPACE

The diffusion of substances in a free medium, such as water or diluted agar, is described by Fick's laws. In contrast to a free medium, diffusion in the ECS of the nervous tissue is hindered by the size of the extracellular clefts, the presence of membranes, fine neuronal and glial processes, macromolecules of the extracellular matrix and charged molecules, and also by cellular uptake. To take these factors into account, it is necessary to modify Fick's original diffusion equations[8,20]. First, diffusion in the CNS is constrained by the restricted volume of the tissue available for the diffusing particles, i.e. by the extracellular space volume fraction (α), which is a dimensionless quantity and is defined as the ratio between the volume of the ECS and the total volume of the tissue (V_{ECS}/V_{TOT}). It is now evident that the ECS in the adult brain amounts to about 20% of the total brain volume, i.e. $\alpha = 0.2$. Second, the free diffusion coefficient (D) in the brain is reduced by the tortuosity factor (λ). ECS tortuosity is defined as $\lambda = (D/ADC)^{0.5}$, where ADC is the apparent diffusion coefficient in the brain. As a result of tortuosity, D is reduced to an apparent diffusion coefficient $ADC = D/\lambda^2$. Thus, any substance diffusing in the ECS is hindered by membrane obstructions, glycoproteins, macromolecules of the extracellular matrix, charged molecules and fine neuronal and glial cell processes (Figure 1a). Third, substances released into the ECS are transported across membranes by non-specific concentration-dependent uptake (k'). In many cases, however, these substances are transported by energy-dependent uptake systems that obey nonlinear kinetics[21]. When these three factors (α, λ and k') are incorporated into Fick's laws, diffusion in the CNS is described fairly satisfactorily[20].

The real-time iontophoretic method is used to determine the ECS diffusion parameters and their dynamic changes in nervous tissue *in vitro* as well as *in vivo*[7,8]. Ion-sensitive microelectrodes (ISMs) are used to measure the diffusion of ions to which the cell membranes are relatively impermeable, such as tetraethylammonium (TEA^+), tetramethylammonium (TMA^+) or choline. These substances are injected into the nervous tissue by pressure, or by iontophoresis from an electrode aligned parallel to a double-barrelled ISM at a fixed distance. Usually, such an electrode array is made by gluing together an iontophoretic pipette and a TMA^+-sensitive ISM with a tip separation of 130–200 μm. In the case of iontophoretic application, the TMA^+ is released into the ECS by applying a current step of +100 nA with a duration of 40–80 s. The released TMA^+ is recorded with the TMA^+-ISM as a diffusion curve, which is then transferred to a computer. Values of the ECS volume, ADC, tortuosity and non-specific cellular uptake are extracted by a non-linear curve-fitting simplex algorithm applied to the diffusion curves (Figure 2).

By introducing the tortuosity factor into diffusion measurements in nervous tissue, it soon became evident that diffusion is not uniform in

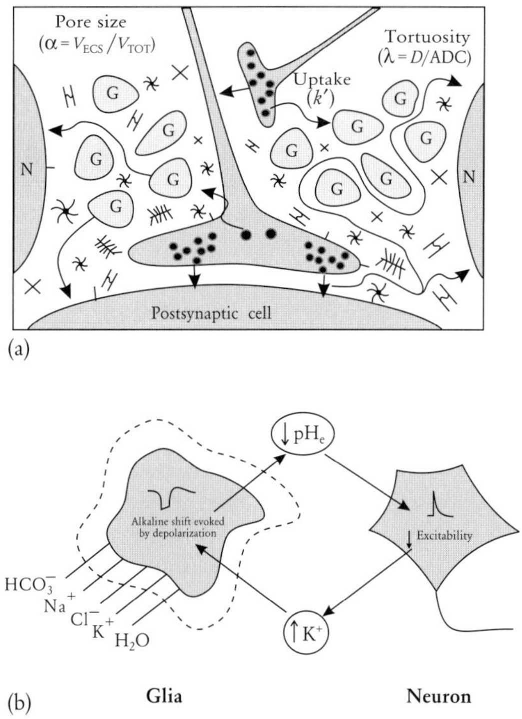

Figure 1 (a) Schematic diagram of central nervous system (CNS) architecture. The CNS architecture is composed of neurons (N), axons, glial cells (G), cellular processes, molecules of the extracellular matrix and intercellular channels between the cells. The architecture affects the movement (diffusion) of substances in the brain, which is critically dependent on channel size, extracellular space tortuosity and cellular uptake (see text for definition of variables). (b) Schematic diagram of the mechanism of non-specific feedback suppressing neuronal excitability. Active neurons release K^+ which accumulates in the extracellular space (ECS) and depolarizes glial cells. This causes an alkaline shift in glial pH_i (intercellular) and an acid shift in pH_e (extracellular). Extracellular acidosis further suppresses neuronal activity. Transmembrane ionic movements result in glial swelling, ECS volume decrease and, therefore, the greater accumulation of ions and neuroactive substances in the ECS

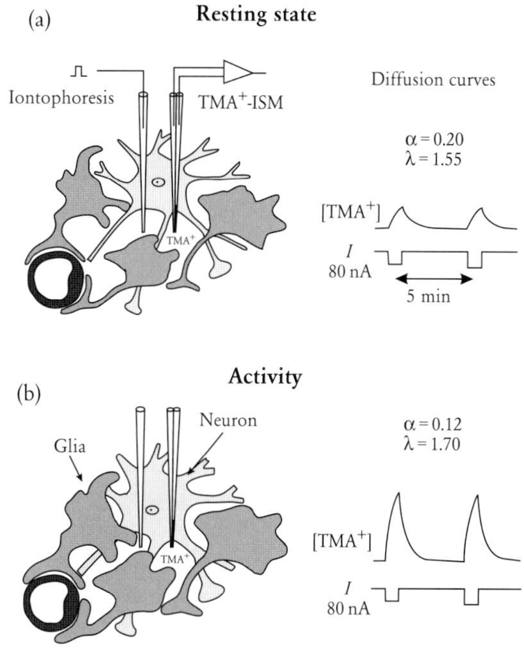

Figure 2 Experimental set-up, tetramethylammonium (TMA^+) diffusion curves and typical extracellular space (ECS) diffusion parameters α (volume fraction) and λ (tortuosity) in the central nervous system (CNS). Schematic diagrams of the experimental arrangement. A TMA^+-selective double-barrelled ion-selective microelectrode (ISM) was glued to a bent iontophoresis microelectrode. Separation between electrode tips was 130–200 μm. Typical TMA^+ diffusion curves obtained in unstimulated brain (a, resting state) and during stimulation (b, activity), evoked by the same iontophoretic current of 80 nA. ECS in unstimulated brain is 20% (volume fraction $\alpha = 0.20$) and tortuosity is about 1.55. When the ECS is smaller owing to cell swelling during activity, the diffusion curves are bigger. ECS volume, e.g. in spinal dorsal horn after tetanic stimulation of the sciatic nerve, may decrease to about 12% ($\alpha = 0.12$) while tortuosity increases ($\lambda = 1.70$)

all directions and is affected by the presence of diffusion barriers, including neuronal and glial processes, myelin sheaths, macromolecules and molecules with fixed negative surface charges. This so-called anisotropic diffusion preferentially channels the movement of substances in the ECS in one direction, (e.g. along axons), and may, therefore, be responsible for a certain degree of specificity in volume transmission. Diffusion anisotropy was found in the CNS in the molecular and granular layer of the cerebellum[22], in the hippocampus[23,24] and in the auditory but not in the somatosensory cortex[25], and a number of studies have revealed that it is present in the myelinated white matter of the corpus callosum or spinal cord[19,26,27]. It was shown that diffusion anisotropy in white matter increases during development. At first, diffusion in unmyelinated tissue is isotropic; it becomes more anisotropic as myelination progresses.

The second method that is also currently used to study ECS volume and geometry is diffusion-weighted magnetic resonance imaging (DW-MRI). DW-MRI provides information only about the apparent diffusion coefficient of water[28-32], and a relationship between an increase in the ADC of water and a decrease in ECS volume fraction has recently been found during brain injury[32] as well as during aging[33].

GLIAL CELLS AND EXTRACELLULAR SPACE DIFFUSION PARAMETERS DURING AGING

All transmembrane ionic shifts, for example K^+, Na^+, Ca^{2+} and H^+, and membrane transport mechanisms such as glutamate uptake, are followed by water movement, thus causing the shrinkage or swelling of neural cells including glia. Glial cells control ionic and volume homeostasis in the CNS by a variety of mechanisms[7,34,35]. Besides the Na^+/K^+ pump, ECS K^+ homeostasis is maintained by three other mechanisms brought about by glia: K^+ spatial buffering, KCl uptake and Ca^{2+}-activated K^+ channels.

Extracellular acid shifts are a consequence of activity-related extracellular K^+ increase; K^+ -induced glial depolarization results in an alkaline shift in glial pH_i (intercellular pH), which leads to the stimulation of classic acid extrusion systems in glial cells. The following non-specific feedback mechanism suppressing neuronal activity has been proposed in the CNS (Figure 1b). Neuronal activity results in the accumulation of $[K^+]_e$ (extracellular K^+); K^+ depolarizes glial cells, and this depolarization induces an alkaline shift in glial pH_i; the glial cells therefore extrude acid; and the acid shifts in pH result in a decrease in neuronal excitability. Furthermore, since the ionic movements are always accompanied by water, this feedback mechanism would be amplified by activity-related glial swelling, which is compensated by ECS volume shrinkage and by increased tortuosity, presumably due to the crowding of ECS matrix molecules and the swelling of fine glial processes. This would result in a greater accumulation of ions and other neuroactive substances in the brain owing to hindrances to their diffusion in the ECS[7].

Neuroactive substances, ions and neurotransmitters released into the ECS during neuronal activity or during pathological states interact not only with neuronal membranes at pre- or postsynaptic sites, but also with extrasynaptic receptors, including those on glial cells. Glial cells respond to such stimulation by the activation of ion channels, second messengers and intracellular metabolic pathways. Simultaneously, the cell volume of glial cells increases, including the swelling and rearrangement of their processes, thus causing dynamic variations in the ECS volume. Glial cells, in addition to their role in the maintenance of extracellular ionic homeostasis, may therefore influence extracellular pathways for the diffusion of neuroactive substances. In the CNS, many pathological processes are accompanied by the loss of nerve cells or their processes, by astrogliosis, manifested as an increase in glial fibrillary acidic protein (GFAP) staining, by demyelination and, in addition, by changes in the extracellular matrix. All these processes lead to changes in CNS architecture and may therefore affect the diffusion of neuroactive substances in the ECS. The mechanisms of the changes in ECS diffusion parameters have been studied during both normal and pathological states such as cell swelling evoked by the application of high K^+ or osmotic stress, astrogliosis induced by trauma (stab wound), gliogenesis blocked by early postnatal X-irradiation, gliosis in tissue grafts, demyelination (experimental autoimmune encephalomyelitis), degeneration and astrogliosis during aging (Figure 3)[10,12,35].

Morphological changes during aging include cell loss, the loss of dendritic processes, demyelination, astrogliosis, swollen astrocytic processes and changes in the extracellular matrix. It is reasonable to assume that there is a significant decrease in the ADC of many neuroactive substances in the aging brain, which accompanies astrogliosis and changes in the extracellular matrix. In aged rats the ECS volume fraction (α) is lower in the cortex, corpus callosum and hippocampus, which correlates with changes in astrocytes and in the extracellular matrix. One of the explanations as to why α in the cortex, corpus callosum and hippocampus of senescent rats is significantly lower than in young adults could

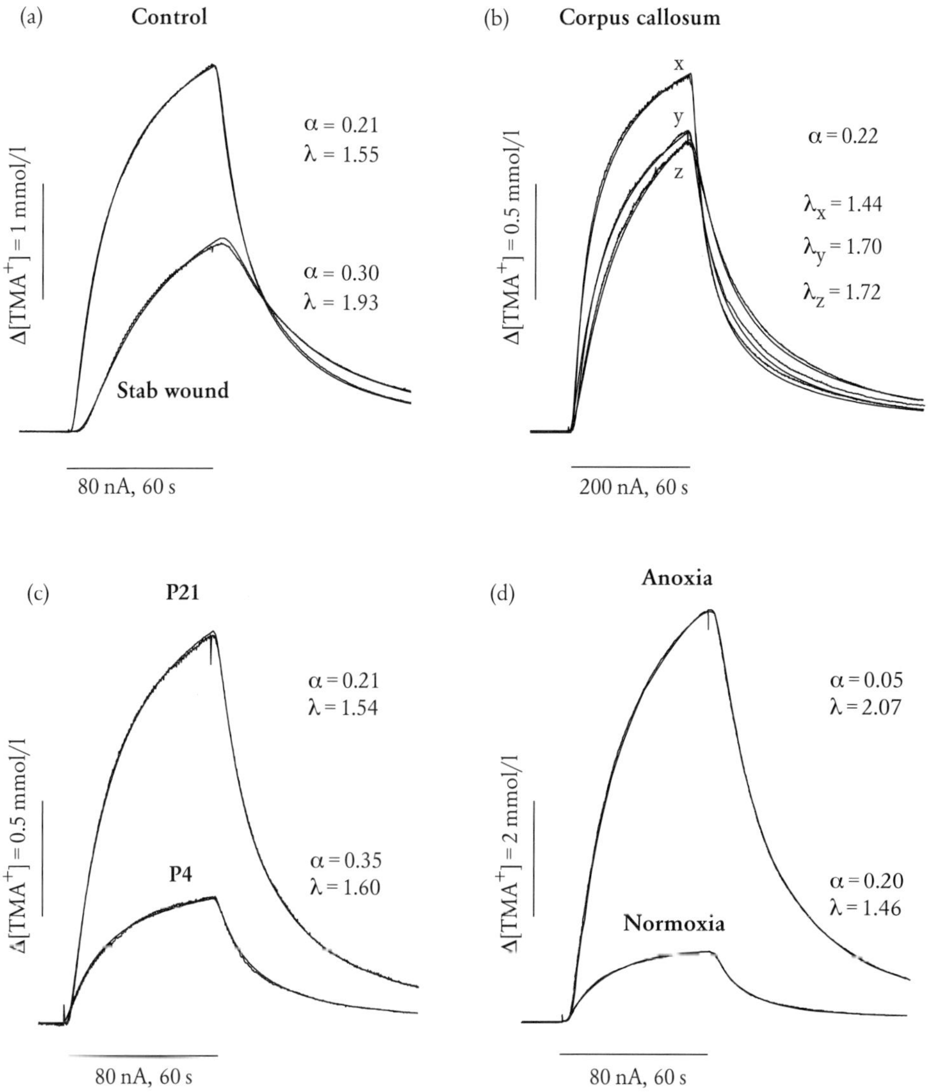

Figure 3 Tetramethylammonium (TMA^+) diffusion curves under different experimental conditions. For each curve, the extracellular space (ECS) diffusion parameters α (volume fraction) and λ (tortuosity) were extracted by appropriate non-linear curve fitting. Experimental and theoretical curves are superimposed in each case. For each figure part the concentration scale is linear. (a) Typical recordings obtained in rat cortex (control). Values of α and λ are increased in the gliotic cortex around a stab wound. Note that the larger is the curve, the smaller is the value of α; a slower rise and decay indicate higher tortuosity. (b) Typical recordings in myelinated corpus callosum of an adult rat. Note that λ has two different values, lower value along the axons (*x*-axis) and higher across the axons (*y*- and *z*-axes). (c) Typical recordings obtained in rat cortex at postnatal days (P) 4 and 21. Note the dramatic decrease in ECS volume during maturation. (d) Typical recordings obtained in adult rat cortex (lamina V) during normoxia and in the same animal about 10 min after cardiac arrest (anoxia)

be astrogliosis. Increased GFAP staining and an increase in the size and fibrous character of astrocytes have been found in the cortex, corpus callosum and hippocampus of senescent rats, which may account for changes in the ECS volume fraction[3,4]. Other changes could account for the observed decreases in λ values and for the disruption of tissue anisotropy. In the hippocampus in CA1 and CA3, as well as in the dentate gyrus, we found changes in the arrangement of fine

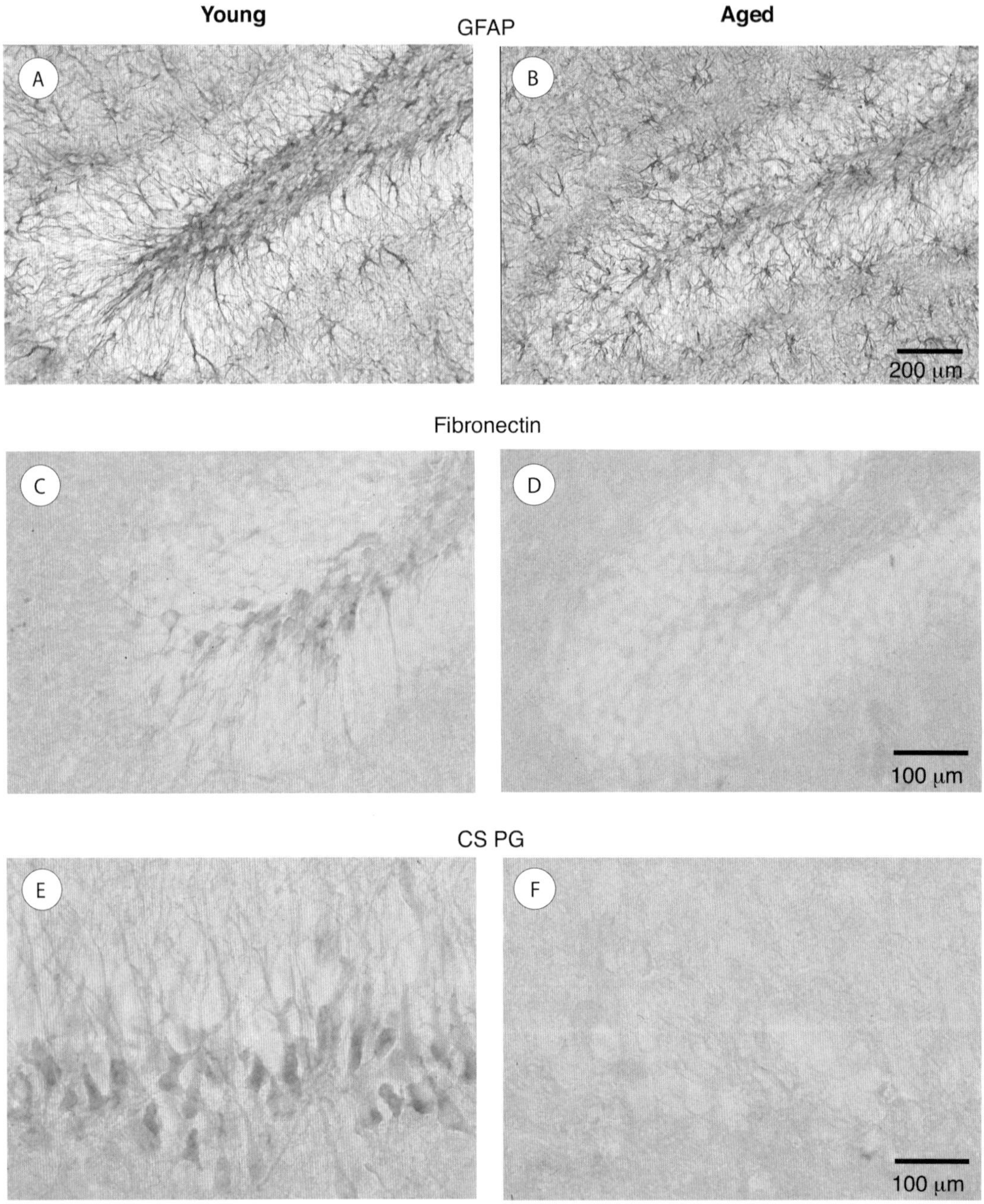

Figure 4 Structural changes in the hippocampus dentate gyrus region of aged rats with memory impairment (rats were tested in a Morris water maze). (a) Astrocytes stained for glial fibrillary acidic protein (GFAP) in a young adult rat; note the radial organization of the astrocytic processes between pyramidal cells (not stained). (b) In an aged rat the radial organization of the astrocytic processes is lost. (c) Staining for fibronectin in a young adult rat shows densely stained cells, apparently due to perineuronal staining around granular cells. (d) In an aged rat the fibronectin staining is lost. (e) Staining for chondroitin sulfate proteoglycans (CSPG) in a young adult rat shows perineuronal nets in the CA1 region. (f) In an aged rat with memory impairment the CSPG staining is lost

astrocytic processes. These are normally organized in parallel in the *x-y* plane (Figure 4a and b), and this organization totally disappears during aging. Moreover, decreased staining for chondroitin sulfate proteoglycans and for fibronectin (Figure 4c–f) suggests a loss of extracellular matrix macromolecules.

The degree of learning deficit during aging correlates with changes in ECS volume, tortuosity and non-specific uptake (Figure 5)[4]. The hippocampus is well known for its role in memory formation, especially declarative memory. It is therefore reasonable to assume that diffusion anisotropy, which leads to a certain degree of specificity in extrasynaptic communication, may play an important role in memory formation. There was a significant difference between mildly and severely behaviorally impaired rats (rats were tested in a Morris water maze), which was particularly apparent in the hippocampus. The ECS in the dentate gyrus of severely impaired rats was significantly smaller than in mildly impaired rats. Also, anisotropy in the hippocampus of severely impaired rats, particularly in the dentate gyrus, was much reduced, while a substantial degree of anisotropy was still present in aged rats with better learning performance (Figure 5). Anisotropy might be important for extrasynaptic transmission by channelling the flux of substances in a preferential direction. Its loss may severely disrupt extrasynaptic communication in the CNS, which has been suggested to play an important role in memory formation[3,8].

Volume fraction is thus decreasing during the entire postnatal life, with the steepest decrease in early postnatal development (Figure 3)[19,36]. The larger ECS (30–45%) in the first days of postnatal development in the rat can be attributed to incomplete neuronal migration, gliogenesis, angiogenesis and the presence of large extracellular matrix proteoglycans, particularly hyaluronic acid, which, owing to the mutual repulsion of its highly negatively charged branches, occupies a great deal of space and holds cells apart from each other. The ensuing decrease in ECS size could be explained by the disappearance of a significant part of the ECS matrix, neuronal migration and the development of dendritic trees, rapid myelination and the proliferation of glia. Some

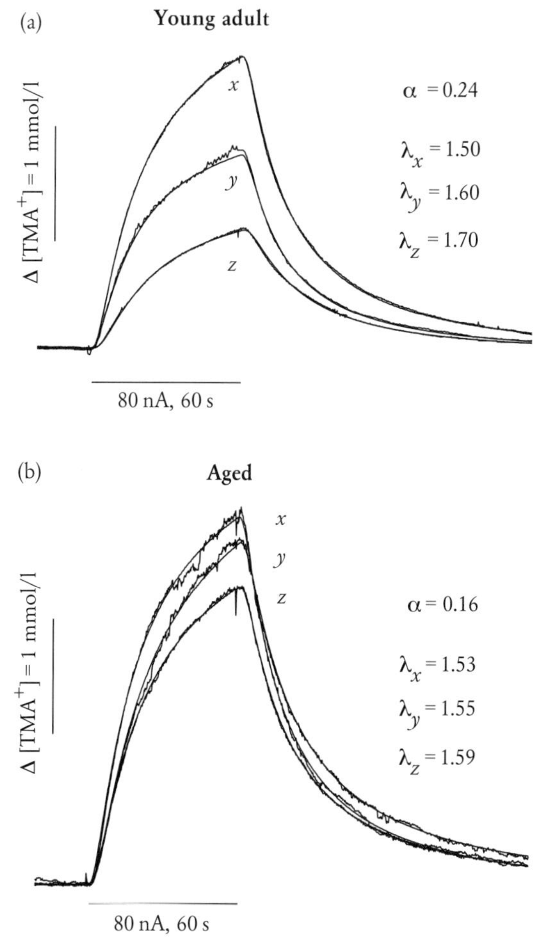

Figure 5 Diffusion parameters in the hippocampus dentate gyrus of a young adult and an aged rat with memory impairment (rats were tested in a Morris water maze). (a) Anisotropic diffusion in the dentate gyrus of a young adult rat. Tetramethylammonium (TMA^+) diffusion curves (concentration-time profiles) were measured along three orthogonal axes (*x* mediolateral, *y* rostrocaudal, *z* dorsoventral). The slower rise in the *z*- than in the *y*-axis and in the *y*- than in the *x*-axis indicates a higher tortuosity and more restricted diffusion. The amplitude of the curves shows that TMA^+ concentration, at approximately the same distance from the tip of the iontophoresis electrode, is much higher along the *x*-axis than along the *y*-axis and even higher than along the *z*-axis (tortuosity λ_x, λ_y, λ_z). Note that the actual extracellular space (ECS) volume fraction α is 0.24 and can be calculated only when measurements are made along the *x*-, *y*- and *z*-axes. (b) Volume fraction decreases to 0.16 and anisotropy is almost lost in an aged rat with memory impairment. Note that the diffusion curves are higher, showing that α is smaller, and their rise and decay time is longer when λ (diffusion barriers) increases

of these processes are also observed during aging. The most important are probably neuronal degeneration, a further loss of extracellular matrix and astrogliosis. Indeed, we observed a decrease of fibronectin and chondroitin sulfate proteoglycans staining in the hippocampus of mildly impaired aged rats and almost a complete loss of staining in severely impaired aged rats (Figure 4c–f). Chondroitin sulfate proteoglycans participate in multiple cellular processes[37,38]. These include axonal outgrowth, axonal branching and synaptogenesis, which are important for the formation of memory traces.

Besides a decrease in ECS volume and changes in diffusion barriers and directionality, a reduction in non-specific TMA^+ uptake was found in aged rats. The underlying mechanism may include transfer into cells or binding to cellular surfaces or to negatively charged molecules of the extracellular matrix. All of these may be reduced during aging. Transfer into cells might decrease due to reduced pinocytosis (stiffer membranes owing to a higher proportion of cholesterol), binding to cellular surfaces due to reduced membrane potential and binding to the extracellular matrix due to its loss.

Because α is lower in aging rats (Figure 5), some differences in the ECS diffusion parameter changes seen during ischemia can be expected in senescent rats. Indeed, the final values of α, λ and k' induced by cardiac arrest are not significantly different between young and aged rats; however, the time course of all the changes is faster in aged animals[3].

It is concluded that the observed changes in ECS diffusion parameters during aging have important functional significance. Anisotropy, which, particularly in the hippocampus and corpus callosum, may help to facilitate the diffusion of neurotransmitters and neuromodulators to regions occupied by their high-affinity extrasynaptical receptors, might have crucial importance for the specificity of signal transmission. The importance of anisotropy for the 'spillover' of glutamate, for 'cross-talk' between synapses and for LTP and LTD has been proposed[14,15]. The observed loss of anisotropy in senescent rats could therefore lead to impaired cortical and, particularly, hippocampal function. The decrease in ECS size could be responsible for the greater susceptibility of the aged brain to pathological events, the poorer outcome of clinical therapy and the more limited recovery of affected tissue after insult.

ACKNOWLEDGEMENTS

This work was supported by grants LN00A065 and J13/98: 11100004 from the Ministry of Education, Youth and Sport of the Czech Republic and AV0Z5039906 from the Academy of Sciences of the Czech Republic.

References

1. Grady CL, Craik FI. Changes in memory processing with age. *Curr Opin Neurobiol* 2000;10:224–31
2. Syková E. Glia and extracellular space diffusion parameters in the injured and aging brain. In de Vellis J, ed. *Neuroglia in the Aging Brain*. Totowa: Humana Press, 2001:77–98
3. Syková E, Mazel T, Šimonová Z. Diffusion constraints and neuron–glia interaction during aging. *Exp Gerontol* 1998;33:837–51
4. Syková E, Mazel T, Hasenöhrl RU, *et al.* Learning deficits in aged rats related to decrease in extracellular volume and loss of diffusion anisotropy in hippocampus. *Hippocampus* 2002;12:469–79
5. Fuxe K, Agnati LF. *Volume Transmission in the Brain. Novel Mechanisms for Neural Transmission*. New York: Raven Press, 1991
6. Agnati LF, Zoli M, Stromberg I, *et al.* Intercellular communication in the brain: wiring versus volume transmission. *Neuroscience* 1995;69:711–26
7. Syková E. The extracellular space in the CNS: its regulation, volume and geometry in normal and pathological neuronal function. *Neuroscientist* 1997; 3:28–41

8. Nicholson C, Syková E. Extracellular space structure revealed by diffusion analysis. *Trends Neurosci* 1998;21:207-15
9. Zoli M, Jansson A, Syková E, *et al.* Intercellular communication in the central nervous system. The emergence of the volume transmission concept and its relevance for neuropsychopharmacology. *Trends Pharmacol Sci* 1999;20:142-50
10. Syková E. Glial diffusion barriers during aging and pathological states. *Prog Brain Res* 2001; 132:339-63
11. Syková E. Plasticity of the extracellular space. In Walz W, ed. *The Neuronal Microenvironment.* Totowa: Humana Press, 2002:57-81
12. Syková E, Mazel T, Vargová L, *et al.* Extracellular space diffusion and pathological states. *Prog Brain Res* 2000;125:155-78
13. Celio MR, Spreafico R, De Biasi S, *et al.* Perineuronal nets: past and present. *Trends Neurosci* 1998;21:510-15
14. Kullmann DM, Erdemli G, Asztely F. LTP of AMPA and NMDA receptor-mediated signals: evidence for presynaptic expression and extrasynaptic glutamate spill-over. *Neuron* 1996;17: 461-74
15. Asztely F, Erdemli G, Kullmann DM. Extrasynaptic glutamate spillover in the hippocampus: dependence on temperature and the role of active glutamate uptake. *Neuron* 1997;18:281-93
16. Danbolt NC. Glutamate uptake. *Prog Neurobiol* 2001;65:1-105
17. Roitbak T, Syková E. Diffusion barriers evoked in the rat cortex by reactive astrogliosis. *Glia* 1999; 28:40-8
18. Syková E, Roitbak T, Mazel T, *et al.* Astrocytes, oligodendroglia, extracellular space volume and geometry in rat fetal brain grafts. *Neuroscience* 1999;91:783-98
19. Voříšbek I, Syková E. Evolution of anisotropic diffusion in the developing rat corpus callosum. *J Neurophysiol* 1997;78:912-19
20. Nicholson C, Phillips JM. Ion diffusion modified by tortuosity and volume fraction in the extracellular microenvironment of the rat cerebellum. *J Physiol (Lond)* 1981;321:225-57
21. Nicholson C. Interaction between diffusion and Michaelis-Menten uptake of dopamine after iontophoresis in striatum. *Biophys J* 1995;68: 1699-715
22. Rice ME, Okada Y, Nicholson C. Anisotropic and heterogeneous diffusion in the turtle cerebellum. *J Neurophysiol* 1993;70:2035-44
23. Pérez-Pinzon MA, Tao L, Nicholson C. Extracellular potassium, volume fraction, and tortuosity in rat hippocampal CA1, CA3 and cortical slices during ischemia. *J Neurophysiol* 1995;74: 565-73
24. Mazel T, Šimonová Z, Syková E. Diffusion heterogeneity and anisotropy in rat hippocampus. *Neuroreport* 1998;9:1299-304
25. Syková E, Mazel T, Roitbak T, *et al.* Morphological changes and diffusion barriers in auditory cortex and hippocampus of aged rats. *Assoc Res Otolaryngol Abstr* 1999;22:117
26. Chvátal A, Berger T, Voříšek I, *et al.* Changes in glial K^+ currents with decreased extracellular volume in developing rat white matter. *J Neurosci Res* 1997; 49:98-106
27. Prokopová Š, Vargová L, Syková E. Heterogeneous and anisotropic diffusion in the developing rat spinal cord. *Neuroreport* 1997;8:3527-32
28. Benveniste H, Hedlund LW, Johnson GA. Mechanism of detection of acute cerebral ischemia in rats by diffusion-weighted magnetic resonance microscopy. *Stroke* 1992;23:746-54
29. Latour LL, Svoboda K, Mitra PP, *et al.* Time-dependent diffusion of water in a biological model system. *Proc Natl Acad Sci USA* 1994;91:1229-33
30. Norris DG, Niendorf T, Leibfritz D. Healthy and infarcted brain tissues studied at short diffusion times: the origins of apparent restriction and the reduction in apparent diffusion coefficient. *NMR Biomed* 1994;7:304-10
31. Van der Toorn A, Syková E, Dijkhuizen RM, *et al.* Dynamic changes in water ADC, energy metabolism, extracellular space volume, and tortuosity in neonatal rat brain during global ischemia. *Magn Reson Med* 1996;36:52-60
32. Voříšek I, Hájek M, Tintěra J, *et al.* Water ADC, extracellular space volume and tortuosity in the rat cortex after traumatic injury. *Magn Reson Med* 2002;48:994-1003
33. Antonova T, Meyer-Luehmann M, Voříšek I, *et al.* Diffusion and extracellular space volume fraction in the brain of APP23 mice: an Alzheimer's disease model. Presented at the *Federation of European Neuroscience Societies Meeting,* Paris, July 2002: abstr 020.1
34. Syková E. Ionic and volume changes in the microenvironment of nerve and receptor cells. In Ottoson D, ed. *Progress in Sensory Physiology.* Heidelberg: Springer-Verlag, 1992:1-167
35. Syková E, Chvátal A. Glial cells and volume transmission in the CNS. *Neurochem Int* 2000;36: 397-409
36. Lehmenkühler A, Syková E, Svoboda J, *et al.* Extracellular space parameters in the rat neocortex and subcortical white matter during postnatal development determined by diffusion analysis. *Neuroscience* 1993;55:339-51
37. Hardington TE, Fosang AJ. Proteoglycans: many forms and many functions. *FASEB J* 1992;6:861-70
38. Margolis RK, Margolis RU. Nervous tissue proteoglycans. *Experientia* 1993;49:429-66

Estrogen regulation of mitochondrial function and impact of the aging process 2

J. Nilsen and R. D. Brinton

Our investigations into estrogen regulation of mitochondrial function grew out of a paradox. Our earlier results demonstrated that pretreatment of neurons with estrogen replacement therapy could either potentiate or attenuate glutamate-induced rise in intracellular Ca^{2+} ($[Ca^{2+}]_i$), depending on the glutamate concentration[1,2]. We knew from our results and those of other laboratories that estrogen induction of memory mechanisms required potentiation of the glutamate *N*-methyl-D-aspartate (NMDA) receptor[3-5]. Initially, one would predict and be concerned that potentiation of the glutamate NMDA receptor function would lead to excitotoxicity. However, a large body of evidence indicated that estrogen was quite effective in protecting against glutamate-induced excitotoxicity[3,6-8]. We sought to understand the mechanism(s) whereby estrogen could both potentiate glutamate NMDA receptor function and yet protect against glutamate-induced excitotoxicity. Pursuing this question, we found that estrogen replacement therapy attenuated glutamate-induced rise in $[Ca^{2+}]_i$[1,2]. What puzzled us about this result was that our experimental paradigm used a prevention model of estrogen exposure, that is, neurons were pretreated with estrogen prior to exposure to glutamate but neurons responded diametrically differently, either potentiating or attenuating glutamate-induced rise in $[Ca^{2+}]_i$, depending on the subsequent exposure to either non-toxic or excitotoxic glutamate concentrations. These data indicated that estrogen exposure proactively activated a mechanism that would protect against excesses in $[Ca^{2+}]_i$. We therefore began to explore what mechanisms would account for the estrogen's proactive protection.

The work presented here is part of a larger conceptual framework of estrogen action in the brain that incorporates a temporal cascade both dependent upon and regulatory of Ca^{2+} signalling. Our working model is a three-tiered temporal cascade composed of first, an initiation mechanism that is Ca^{2+} dependent, second, a propagation phase that enhances Ca^{2+} signalling cascades and finally, a third phase of proactive adaptation that protects against excesses in $[Ca^{2+}]_i$ (Figure 1). The focus of our recent work is on the third phase, that of proactive adaptation. We use the term proactive adaptation to represent two conditions: estrogen induction of a protected cellular state, and a broad spectrum defense against multiple and seemingly unrelated toxic agents.

ESTROGEN-INDUCED NEUROPROTECTION: CURRENT MODELS AND REMAINING CHALLENGES

Estrogen treatment can protect against a wide range of toxic insults, including free radical generators[9-11], excitotoxicity[3,12,13], β-amyloid-induced toxicity[3] and ischemia[6,7]. Estrogen replacement therapy (ERT) is associated with numerous health benefits, including decreased incidence of osteoporosis[14] and reduced risk of Alzheimer's disease (AD)[15-18]. In laboratory animals, estradiol (E_2) exposure dramatically reduced mortality and improved neurological outcome following middle cerebral artery (MCA) occlusion and common carotid artery (CCA) occlusion models[19-22]. Results of animal experiments are paralleled by clinical observations indicating that E_2 exposure decreases the neuronal damage from stroke in humans[22].

Estrogen neuroprotective effects are multi-faceted, and encompass mechanisms that range from the chemical to the biochemical to the genomic and fall within three broad mechanistic

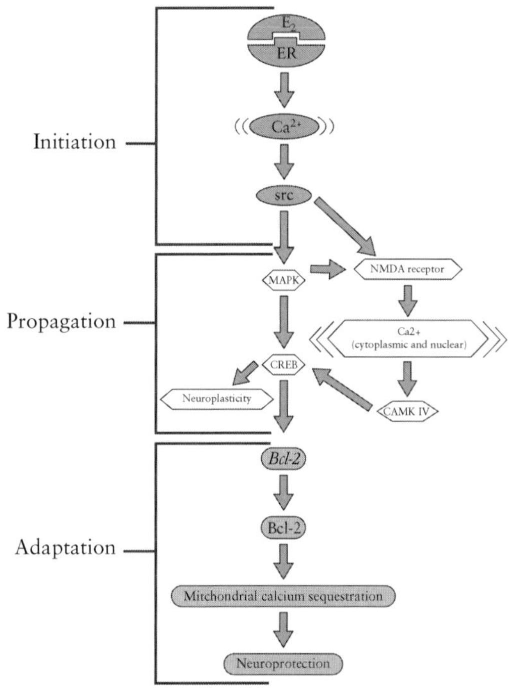

Figure 1 Conceptual model of estrogen action in the brain. The initiation stage of estrogen action is mediated by an increase in intracellular calcium. The propagation of the estrogen signal is mediated by alterations in signal transduction. The protective adaptation is the end result of these signal cascades coupled with alterations in gene expression, which culminate in estrogen-induced protection against calcium excess. E_2, estradiol; ER, estrogen receptor; MAPK, mitogen-activated protein kinase; CREB, cyclic adenosine monophosphate (cAMP) response element binding protein; NMDA, *N*-methyl-D-aspartate; CAMK, calcium/calmodulin dependent kinase

categories, antioxidant, defense and viability[10,23]. To what extent each of these levels of action leads to the overall neuroprotective effect is not fully determined; however, each appears to make a significant if not obligatory impact on the neuroprotective effects of estrogens. It is not yet clear whether there is one unifying neuroprotective cascade induced by estrogen or whether estrogen induces multiple mechanisms that are selectively neuroprotective against different neurotoxins, or whether it is a combination of the two. The hypothesis we put forth is that estrogen regulation of mitochondrial calcium sequestration and calcium load tolerability serve as a unifying neuroprotective mechanism for insults caused by dysregulation of calcium homeostasis.

Current mechanistic models of estrogen-induced neuroprotection are limited in mechanistic detail. The cellular effects of estrogens include activation of nuclear estrogen receptors (ERs), increased expression of antiapoptotic proteins, activation of second-messenger cascades, alterations of glutaminergic activation, regulation of intracellular calcium homeostasis and antioxidant activity. While E_2 activation of mitogen-activated protein kinase (MAPK) signalling has been investigated in substantial detail[12,20,21,24-27], most estrogen-inducible survival strategies remain as isolated and independent cascades[12,24,25,28]. It is unknown whether or how these pathways interact with one another, or which are necessary for E_2-mediated neuroprotection in one or all of the model systems.

At the estrogen receptor (ER) level, the estrogen–ER complex can associate with estrogen responsive elements (EREs), and functions as an enhancer for ERE-containing genes, including the neurotrophin brain-derived neurotrophic factor (BDNF)[29-31] and the antiapoptotic proteins Bcl-2 and Bcl-x_L[2,32-37]. There exist two different receptor subtypes, ERα and ERβ[38], which can differentially regulate gene expression[39]. Currently, the question of which estrogen receptor, ERα or ERβ, is required for neuroprotection remains unresolved. Both *in vitro* and *in vivo* reports indicate that ERα, but not ERβ, is required for the neuroprotective effects of E_2[36,40,41]. Similarly, E_2 up-regulated *bcl-2* mRNA expression in hypothalamic cell lines expressing both ERα and ERβ, but not in hypothalamic cell lines expressing only ERβ, indicating that only the ERα subtype was responsible for the increased *bcl-2* expression[36]. In contrast, ERα and ERβ both mediate E_2-induced MAPK activation[42,43]. The weight of the evidence favors a definite role of ERα in estrogen-induced neuroprotection with a possible, but not yet proven role for ERβ. The existing biochemical and immunocytochemical data relevant to the localization of ER increasingly point to a membrane site of action utilizing the same receptor protein as that found in the nucleus[26,43-47].

One model of estrogen neuroprotection proposed a reciprocal and dependent relationship between ER and receptors for growth factors such as nerve growth factor (NGF) and BDNF[31,48]. In this model, E_2 interaction with neurotrophins is mediated by a reciprocal regulation of ERs and neurotrophin receptors, both p75 and trkA, by their ligands[48], and by convergent activation of the MAPK pathway[12,13,42]. However, Aggarwal and Gibbs found that E_2 did not reverse the effects of lesions on cholinergic neuron survival, suggesting that, *in vivo*, E_2 does not promote neurotrophin action that would lead to increased cholinergic neuron survival[49].

Singer and colleagues have provided evidence that activation of the MAPK pathway is necessary for E_2-induced neuroprotection[12]. Phosphorylation of one MAPK substrate, cyclic adenosine monophosphate (cAMP) response element binding protein (CREB), is associated with increased resistance to ischemic injury[50], and CREB is activated in response to E_2[26,51]. It should be noted that CREB can be activated by pathways other than the MAPK pathway[52–54], but it does provide a possible convergence point for multiple E_2-mediated signalling events.

Maintenance of $[Ca^{2+}]_i$ homeostasis may be a component of E_2-mediated neuroprotection. E_2 treatment attenuated the increase in $[Ca^{2+}]_i$ associated with gp-120-mediated toxicity by reducing the number of neurons that responded to gp-120 with increased $[Ca^{2+}]_i$[55]. This is in contrast to the estrogen-induced attenuation of the increase in $[Ca^{2+}]_i$ associated with excitotoxic glutamate exposure, in which estrogens did not alter the number of neurons that responded to glutamate[1]. Although researchers have proposed a direct antioxidant activity of estrogens[56–58] and E_2-mediated alterations of the mitochondrial Na^+/K^+-adenosine triphosphatase (ATPase) activity[59,60] as mechanisms for E_2-mediated neuroprotection, these effects require concentrations of estrogens of at least 1–10 μmol/l[56–59,61]. Thus, these effects generated at micromolar concentrations of E_2 should not impact on our model system, which relies on lower (nmol/l) concentrations of E_2, as is consistent with numerous reports of *in vitro* and *in vivo* E_2-mediated neuroprotection[3,6,8,28,32,33].

To summarize, the current body of knowledge strongly supports a neuroprotective action of E_2. The estrogen receptor most likely to mediate this neuroprotective effect is the α subtype. Calcium signalling and the MAPK and Bcl-2 signalling pathways appear to be pivotal to the neuroprotective action of E_2.

CALCIUM, GLUTAMATE-INDUCED EXCITOTOXICITY AND ESTROGEN-INDUCED NEUROPROTECTION

Calcium is a ubiquitous intracellular signal responsible for controlling numerous cellular processes[62]. Exceeding the normal spatial and temporal boundaries for Ca^{2+} can result in cell death through both necrosis and apoptosis. Loss of $[Ca^{2+}]_i$ homeostasis is implicated in several brain disorders, including stroke and severe epileptic seizures, and in the pathogenesis of Alzheimer's disease (AD)[63,64]. A major contributor to the loss in Ca^{2+} homeostasis in these neurological disorders is glutamate excitotoxicity[65–67]. Glutamate excitotoxicity results from energy depletion, overactivation of glutamate receptors, excessive calcium influx and oxidative stress[68–72]. Glutamate-dependent cell death occurs through Ca^{2+} influx through the NMDA receptor, as evidenced by prevention of neuronal death by removal of extracellular Ca^{2+} or addition of glutamate NMDA receptor antagonists[73–78].

Findings from our laboratory have provided evidence that maintenance of intracellular Ca^{2+} homeostasis may be a component of E_2-mediated neuroprotection. Hippocampal neurons pretreated with estrogens and then exposed to excitotoxic glutamate respond with an attenuated rise in $[Ca^{2+}]_i$ and increased survival relative to untreated neurons[1,3,45]. Such attenuation occurs without an alteration in the number of neurons that respond to glutamate[1]. This is in contrast to the estrogen-induced attenuation of the increase in $[Ca^{2+}]_i$ associated with gp-120-mediated toxicity, in which the number of neurons responding to gp-120 with increased $[Ca^{2+}]_i$ is reduced[55]. The most parsimonious explanation for this effect is that E_2 inhibits the glutamate response, as previously reported[79]. However, such an explanation is at odds with reports that E_2 potentiates NMDA receptor function. E_2 increases the amplitude of NMDA-mediated excitatory postsynaptic potentials (EPSPs)[80]. E_2 also significantly increases long-term potentiation, a cellular model of learning and memory that is dependent upon NMDA receptors[80]. Furthermore, we have shown that E_2 can exert a dual paradoxical effect upon glutamate-induced $[Ca^{2+}]_i$ rise. In contrast to E_2-induced attenuation of the Ca^{2+} response to excitotoxic glutamate, in the presence of synaptically relevant concentrations of glutamate, estrogens potentiated NMDA receptor-dependent glutamate-induced $[Ca^{2+}]_i$ rise[1]. Because NMDA receptor-mediated rise in $[Ca^{2+}]_i$ can be neurotoxic, one might anticipate that potentiation of NMDA receptor function would be deleterious for neuronal survival, but in fact the opposite was found. Estrogen treatment that potentiated the glutamate-induced $[Ca^{2+}]_i$ rise was neuroprotective and also attenuated the excitotoxic glutamate-induced $[Ca^{2+}]_i$ rise[1].

Further ruling out inhibition of the glutamate receptor as a mechanism of E_2-induced attenuation of excitotoxic glutamate rise in $[Ca^{2+}]_i$, we have shown that E_2 potentiates $^{45}Ca^{2+}$ uptake in response to both low (25 μmol/l) and excitotoxic (200 μmol/l) concentrations of glutamate[2]. Additionally, when using the low-affinity Ca^{2+} indicator Fura4F to measure $[Ca^{2+}]_i$ in response to excitotoxic glutamate, there is an initial peak in $[Ca^{2+}]_i$ followed by a rapid decline to steady-state levels. The initial peak is larger and the latter plateau is lower in E_2-treated neurons than in control neurons[2]. These results indicate two important features. First, E_2 potentiates the rise in $[Ca^{2+}]_i$ induced by glutamate irrespective of glutamate concentration. Second, the mechanism of E_2-induced attenuation of excitotoxic glutamate rise in $[Ca^{2+}]_i$ is downstream to the glutamate receptor, indicating that estrogen-induced reduction in $[Ca^{2+}]_i$ following exposure to excitotoxic glutamate is due to a buffering or sequestration mechanism downstream of Ca^{2+} influx.

REGULATION OF MITOCHONDRIAL CALCIUM UPTAKE

Calcium-induced neurotoxicity is complex, as exemplified by glutamate-induced neurotoxicity which correlates with the Ca^{2+} load measured by $^{45}Ca^{2+}$ uptake, but not with free $[Ca^{2+}]_i$ measured by the fluorescent Ca^{2+} indicator Fura2[75], suggesting a role of subcellular Ca^{2+} sequestration. Owing to the large capacity for Ca^{2+}, mitochondria play a central role in shaping Ca^{2+} transient in neurons. Ca^{2+} uptake by mitochondria occurs above a threshold of cytosolic Ca^{2+}, and is only slowly released, leading to a net accumulation of mitochondrial calcium ($[Ca^{2+}]_m$) and an alteration of physiological $[Ca^{2+}]_i$ transients[81,82]. Since in this way mitochondrial Ca^{2+} uptake limits the glutamate-induced rise in $[Ca2+]_i$[83], a potential mechanism for E_2 attenuation of $[Ca^{2+}]_i$ rise is increased mitochondrial sequestration of Ca^{2+}. Supporting a role for E_2 in the modulation of mitochondrial Ca^{2+} cycling, mitochondria isolated from the liver treated with E_2 show enhanced respiratory substrate-dependent binding of Ca^{2+} compared with mitochondria from control rats[84,85].

Recently, we have shown that E_2-induced attenuation of the rise in bulk free $[Ca^{2+}]_i$ induced by excitotoxic glutamate is dependent upon mitochondrial sequestration of Ca^{2+}. Mitochondrial inhibitors, either a combination of rotenone, to inhibit the respiratory chain at complex I, and oligomycin, to inhibit mitochondrial ATP synthase, or antimycin, to inhibit the respiratory chain at complex III, completely depolarize *in situ* mitochondria, effectively blocking mitochondrial Ca^{2+} accumulation[86,87]. The E_2-induced attenuation of the rise in bulk free $[Ca^{2+}]_i$ is blocked by the addition of these mitochondrial inhibitors[2]. Further supporting a model of E_2-induced mitochondrial sequestration of Ca^{2+}, we demonstrated that E_2-treatment resulted in increased mitochondrial Ca^{2+} sequestration in intact neurons following exposure to excitotoxic glutamate. Maintenance of $[Ca^{2+}]_m$ levels is dependent upon the proton gradient across the inner membrane, allowing one to employ the protonophore carbonyl cyanide 4-(trifluoromethoxy) phenylhydrazone (FCCP) as a tool to dissipate the electrochemical gradient, resulting in release of mitochondrial Ca^{2+} uptake[87-89]. The release of $[Ca^{2+}]_m$ is manifested as an increase in $[Ca^{2+}]_i$, which can be detected by calcium indicator dyes[88]. Administration of carbonyl cyanide 4-(trifluoromethoxy) phenylhydrazone (FCCP) following an excitotoxic glutamate stimulus resulted in a significantly greater release of mitochondrial Ca^{2+} stores from E_2-treated cells than from control cells[2]. These data indicate that E_2-induced increase in mitochondrial Ca^{2+} sequestration is coupled with an increased $[Ca^{2+}]_m$ load.

These data were validated by direct measurements of $[Ca^{2+}]_m$ using the mitochondrial-specific, Ca^{2+}-sensitive dye RhodFF. Hippocampal neurons pretreated with estradiol showed a larger increase in RhodFF fluorescence in response to excitotoxic glutamate than control neurons (Figure 2). When neuronal Ca^{2+} was measured simultaneously in the cytosol and the mitochondria using Fura4F and RhodFF, respectively, it was apparent that the E_2-mediated attenuation of $[Ca^{2+}]_i$ was correlated with a significant increase in $[Ca^{2+}]_m$, compared with control (Figure 3).

Because of the relatively large capacity for Ca^{2+}, mitochondrial Ca^{2+} uptake could be neuroprotective at low levels of insult by removing calcium from the cytoplasm[82,90,91]. However, high mitochondrial calcium levels ($[Ca^{2+}]_m$) exert detrimental effects, as high $[Ca^{2+}]_m$ results in both enhanced reactive oxygen species (ROS) production and mitochondrial membrane depolarization[64,92-94]. These excessive loads of $[Ca^{2+}]_m$, which lead to mitochondrial dysfunction, are thought to underlie cell death in response to excitotoxicity[75,95]. In fact, blockade of mitochondrial calcium uptake can prevent excitotoxic cell death[86,96].

Although mitochondria exert a vital function in glutamate-induced neurotoxicity, there is disagreement as to the relative role of different intracellular organelles in buffering the cytosolic free Ca^{2+} and in the concentration of extra-mitochondrial free Ca^{2+} at which mitochondria will buffer Ca^{2+}. Calcium buffered in mitochondria[97,98] has been found to account for 60–80% of the total cell Ca^{2+}. In contrast, using permeabilized cells or isolated mitochondria, uptake into a non-mitochondrial pool had a much higher affinity for Ca^{2+} than the mitochondria, so that mitochondrial calcium content was very low[99-102]. Under these conditions in the presence of physiological levels of free Mg^{2+}, mitochondria from neurons will buffer extra-mitochondrial free Ca^{2+} at 0.6–1 μmol/l[81,97,103]. Based on these findings, the current thinking[87,104-106] is that mitochondria are active regulators of neuronal Ca^{2+} homeostasis especially at near toxic levels of extramitochondrial free Ca^{2+}.

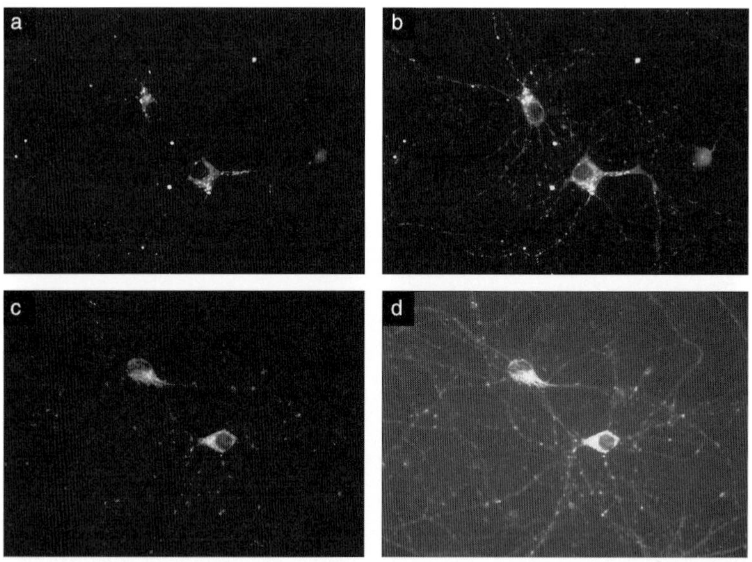

Figure 2 Estrogen potentiates mitochondrial calcium sequestration induced by excitotoxic glutamate. Hippocampal neurons were treated with 17β-estradiol (10 ng/ml) (c, d) or vehicle control (a, b) for 48 h prior to excitotoxic glutamate (200 μmol/l) exposure (b, d). Cytosolic Ca^{2+} and mitochondrial Ca^{2+} were visualized by Fura4F and RhodFF, respectively. Image shows estrogen-mediated attenuation of the glutamate-induced rise in intracellular Ca^{2+} and potentiation of the glutamate-induced rise in mitochondrial Ca^{2+}

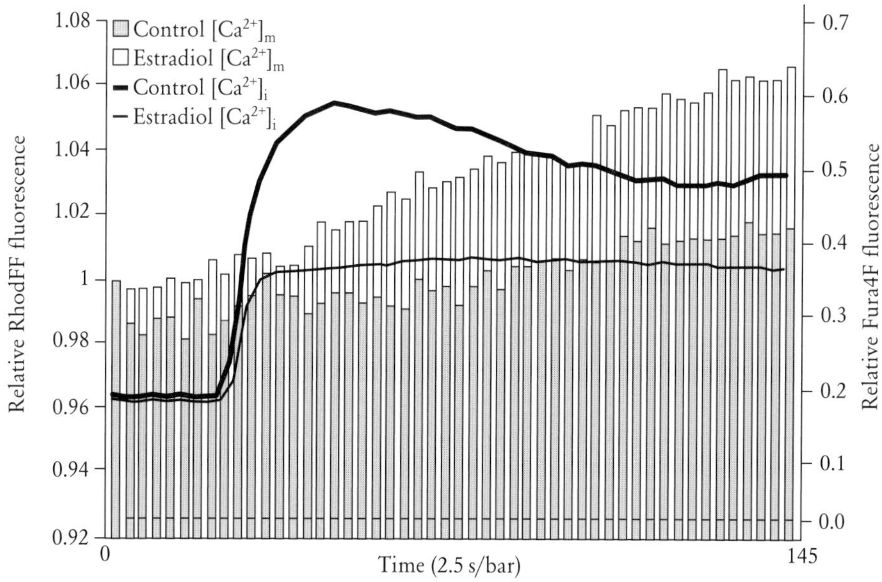

Figure 3 Estrogen attenuates cytosolic calcium and potentiates mitochondrial calcium induced by excitotoxic glutamate. Hippocampal neurons were treated with 17β-estradiol (10 ng/ml) or vehicle control for 48 h prior to excitotoxic glutamate (200 μmol/l) exposure. Cytosolic Ca^{2+} (curves) and mitochondrial Ca^{2+} (bars) were visualized by Fura4F and RhodFF, respectively. Data represent mean of at least ten neurons per condition per coverslip. Data are representative of four independent experiments with three coverslips per condition per experiment

Increased $[Ca^{2+}]_m$ could underlie the E_2-induced attenuation of the $[Ca^{2+}]_i$ rise; however, since excessive loads of $[Ca^{2+}]_m$ lead to mitochondrial dysfunction, the increased $[Ca^{2+}]_m$ loads induced by E_2 treatment would be expected to lead to increased cell death, not cell survival. Paradoxically, E_2 protects against glutamate-induced excitotoxicity[8,45]. Thus, if E_2 is acting to increase mitochondrial sequestration, two mechanisms must be induced. First, the threshold for calcium uptake by mitochondria has to be lowered to achieve the increase in sequestration. Second, to protect against Ca^{2+}-induced respiratory injury and mitochondria dysfunction, an increase in mitochondrial calcium load tolerability must occur.

MITOCHONDRIAL CALCIUM LOAD TOLERABILITY AND E_2 REGULATION OF Bcl-2

The magnitude of Ca^{2+} accumulation by mitochondria can be altered by the antiapoptotic protein Bcl-2[107-109]. Bcl-2 is localized to the mitochondrial membrane, and its expression has been shown to enhance mitochondrial Ca^{2+} sequestration significantly[108]. Bcl-2 has been identified as an E_2-responsive gene in reproductive tissues and brain[34,36,110]. E_2 may directly up-regulate this survival factor through receptor-mediated interactions with regions of the *bcl-2* promoter, which contains several putative estrogen-responsive sites, or by indirect pathways[110]. E_2 can activate transcription of a reporter gene driven by a distal region of the *bcl-2* promoter through an ERα–SP1 interaction in breast cancer cells[111]. In the hypothalamus, *bcl-2* is elevated in E_2-treated and estrous rats[34]. Furthermore, *bcl-2* is elevated with E_2 treatment in $ER\alpha^+/ER\beta^+$, but not in $ER\alpha^-/ER\beta^+$ neuronal cell lines[36]. We have shown that E_2 significantly up-regulates Bcl-2 expression in primary cultured hippocampal neurons, which will be used in the studies proposed herein[35].

In addition to increasing the magnitude of Ca^{2+} sequestered by mitochondria, Bcl-2 enhances the tolerability of mitochondria for increased levels of $[Ca^{2+}]_i$ that otherwise result in dissipation of mitochondrial function ($\Delta\Psi_m$) and cell death[112]. Consistent with an increase in mitochondrial Ca^{2+} load tolerability, Mattson and colleagues showed that a supraphysiological concentration of E_2 (10 µmol/l) preserved $\Delta\Psi_m$ in PC12 cells expressing mutant presenilin that were exposed to β-amyloid[113]. We propose that by increasing $[Ca^{2+}]_m$ uptake capacity, and Bcl-2-induced resistance to Ca^{2+}-induced respiratory inhibition, E_2 limits the loss of viability initiated by excitotoxic glutamate. However, it is currently unknown what impact other members of the Bcl-2 family will have on this effect.

The Bcl-2 family of proteins that controls apoptosis is divided into three subfamilies[114]. The subfamily including Bcl-2 and Bcl-x_L inhibits apoptosis, whereas the Bax subfamily consisting of Bax and Bak as well as the BH3-only subfamily including Bid and Bad promote apoptosis. Interestingly, members of the Bcl-2 family with opposing functions can form homo- and heterodimers[115]. Bcl-2 can react with Bax to form Bcl-2 : Bax heterodimers, which, in contrast to Bax : Bax homodimers, are devoid of pro-cell death effects. Bad is another proapoptotic Bcl-2 family member[116]. Bad can displace Bcl-2 from the harmless Bcl-2 : Bax heterodimer, favoring the formation of Bax : Bax dimers, which, in turn, promote cell death[117]. The protein expression level of one or more of the family members can impact upon the balance of anti-/pro-apoptotic regulators, and thus the probability of neuronal cell death. These observations emphasize the complexity and multilevelled nature of the interactions existing among the Bcl-2 family members.

Multiple signalling pathways that impact on Bcl-2 expression have been identified as necessary for E_2-induced neuroprotection. For example, E_2 neuroprotection against glutamate excitotoxicity is dependent upon MAPK activation[12,13,42,118], and E_2-induced attenuation of the $[Ca^{2+}]_i$ rise induced by excitotoxic glutamate is dependent upon active MAPK[1]. The MAPK/extracellular signal-related kinase (ERK) pathway activates CREB, which can regulate *bcl-2* gene expression[119]. Synchronous with E_2 activation of MAPK/ERK, E_2 activates the Akt signalling pathway[24,120], which lies upstream of Bad phosphorylation[121]. Unphosphorylated Bad acts as a potent proapoptotic effector by displacing Bcl-2 from the harmless Bcl-2 : Bax heterodimer, favoring the formation of Bax : Bax dimers, which, in turn, promote cell death[117]. Conversely, phosphorylated Bad is devoid of apoptotic activity[121]. We propose that E_2 regulates Bcl-2 family protein content and function by synchronous activation of the MAPK/ERK and Akt signalling pathways.

As all of these studies had been performed in embryonic neurons and neurodegeneration is an age-related disease, it was important to determine whether the effects occurred in aged neurons. Neurons from aged rats (23–24 months) are much more susceptible to glutamate-induced Ca^{2+} dysregulation following repeated pulses of glutamate. Whereas embryonic neurons were able to buffer Ca^{2+} back to baseline, aged neurons were unable to buffer adequately the Ca^{2+} influxes[122]. The ability of neurons from middle-aged female rats (10–12 months) to buffer Ca^{2+} was intermediate between that of embryonic and aged neurons. Estrogen treatment reversed the age-related Ca^{2+}

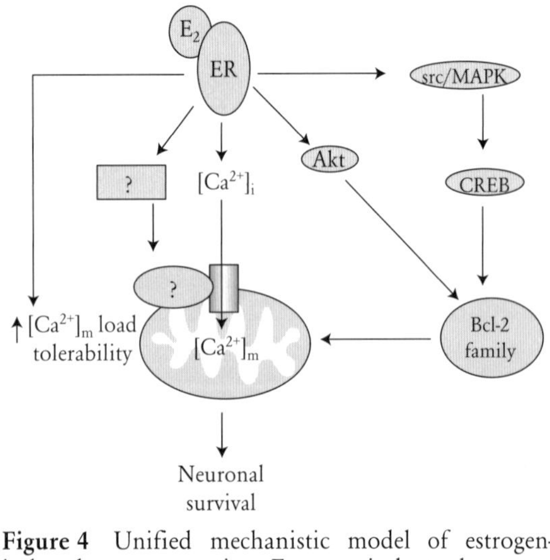

Figure 4 Unified mechanistic model of estrogen-induced neuroprotection. Estrogen induces the potentiation of Ca^{2+} influx, and lowers the set-point for mitochondrial Ca^{2+} sequestration, which, in the presence of excessive Ca^{2+}, leads to an attenuation of bulk free intracellular Ca^{2+} ($[Ca^{2+}]_i$). This increased mitochondrial Ca^{2+} ($[Ca^{2+}]_m$) load is offset by src/mitogen-activated protein kinase (MAPK) and Akt signalling pathway-dependent alterations in the expression of Bcl-2 family proteins that result in increased neuronal survival. E_2, estradiol; ER, estrogen receptor; CREB, cAMP response element binding protein

dysregulation, making aged neurons respond like middle-aged neurons[122]. In addition, as with embryonic neurons, estrogen was neuroprotective against glutamate excitotoxicity in aged neurons[122].

SUMMARY

We propose a unified mechanistic model of estrogen-induced neuroprotection that incorporates both novel mechanisms of estrogen action and several existing estrogen-inducible pathways (Figure 4). This model entails the potentiation of Ca^{2+} influx, which leads to increased cognitive abilities. In the presence of excessive levels of Ca^{2+}, estrogen induces an increased mitochondrial sequestration of Ca^{2+}, which leads to an attenuation of the rise in bulk free $[Ca^{2+}]_i$. This increased $[Ca^{2+}]_m$ load is offset by src/MAPK and Akt signalling pathway-dependent alterations in Bcl-2 family protein expression that result in increased neuronal survival.

Our concept that mitochondrial function is the ultimate target of multiple estrogen-inducible signalling cascades, MAPK–CREB, Akt and Bcl-2, unifies many seemingly disparate findings into a coherent mechanistic logic for promoting neuron survival (Figure 5). This model fits within an overall conceptual framework of a three-tiered cascade of E_2-induced signalling that begins with the initiation phase, progresses to the propagation phase and concludes with the proactive adaptation phase (Figure 1). This unified concept of proactive adaptation could provide a mechanistic understanding for estrogen-induced protection against calcium-associated degenerative insults specifically, while opening the possibility that this same pathway for promoting survival could generalize to estrogen protection against other toxic insults in which mitochondrial function is key. Moreover, these findings derived from neuronal systems could provide a mechanistic framework for understanding estrogen action in other organ systems where estrogen has been found to be protective against toxic insults.

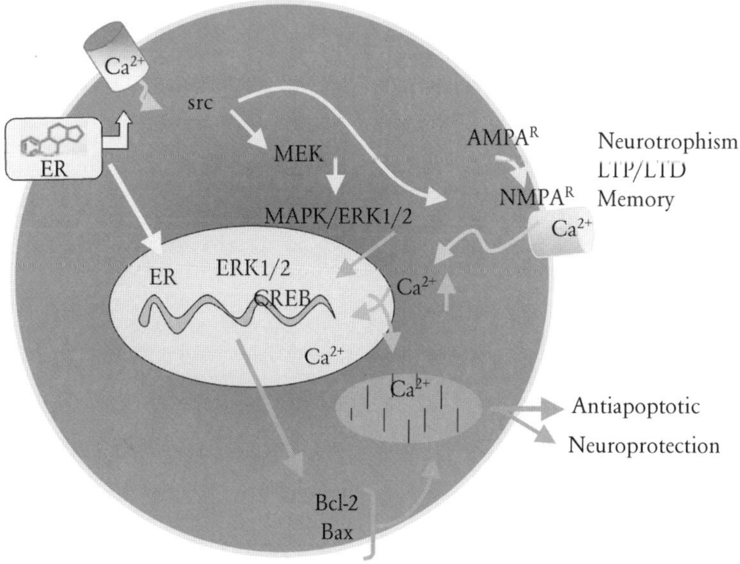

Figure 5 Estrogen-induced signalling cascade required for activation of memory and neuroprotection. The initiation stage of estrogen action is mediated by an increase in intracellular calcium, which propagates through the src/mitogen-activated protein kinase (MAPK) pathway to potentiate α-amino-3-hydroxy-5-methyl-4-isoxazole propionic acid (AMPA) and *N*-methyl-D-aspartate (NMDA) receptors. The potentiated Ca^{2+} signalling couples with estrogen receptor (ER) mediated gene transcription and the src/MAPK pathway through cAMP response element binding protein (CREB) to induce proactive adaptation. Proactive adaptation entails alteration in the expression/function of the Bcl-2 family proteins resulting in protection against toxic insults. ERK, extracellular signal-related kinase; MEK, MAP kinase kinase; LTP, long-term potentiation; LTD, long-term depression

From a clinical perspective, the health benefits and risks of estrogen replacement therapy (ERT) remain a topic of controversy[123,124]. Elucidation of the sites and targets of estrogen action should have a clear impact on both the use of estrogen replacement therapy for the prevention of neurodegenerative disease and the future design of target specific estrogens.

ACKNOWLEDGEMENTS

This study was supported by grants from the National Institutes of Aging (PO1 AG1475: Project 2), the Kenneth T. and Eileen L. Norris Foundation and the L. K. Whittier Foundation (R.D.B.) and from the Alzheimer's Association (NIRG-01-2626) (J.N.).

References

1. Nilsen J, Chen S, Brinton RD. Dual action of estrogen on glutamate-induced calcium signaling: mechanisms requiring the interaction between estrogen receptors and src/mitogen activated protein kinase pathway. *Brain Res* 2002;903: 216–34
2. Nilsen J, Brinton RD. Mechanism of estrogen-mediated neuroprotection: regulation of mitochondrial calcium and Bcl-2 expression. *Proc Natl Acad Sci USA* 2003;100:2842–7
3. Brinton RD, Chen S, Montoya M, *et al.* The Women's Health Initiative estrogen replacement therapy is neurotrophic and neuroprotective. *Neurobiol Aging* 2000;21:475–96
4. Woolley CS, McEwen BS. Estradiol regulates hippocampal dendritic spine density via an *N*-methyl-D-aspartate receptor-dependent mechanism. *J Neurosci* 1994;14:7680–7
5. Adams MM, Fink SE, Shan RA, *et al.* Estrogen and aging affect the subcellular distribution of estrogen receptor-α in the hippocampus of female rats. *J Neurosci* 2002;22:3608–14
6. Dubal DB, Kashon ML, Pettigrew LC, *et al.* Estradiol protects against ischemic injury. *J Cereb Blood Flow Metab* 1998;18:1253–8
7. Green PS, Simpkins JW. Neuroprotective effects of estrogens: potential mechanisms of action. *Int J Dev Neurosci* 2000;18:347–58
8. Singer CA, Rogers KL, Strickland TM, Dorsa DM. Estrogen protects primary cortical neurons from glutamate toxicity. *Neurosci Lett* 1996;212:13–16
9. Behl C, Holsboer F. The female sex hormone oestrogen as a neuroprotectant. *Trends Pharmacol Sci* 1999;20:441–4
10. Brinton RD, Chen S, Montoya M, Hsieh D, Minaya J. The estrogen replacement therapy of the Women's Health Initiative promotes the cellular mechanisms of memory and neuronal survival in neurons vulnerable to Alzheimer's disease. *Maturitas* 2000;34(Suppl 2):S35–52
11. Green PS, Gordon K, Simpkins JW. Phenolic A ring requirement for the neuroprotective effects of steroids. *J Steroid Biochem Mol Biol* 1997; 63:229–35
12. Singer CA, Figueroa-Masot XA, Batchelor RH, Dorsa DM. The mitogen-activated protein kinase pathway mediates estrogen neuroprotection after glutamate toxicity in primary cortical neurons. *J Neurosci* 1999;19:2455–63
13. Singh M, Setalo G Jr, Guan X, Warren M, Toran-Allerand CD. Estrogen-induced activation of mitogen-activated protein kinase in cerebral cortical explants: convergence of estrogen and neurotrophin signaling pathways. *J Neurosci* 1999;19:1179–88
14. Unnikrishnan AG, Rajaratnam S. An approach to postmenopausal osteoporosis. *Natl Med J India* 2000;13:145–6
15. Yaffe K, Sawaya G, Lieberburg I, Grady D. Estrogen therapy in postmenopausal women: effects on cognitive function and dementia. *J Am Med Assoc* 1998;279:688–95
16. Henderson VW. The epidemiology of estrogen replacement therapy and Alzheimer's disease. *Neurology* 1997;48:S27–35
17. Tang MX, Jacobs D, Stern Y, *et al.* Effect of oestrogen during menopause on risk and age at onset of Alzheimer's disease. *Lancet* 1996;348: 429–32
18. Zandi PP, Carlson MC, Plassman BL, *et al.* Hormone replacement therapy and incidence of Alzheimer disease in older women: the Cache County Study. *J Am Med Assoc* 2002;288:2123–9
19. Hawk T, Zhang YQ, Rajakumar G, Day AL, Simpkins JW. Testosterone increases and estradiol decreases middle cerebral artery

occlusion lesion size in male rats. *Brain Res* 1998; 796:296–8
20. Endoh H, Sasaki H, Maruyama K, *et al.* Rapid activation of MAP kinase by estrogen in the bone cell line. *Biochem Biophys Res Commun* 1997;235: 99–102
21. Improta-Brears T, Whorton AR, Codazzi F, *et al.* Estrogen-induced activation of mitogen-activated protein kinase requires mobilization of intracellular calcium. *Proc Natl Acad Sci USA* 1999;96:4686–91
22. Schmidt R, Fazekas F, Reinhart B, *et al.* Estrogen replacement therapy in older women: a neuropsychological and brain MRI study. *J Am Geriatr Soc* 1996;44:1307–13
23. Behl C. *Estrogen - Mystery Drug for the Brain? The Neuroprotective Activities of the Female Sex Hormone.* Vienna: Springer, 2001:228
24. Singh M. Ovarian hormones elicit phosphorylation of Akt and extracellular-signal regulated kinase in explants of the cerebral cortex. *Endocrine* 2001;14:407–15
25. Wade CB, Robinson S, Shapiro RA, Dorsa DM. Estrogen receptor (ER)α and ERβ exhibit unique pharmacologic properties when coupled to activation of the mitogen-activated protein kinase pathway. *Endocrinology* 2001;142:2336–42
26. Watters JJ, Campbell JS, Cunningham MJ, Krebs EG, Dorsa DM. Rapid membrane effects of steroids in neuroblastoma cells: effects of estrogen on mitogen activated protein kinase signalling cascade and *c-fos* immediate early gene transcription. *Endocrinology* 1997;138:4030–3
27. Nethrapalli IS, Singh M, Guan X, *et al.* Estradiol (E_2) elicits SRC phosphorylation in the mouse neocortex: the initial event in E_2 activation of the MAPK cascade? *Endocrinology* 2001;142:5145–8
28. Wise PM, Dubal DB, Wilson ME, *et al.* Estradiol is a protective factor in the adult and aging brain: understanding of mechanisms derived from *in vivo* and *in vitro* studies. *Brain Res Brain Res Rev* 2001;37:313–19
29. Gibbs RB. Treatment with estrogen and progesterone affects relative levels of brain-derived neurotrophic factor mRNA and protein in different regions of the adult rat brain. *Brain Res* 1999;844:20–7
30. Singh M, Meyer EM, Simpkins JW. The effect of ovariectomy and estradiol replacement on brain-derived neurotrophic factor messenger ribonucleic acid expression in cortical and hippocampal brain regions of female Sprague-Dawley rats. *Endocrinology* 1995;136:2320–4
31. Sohrabji F, Miranda RC, Toran-Allerand CD. Identification of a putative estrogen response element in the gene encoding brain-derived neurotrophic factor. *Proc Natl Acad Sci USA* 1995; 92:11110–14
32. Pike CJ. Estrogen modulates neuronal Bcl-x_L expression and β-amyloid-induced apoptosis: relevance to Alzheimer's disease. *J Neurochem* 1999;72:1552–63
33. Dubal DB, Shughrue PJ, Wilson ME, Merchenthaler I, Wise PM. Estradiol modulates *bcl-2* in cerebral ischemia: a potential role for estrogen receptors. *J Neurosci* 1999;19:6385–93
34. Garcia-Segura LM, Cardona-Gomez P, Naftolin F, Chowen JA. Estradiol upregulates Bcl-2 expression in adult brain neurons. *Neuroreport* 1998; 9:593–7
35. Nilsen J, Brinton RD. Impact of progestins on estrogen-induced neuroprotection: synergy by progesterone and 19-norprogesterone and antagonism by medroxyprogesterone acetate. *Endocrinology* 2002;143:205–12
36. Nilsen J, Mor G, Naftolin F. Estrogen-regulated developmental neuronal apoptosis is determined by estrogen receptor subtype and the Fas/Fas ligand system. *J Neurobiol* 2000;43:64–78
37. Singer CA, Rogers KL, Dorsa DM. Modulation of Bcl-2 expression: a potential component of estrogen protection in NT2 neurons. *Neuroreport* 1998;9:2565–8
38. Kuiper GG, Enmark E, Pelto-Huikko M, Nilsson S, Gustafsson JA. Cloning of a novel receptor expressed in rat prostate and ovary. *Proc Natl Acad Sci USA* 1996;93:5925–30
39. Paech K, Webb P, Kuiper GGJM, *et al.* Differential ligand activation of estrogen recptors ERα and ERβ at AP1 sites. *Science* 1997;277:1508–10
40. Kim H, Bang OY, Jung MW, *et al.* Neuroprotective effects of estrogen against β-amyloid toxicity are mediated by estrogen receptors in cultured neuronal cells. *Neurosci Lett* 2001;302:58–62
41. Dubal DB, Zhu H, Yu J, *et al.* Estrogen receptor α, not β, is a critical link in estradiol-mediated protection against brain injury. *Proc Natl Acad Sci USA* 2001;98:1952–7
42. Singh M, Setalo G Jr, Guan X, Frail DE, Toran-Allerand CD. Estrogen-induced activation of the mitogen-activated protein kinase cascade in the cerebral cortex of estrogen receptor-α knock-out mice. *J Neurosci* 2000;20:1694–700
43. Fretland JL, Mize AL, Dorsa DM. Initiation of rapid signaling pathways at the plasma membrane by estrogen in HT22 cells stably expressing ERα or ERβ. *Soc Neurosci* 2002;Abstr 272.15
44. Nilsen J, Brinton RD. A unifying mechanism of estrogen-mediated neuroprotection: convergence on mitochondrial function. In Schneider HPG, ed. *Menopause: The State of the Art - In Research and Management.* London, UK: Parthenon Publishing 2003:178–85
45. Brinton RD. Cellular and molecular mechanisms of estrogen regulation of memory function and neuroprotection against Alzheimer's disease:

recent insights and remaining challenges. *Learn Mem* 2001;8:121–33
46. McEwen B, Akama K, Alves S, *et al.* Tracking the estrogen receptor in neurons: implications for estrogen-induced synapse formation. *Proc Natl Acad Sci USA* 2001;98:7093–100
47. Milner TA, McEwen BS, Hayashi S, *et al.* Ultrastructural evidence that hippocampal α estrogen receptors are located at extranuclear sites. *J Comp Neurol* 2001;429:355–71
48. Toran-Allerand CD. The estrogen/neurotrophin connection during neural development: is colocalization of estrogen receptors with the neurotrophins and their receptors biologically relevant? *Dev Neurosci* 1996;18:36–48
49. Aggarwal P, Gibbs RB. Estrogen replacement does not prevent the loss of choline acetyltransferase-positive cells in the basal forebrain following either neurochemical or mechanical lesions. *Brain Res* 2000;882:75–85
50. Walton M, Sirimanne E, Williams C, Gluckman P, Dragunow M. The role of the cyclic AMP-responsive element binding protein (CREB) in hypoxic-ischemic brain damage and repair. *Brain Res Mol Brain Res* 1996;43:21–9
51. Zhou Y, Watters JJ, Dorsa DM. Estrogen rapidly induces the phosphorylation of the cAMP response element binding protein in rat brain. *Endocrinology* 1996;137:2163–6
52. Sheng M, McFadden G, Greenberg ME. Membrane depolarization and calcium induce *c-fos* transcription via phosphorylation of transcription factor CREB. *Neuron* 1990;4:571–82
53. Moore AN, Waxham MN, Dash PK. Neuronal activity increases the phosphorylation of the transcription factor cAMP response element-binding protein (CREB) in rat hippocampus and cortex. *J Biol Chem* 1996;271:14214–20
54. Dash PK, Karl KA, Colicos MA, Prywes R, Kandel ER. cAMP response element-binding protein is activated by Ca^{2+}/calmodulin- as well as cAMP-dependent protein kinase. *Proc Natl Acad Sci USA* 1991;88:5061–5
55. Brooke S, Chan R, Howard S, Sapolsky R. Endocrine modulation of the neurotoxicity of gp120: implications for AIDS-related dementia complex. *Proc Natl Acad Sci USA* 1997;94:9457–62
56. Nakano M, Sugioka K, Naito I, Takekoshi S, Niki E. Novel and potent biological antioxidants on membrane phospholipid peroxidation: 2-hydroxy estrone and 2-hydroxy estradiol. *Biochem Biophys Res Commun* 1987;142:919–24
57. Mukai K, Daifuku K, Yokoyama S, Nakano M. Stopped-flow investigation of antioxidant activity of estrogens in solution. *Biochim Biophys Acta* 1990;1035:348–52
58. Behl C, Skutella T, Lezoualc'h F, *et al.* Neuroprotection against oxidative stress by estrogens: structure-activity relationship. *Mol Pharmacol* 1997;51:535–41
59. Keller JN, Germeyer A, Begley JG, Mattson MP. 17β-Estradiol attenuates oxidative impairment of synaptic Na+/K+-ATPase activity, glucose transport, and glutamate transport induced by amyloid β-peptide and iron. *J Neurosci Res* 1997;50:522–30
60. Zheng J, Ramirez VD. Rapid inhibition of rat brain mitochondrial proton F0F1-ATPase activity by estrogens: comparison with Na^+,K^+-ATPase of porcine cortex. *Eur J Pharmacol* 1999;368:95–102
61. Behl C, Widmann M, Trapp T, Holsboer F. 17-β Estradiol protects neurons from oxidative stress-induced cell death *in vitro*. *Biochem Biophys Res Commun* 1995;216:473–82
62. Berridge MJ, Lipp P, Bootman MD. The versatility and universality of calcium signalling. *Nat Rev Mol Cell Biol* 2000;1:11–21
63. Mattson MP. Calcium as sculptor and destroyer of neural circuitry. *Exp Gerontol* 1992;27:29–49
64. White RJ, Reynolds IJ. Mitochondrial depolarization in glutamate-stimulated neurons: an early signal specific to excitotoxin exposure. *J Neurosci* 1996;16:5688–97
65. Greenamyre JT, Young AB. Excitatory amino acids and Alzheimer's disease. *Neurobiol Aging* 1989;10:593–602
66. Brorson JR, Bindokas VP, Iwama T, *et al.* The Ca^{2+} influx induced by β-amyloid peptide 25–35 in cultured hippocampal neurons results from network excitation. *J Neurobiol* 1995;26:325–38
67. Beal MF. Does impairment of energy metabolism result in excitotoxic neuronal death in neurodegenerative illnesses? *Ann Neurol* 1992;31: 119–30
68. Choi DW. Ischemia-induced neuronal apoptosis. *Curr Opin Neurobiol* 1996;6:667–72
69. Choi DW. Glutamate neurotoxicity and diseases of the nervous system. *Neuron* 1988;1:623–34
70. Choi DW, Rothman SM. The role of glutamate neurotoxicity in hypoxic-ischemic neuronal death. *Annu Rev Neurosci* 1990;13:171–82
71. Beal MF. Mechanisms of excitotoxicity in neurologic diseases. *FASEB J* 1992;6:3338–44
72. Beal MF. Mitochondrial dysfunction in neurodegenerative diseases. *Biochim Biophys Acta* 1998;1366:211–23
73. Choi DW. Ionic dependence of glutamate neurotoxicity. *J Neurosci* 1987;7:369–79
74. Goldberg MP, Weiss JH, Pham PC, Choi DW. *N*-methyl-D-aspartate receptors mediate hypoxic neuronal injury in cortical culture. *J Pharmacol Exp Ther* 1987;243:784–91
75. Hartley DM, Kurth MC, Bjerkness L, Weiss JH, Choi DW. Glutamate receptor-induced $^{45}Ca^{2+}$ accumulation in cortical cell culture correlates with subsequent neuronal degeneration. *J Neurosci* 1993;13:1993–2000

76. Randall RD, Thayer SA. Glutamate-induced calcium transient triggers delayed calcium overload and neurotoxicity in rat hippocampal neurons. *J Neurosci* 1992;12:1882–95
77. Rothman SM, Olney JW. Glutamate and the pathophysiology of hypoxic-ischemic brain damage. *Ann Neurol* 1986;19:105–11
78. Tymianski M, Wallace MC, Spigelman I, *et al.* Cell-permeant Ca^{2+} chelators reduce early excitotoxic and ischemic neuronal injury *in vitro* and *in vivo*. *Neuron* 1993;11:221–35
79. Weaver CE, Park-Chung M, Gibbs TT, Farb DH. 17β-Estradiol protects against NMDA-induced excitotoxicity by direct inhibition of NMDA receptors. *Brain Res* 1997;761:338–41
80. Foy MR, Xu J, Xie X, *et al.* 17β-Estradiol enhances NMDA receptor-mediated EPSPs and long-term potentiation. *J Neurophysiol* 1999;81:925–9
81. Nicholls DG. The regulation of extramitochondrial free calcium ion concentration by rat liver mitochondria. *Biochem J* 1978;176:463–74
82. Nicholls D, Akerman K. Mitochondrial calcium transport. *Biochim Biophys Acta* 1982;683:57–88
83. Khodorov B, Pinelis V, Storozhevykh T, Yuravichus A, Khaspekhov L. Blockade of mitochondrial Ca^{2+} uptake by mitochondrial inhibitors amplifies the glutamate-induced calcium response in cultured cerebellar granule cells. *FEBS Lett* 1999;458:162–6
84. Kimberg DV, Goldstein SA. Binding of calcium by liver mitochondria of rats treated with steroid hormones. *J Biol Chem* 1966;241:95–103
85. Kimberg DV, Goldstein SA. Binding of calcium by liver mitochondria: an effect of steroid hormones in vitamin D-depleted and parathyroidectomized rats. *Endocrinology* 1967;80:89–98
86. Budd SL, Nicholls DG. Mitochondria, calcium regulation, and acute glutamate excitotoxicity in cultured cerebellar granule cells. *J Neurochem* 1996;67:2282–91
87. Wang GJ, Thayer SA. Sequestration of glutamate-induced Ca^{2+} loads by mitochondria in cultured rat hippocampal neurons. *J Neurophysiol* 1996; 76:1611–21
88. Brocard JB, Tassetto M, Reynolds IJ. Quantitative evaluation of mitochondrial calcium content in rat cortical neurones following a glutamate stimulus. *J Physiol* 2001;531:793–805
89. Budd SL, Nicholls DG. A reevaluation of the role of mitochondria in neuronal Ca^{2+} homeostasis. *J Neurochem* 1996;66:403–11
90. Gunter TE, Gunter KK, Sheu SS, Gavin CE. Mitochondrial calcium transport: physiological and pathological relevance. *Am J Physiol* 1994;267: C313–39
91. Gunter TE, Pfeiffer DR. Mechanisms by which mitochondria transport calcium. *Am J Physiol* 1990;258:C755–86
92. Dugan LL, Sensi SL, Canzoniero LM, *et al.* Mitochondrial production of reactive oxygen species in cortical neurons following exposure to *N*-methyl-D-aspartate. *J Neurosci* 1995;15:6377–88
93. Reynolds IJ, Hastings TG. Glutamate induces the production of reactive oxygen species in cultured forebrain neurons following NMDA receptor activation. *J Neurosci* 1995;15:3318–27
94. Schinder AF, Olson EC, Spitzer NC, Montal M. Mitochondrial dysfunction is a primary event in glutamate neurotoxicity. *J Neurosci* 1996;16: 6125–33
95. McCormack JG, Denton RM. Mitochondrial Ca^{2+} transport and the role of intramitochondrial Ca^{2+} in the regulation of energy metabolism. *Dev Neurosci* 1993;15:165–73
96. Stout AK, Raphael HM, Kanterewicz BI, Klann E, Reynolds IJ. Glutamate-induced neuron death requires mitochondrial calcium uptake. *Nat Neurosci* 1998;1:366–73
97. Joseph SK, Coll KE, Cooper RH, Marks JS, Williamson JR. Mechanisms underlying calcium homeostasis in isolated hepatocytes. *J Biol Chem* 1983;258:731–41
98. Murphy E, Coll K, Rich TL, Williamson JR. Hormonal effects on calcium homeostasis in isolated hepatocytes. *J Biol Chem* 1980;255:6600–8
99. Burgess GM, McKinney JS, Fabiato A, Leslie BA, Putney JW Jr. Calcium pools in saponin-permeabilized guinea pig hepatocytes. *J Biol Chem* 1983;258:15336–45
100. Blaustein MP, Ratzlaff RW, Kendrick NC, Schweitzer ES. Calcium buffering in presynaptic nerve terminals. I. Evidence for involvement of a nonmitochondrial ATP-dependent sequestration mechanism. *J Gen Physiol* 1978;72:15–41
101. Blaustein MP, Ratzlaff RW, Schweitzer ES. Calcium buffering in presynaptic nerve terminals. II. Kinetic properties of the nonmitochondrial Ca sequestration mechanism. *J Gen Physiol* 1978; 72:43–66
102. Schweitzer ES, Blaustein MP. Calcium buffering in presynaptic nerve terminals. Free calcium levels measured with arsenazo III. *Biochim Biophys Acta* 1980;600:912–21
103. Becker GL. Steady state regulation of extramitochondrial Ca^{2+} by rat liver mitochondria: effects of Mg^{2+} and ATP. *Biochim Biophys Acta* 1980;591:234–9
104. White RJ, Reynolds IJ. Mitochondria accumulate Ca^{2+} following intense glutamate stimulation of cultured rat forebrain neurones. *J Physiol* 1997; 498:31–47
105. Pozzan T, Magalhaes P, Rizzuto R. The comeback of mitochondria to calcium signalling. *Cell Calcium* 2000;28:279–83
106. Duchen MR. Mitochondria and calcium: from cell signalling to cell death. *J Physiol* 2000;529: 57–68

107. Kluck RM, Bossy-Wetzel E, Green DR, Newmeyer DD. The release of cytochrome c from mitochondria: a primary site for Bcl-2 regulation of apoptosis. *Science* 1997;275:1132–6
108. Murphy AN, Bredesen DE, Cortopassi G, Wang E, Fiskum G. Bcl-2 potentiates the maximal calcium uptake capacity of neural cell mitochondria. *Proc Natl Acad Sci USA* 1996;93:9893–8
109. Murphy AN. Ca(2+)-mediated mitochondrial dysfunction and the protective effects of Bcl-2. *Ann NY Acad Sci* 1999;893:19–32
110. Teixeira C, Reed JC, Pratt MA. Estrogen promotes chemotherapeutic drug resistance by a mechanism involving Bcl-2 proto-oncogene expression in human breast cancer cells. *Cancer Res* 1995; 55:3902–7
111. Dong L, Wang W, Wang F, *et al.* Mechanisms of transcriptional activation of *bcl-2* gene expression by 17β-estradiol in breast cancer cells. *J Biol Chem* 1999;274:32099–107
112. Zhu L, Ling S, Yu XD, *et al.* Modulation of mitochondrial Ca(2+) homeostasis by Bcl-2. *J Biol Chem* 1999;274:33267–73
113. Mattson MP, Robinson N, Guo Q. Estrogens stabilize mitochondrial function and protect neural cells against the pro-apoptotic action of mutant presenilin-1. *Neuroreport* 1997;8: 3817–21
114. Gross A, McDonnell JM, Korsmeyer SJ. Bcl-2 family members and the mitochondria in apoptosis. *Genes Dev* 1999;13:1899–911
115. Oltvai ZN, Milliman CL, Korsmeyer SJ. Bcl-2 heterodimerizes *in vivo* with a conserved homolog, Bax, that accelerates programmed cell death. *Cell* 1993;74:609–19
116. Merry DE, Korsmeyer SJ. Bcl-2 gene family in the nervous system. *Annu Rev Neurosci* 1997; 20:245–67
117. Yang E, Korsmeyer SJ. Molecular thanatopsis: a discourse on the Bcl2 family and cell death. *Blood* 1996;88:386–401
118. Bi R, Broutman G, Foy MR, Thompson RF, Baudry M. The tyrosine kinase and mitogen-activated protein kinase pathways mediate multiple effects of estrogen in hippocampus. *Proc Natl Acad Sci USA* 2000;97:3602–7
119. Finkbeiner S. CREB couples neurotrophin signals to survival messages. *Neuron* 2000;25:11–14
120. Honda K, *et al.* Nongenomic antiapoptotic signal transduction by estrogen in cultured cortical neurons. *J Neurosci Res* 2001;64:466–75
121. Yano S, Tokumitsu H, Soderling TR. Calcium promotes cell survival through CaM-K kinase activation of the protein-kinase-B pathway. *Nature (London)* 1998;396:584–7
122. Brewer GJ, Reichensperger JD, Brinton RD. Age-related estrogen regulation of Ca^{2+} dynamics in hippocampal neurons. *Soc Neurosci Abstr* 2002; 73:272.7
123. Genazzani AR, Gambacciani M. A personal initiative for women's health: to challenge the Women's Health Initiative. *Gynecol Endocrinol* 2002;16:255–7
124. Resnick SM, Henderson VW. Hormone therapy and risk of Alzheimer disease: a critical time. *J Am Med Assoc* 2002;288:2170–2

The immune system, estrogen and brain aging 3

I. Silva, G. Mor, I. Bechmann and F. Naftolin

INTRODUCTION

Today, women are living an increasing portion of their lives in the post-reproductive period, when the circulating estrogen level is low. In part, the above is due to a dramatic increase in life expectancy. This longer exposure to low circulating estrogen creates new challenges, one of which is the prevention and repair of damage to the aging brain.

In the early 20th century, Ramon y Cajal[1] suggested that brain cells are capable of morphological changes in response to their environment. Since then, gonadal steroids have become known to play important roles in determining and modulating cell number and size, neuronal morphology and synaptic density of sex steroid-responsive structures in the central nervous system (CNS), during both development and adulthood. Furthermore, sex steroids have been shown to regulate the number and action of the cells in the glial compartments (astroglia, microglia and oligodendroglia) of the brain.

These sex steroid effects may be direct or indirect. Generally, they include diverse responses such as the increased expression of neurotrophic factors and their receptors.

Only one in ten brain cells is a neuron; the other nine are in the glial compartment and are responsible for maintaining the microenvironment around neurons, and guiding neuronal projections or processes to other neurons so that messages can be passed in the form of close connections called synapses. Estrogen may act directly on neurons and glial cells via intracellular estrogen receptors (ERs), or indirectly by inducing the expression of cytokines and growth factors in other, ER-bearing cells.

ESTROGEN AND NEURONS

The effects of estrogens on neurons have been widely studied and reported. For the purposes of this chapter, it is necessary only to point out that we and others have shown direct effects of estrogens on the developmental proliferation of neurons *in vitro* and *in vivo*, as well as estrogen's regulation of the number and extent of neural processes and synaptic connections[2]. Although the following concentrates on the role of the glia in maintaining the microenvironment so that the neuronal cells and their processes can remain vital and active, intrinsic factors related to neuronal function and the direct effects of both aging and insults on the neurons should not be discounted[3].

ESTROGEN AND GLIA

There are two general classes of glia in the CNS, the macroglia cells (astrocytes and oligodendrocytes) and microglia.

Oligodendrocytes

Oligodendrocytes are responsible for myelination in the CNS. They are affected by the demyelinating diseases, some of which appear to have an immunological basis[4]. There is developing evidence that B ring-unsaturated androgens and progestins (neurosteroids) are formed by the oligodendroglia, and can regulate myelination[5]. While there is not yet evidence regarding the role of these compounds in the pathophysiology of diseases such as multiple sclerosis, the above seems a possibility.

Astroglia

Astroglia are the most numerous cells in the brain. They have distinct relationships with structures in the brain that indicate specific functions. For example, the glia limitans wrap processes around brain blood vessels and appear to have a gating function for the passage of molecules and cells into and out of the brain. Types 1 and 2 astrocytes ensheath neurons and regulate the micro-environment of the synaptic and non-synaptic areas of the neurons[6]. Recently, it has been appreciated that the astroglia form a network of (slower) calcium flux-mediated conduction in the brain[6].

In a cellular context, the astroglia have been shown to express both estrogen synthetase (aromatase) and ER under stressful conditions. Thus, they are sensitive to indirect (via, for example, cytokines and growth factors) and direct effects of estrogen that affect their shape and function[7]. Among these roles are immune and non-immune responses to injury. In this regard it is of particular importance that astroglia express immune proteins (see below).

Microglia

Microglia are cellular equivalents of the macrophages of the brain. They constitute master cells in the brain's immune response[3,8].

Recent studies have made it clear that regulation by the immune system is critical in homeostasis and disease in all tissues, including the brain. This chapter draws on general principles of immunobiology, including studies of estrogen formation and action in immunocytes, plus data gathered in studies of the brain, to present a comprehensive view of the relationship between estrogen and the immune system in the very special conditions of the CNS. These include particular constraints on the brain: unyielding space, and dense membranes that house the brain in place with little replacement if any of neurons are lost due to brain swelling. Finally, vulnerable neural fibers pass through distant and apparently unrelated parts of the CNS. If those areas are undergoing immune responses, this could result in soma or fiber damage. Thus, it is important to regulate the amount of inflammation, edema and release of toxic compounds into the area of immune responses in the brain, to avoid dangerous brain shifts and collateral damage to sensitive neurons and neuronal processes.

IMMUNE RESPONSES AND THE BRAIN

Homeostasis versus disease

As in the rest of the body, there is a constant need for cleaning and repair of the cellular machinery and intercellular spaces of the brain. This is in part accomplished by the immune system. We have reviewed this action elsewhere[9,10]. In essence, the primary cells involved are the macrophages of the brain, which are known as microglial cells[8]. These cells constantly patrol the entire brain, adjusting the microenvironment, removing waste products, etc. They have different phenotypes and activities as seen in Figure 1. The microglia are under endocrine and humoral control, the former via hormonal receptors in/on the microglia and the latter via cytokines known as chemokines that are made by nearby cells[11]. These humoral substances also modulate the tone of the immune system between a dominance of cellular (TH1 type) and humoral (TH2) immune responses[12].

Proinflammation

Esch and Stefano have proposed that, during the homeostatic period, the immune system is regulated by 'proinflammation'. This is a humorally regulated state in which the principal immune cells adjust the balance of the immune system so that they can perform their homeostatic functions while retaining their immune tone capability for immediate responses required of the immune system when it is abruptly challenged. Adrenocorticosteroids and other stress hormones plus cytokines regulate proinflammation[13].

MICROGLIAL CELLS

We have shown that microglial cells patrol the brain under the control of estrogen (Williams and colleagues, unpublished data). During an immune challenge in the brain, microglial cells respond in a manner concordant with the systemic immune system's responses[14,15]. This includes

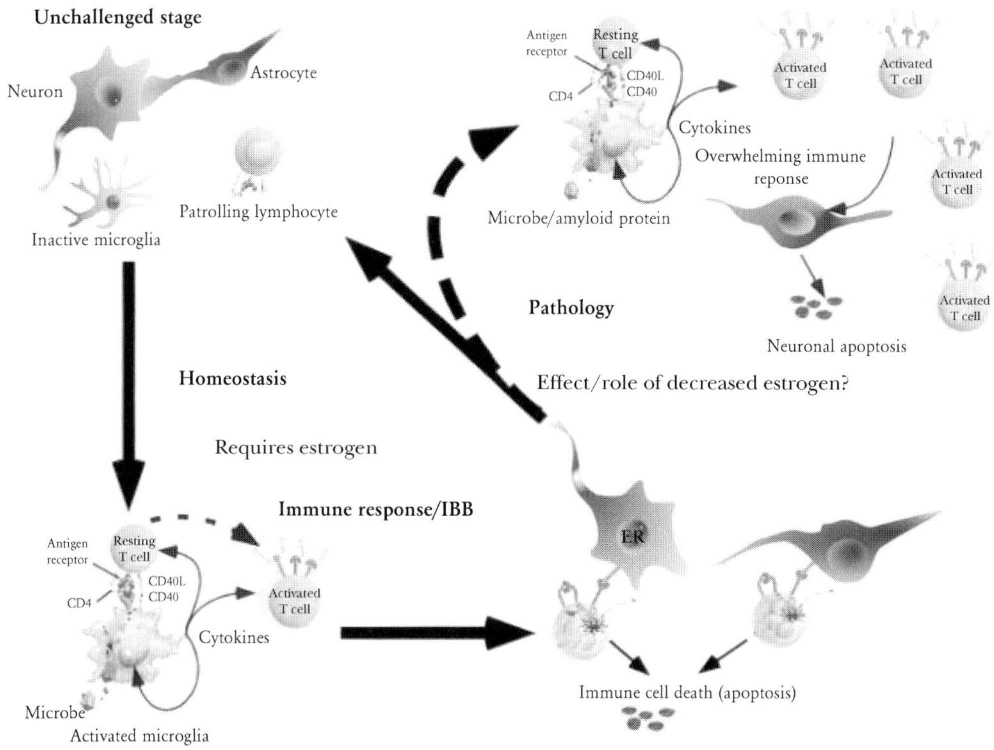

Figure 1 Hypothesis of the role of estrogen in immune-regulated homeostasis and pathology in the brain deriving from the immune-brain barrier (IBB). Homeostasis in the brain is maintained by functional balance between the induced immune response and apoptosis of activated cells. Estrogen plays a key role in brain-immune homeostasis by regulating microglia activation, CD40 and Fas ligand (FasL). The result is the maintenance of a controlled inflammatory response to injury or noxious stimuli. Pathology occurs in the absence of estrogen action because of compromised elements of the IBB and/or in the presence of overwhelming injury or noxious substances. ER, estrogen receptor. Modified from reference 3

proliferation, activation of other immunocytes and glial activation. These responses include gliosis that may lead to scarring, as well as the stripping of synapses during inflammation[7].

Regulation of microglia by estrogen

The regulation of microglia by estrogen and its results are central issues in the aging brain. Monocytes have been shown to contain estrogen synthetase (aromatase) and form estrogen from (circulatory) androgens[16]. This remains to be shown in microglia, but estrogen is available in the brain from neighboring neurons[17], reactive glia[18] and circulation[19]. Moreover, the microglia are responsive to estrogens. Microglia express the estrogen receptor β (ERβ)[10]. This allows speculation that microglia and their products mediate certain effects of estrogen on immunological and brain function. Important effects on brain function of estrogen-regulated products such as cytokines and nitric oxide have been reported[20,21].

PAST PROINFLAMMATION

The brain is an unusually complex and diverse organ that receives input from all senses, functions at varying levels of intensity and is subject to challenges from both internal and external sources. These challenges may be from trauma, hypoxia and brain metabolites, as well as from infectious agents. In contrast to most organs, the brain is constrained in unusual ways that arise from its protected (constraining) location, its great metabolic flux and the blood flow needed to maintain brain function and cerebrospinal fluid in which the brain is suspended and with which it is bathed. The brain is in the rigid cranium, and is held compartmentalized in rigid membranous supports that, in dictating the total volume of their contents, also allow the sacrifice of non-edematous tissue to pressure created by the growth of areas of brain swelling from inflammation, trauma, etc. The brain cannot easily accommodate edema, position shifts or displacement, as can other organs.

Neurons are the brain's most important and delicate cells. They are generally not replaceable. Furthermore, they have vulnerable, distant extensions (processes) and are suspended in a matrix of other brain cells, mainly the astroglia. The latter are themselves subject to injury and response characteristics that are not always consonant with the maintenance of the neuronal components in their midst[22-24]. These issues are in play on a moment-to-moment basis as well as being cumulative[22]. It is therefore necessary that inflammation and collateral damage arising in the brain be controlled.

Immune checkpoint proteins

Protection against premature or overly zealous immunoreactions is afforded by the brain's system of immune proteins, especially the Fas (CD95)–Fas ligand (FasL, CD95L) and CD40–CD40 ligand (CD40L) systems[3,8-10]. These are enabling proteins that regulate the extent of the immune response, thereby countering proinflammation's tone and actual immune reactions to ensure that a false triggering or overzealous response by the brain's immune system will not result in excessive edema, process loss or neuronal loss, etc. In regulating the expression of immune checkpoint proteins, estrogen hinders the activation of immunocytes. This automatically places more of the response in the province of the local inflammatory cells, thereby circumscribing the immune reaction to cause less collateral damage. For example, estrogen induces the expression of FasL by brain immunocytes and this results in apoptosis of cells activated by antigen-presenting cells (APCs) such as infiltrating lymphocytes[9,25]. These lymphocytes are therefore unable to induce antigen-specific immunity in response to the insult, an important mechanism of immune tolerance[26]. Microglia and astrocytes in the area are present to deal with the insult. A similar scenario is triggered in the presence of estrogen if the pro-proliferation signal transduction pathway from CD40 is not activated after local insult. In our *in vitro* work, we have shown that estrogen down-regulates the expression of CD40 in microglia in culture (unpublished data). Although the CD40-suppressing effect of estrogen remains to be demonstrated *in vivo*, the results are promising in that this will eventuate in the description of a symmetrical (apoptosis and proliferation) immune suppression by estrogen. This means that estrogen causes less superoxide release, phagocytosis and immunological nitric oxide synthase (iNOS) expression[27], both directly and via the effects of FasL and CD40.

We recently showed that in estrogen-treated primates there is an inverse relationship between estrogen levels and the movement of microglia in the cerebellum. The cerebellum of normally cycling rats at proestrus, when estrogen levels peak, contains few microglial cells, while in diestrus these cells are abundant in the molecular and granular layers and tend to increase in the Purkinje layer. Thus, it appears that a low estrogen level is associated with a swarming of microglia to the Purkinje layer and surrounding areas, passing through the white matter and showing changes associated with microglia activation (Williams and colleagues, unpublished data).

ESTROGEN AND ASTROCYTES

Proliferation

Astrocytes are often involved in immune responses to insult in the brain, including proliferation, so-called gliosis[7,22]. Recently, the expression of estrogen receptors by astrocytes under stress has been reported[7]. While estrogen does not affect astroglia in primary cultures, astrocytes in human temporal cortex slice preparations retract their processes. It is not known whether this response of human astroglia to estradiol requires ER, but it occurs in minutes, indicating that it may be non-genomic (unpublished data). The occurrence of gliosis and an estrogen effect in astroglia indicate that the usual mechanism of injury-induced proliferation via the activation of the

CD40 pathway may be under way. This possibility is currently under study.

Protective effects

Neuroprotective effects of estradiol and raloxifene have been shown. The cells that are protected express estrogen receptors[7,28]. We are currently examining the possibility of estradiol's protective effects on astroglia.

IMMUNE–BRAIN BARRIER

The presence of an immune-brain barrier (IBB) has been proposed as a mechanism that could mitigate the brain's response to injury. This would avoid undue inflammation and collateral damage to neurons and neuronal processes[9]. The IBB depends on the action of immune checkpoint proteins to avoid overexuberant immune reactions in the brain[22]. We have discussed the difference between the homeostasis that is normally maintained by the immune system and disease, which may arise during immune responses to injury, etc. The IBB modulates the brain's immune activity to ensure that the escalation from homeostasis (which is performed by local immunocytes) to a TH1 or TH2 immune response (which requires interplay with other immunocytes) is neither haphazard nor greater than required[10]. Recently, we have focused on two of the checkpoint proteins, FasL and CD40, that are called into play when there is brain injury or other insult.

The Fas (receptor)–Fas ligand (FasL) system is a system that protects against inappropriate activation of immunocytes and other cells by apoptosis. Fas is a cell surface receptor that is extruded from cells of the CNS (see above) under conditions of stress, and during immune activation in the presence of antigen-presenting cell (APCs). Activation of Fas by the binding of FasL triggers a signal transduction pathway that eventuates in caspase-dependent apoptosis[29].

FasL is expressed by astrocytes, neurons and microglia. As one of the stimuli for FasL expression, estrogen restrains the reaction to injury by increasing apoptosis among the incoming, activated immunocytes during antigen presentation. The result is that the antigen-specific immune response is curtailed or aborted. This leaves the local innate immunocytes, especially the microglia, to deal with the noxious stimulus. This minimizes the collateral damage to nearby neurons or processes. This portion of the IBB has been well studied and described[9,10].

The second immune checkpoint protein system is CD40 (receptor)–CD40 ligand (CD40L). In contradistinction to the Fas–FasL system, activation of CD40 leads to proliferation of the cells that are responding during immune activation, and therefore a greater immune response. CD40L present on APCs must bind to CD40 on the incoming glial immunocytes and leukocytes for this proliferation to occur. Using *in vitro* techniques we have shown that estradiol decreases the expression of CD40 by microglia (Silva, unpublished data). Thus, estradiol controls two of the vital proteins making up the IBB (Figure 2).

Estrogen treatment has been shown to be neuroprotective in acute and chronic models of brain hypoxia/asphyxia, injury and stress[22,28,30]. In clinical settings, estrogen treatment is associated with delay of dystrophic brain diseases such as Alzheimer's dementia. It is possible that the IBB represents one of the routes of estrogen's protection against brain disease.

CONCLUSION

The mechanisms of estrogen-induced neuroprotection are currently under study. There are functional and morphological links between homeostatic and potentially disease-producing responses by brain cells. Estrogen affects normal brain function, the brain's vasculature, its repair mechanisms and the brain's management of inflammation. Estrogen's role in brain protection involves more systems than are generally appreciated. These include the cellular regulation of neuroactive substances, hormones, cytokines and growth factors and brain proteins that play individual roles in neuroprotection.

In addition to the cellular neuroprotective effects of estrogen, there are broader, systemic brain-protective actions of estrogen that, for example, are exerted via regulation of the immune system. This chapter concentrates on estrogen's regulation of the immune system allowing

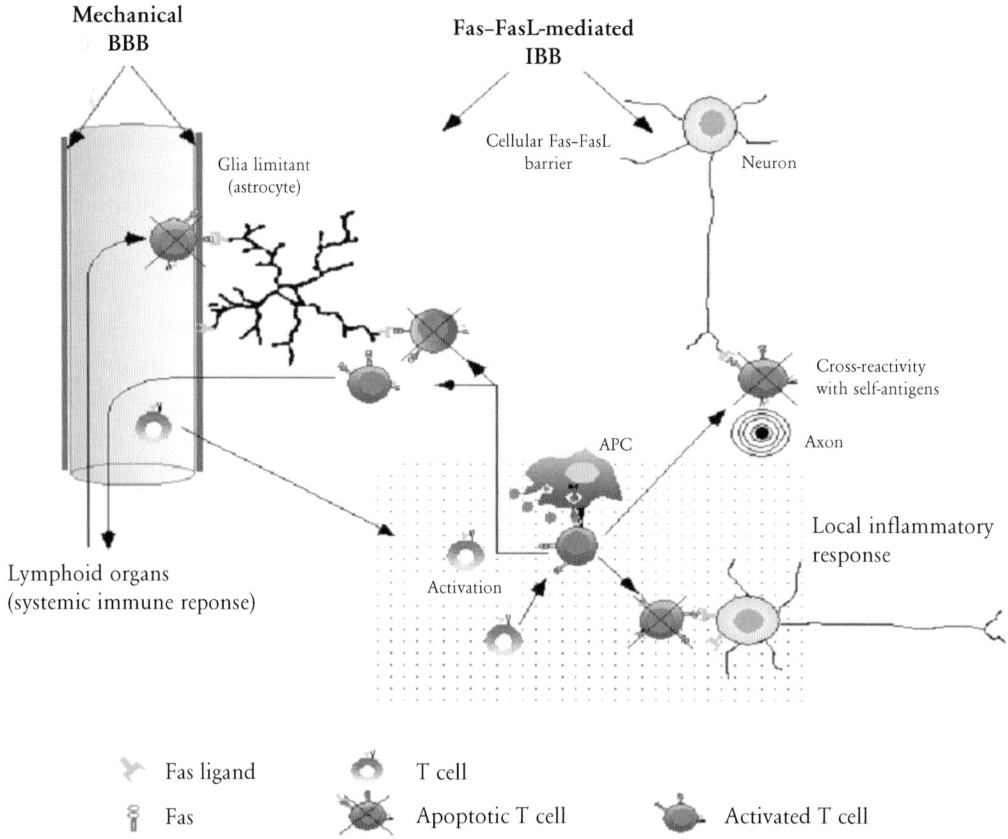

Figure 2 The immune-brain barrier (IBB). The IBB furnishes a means of regulating the immune response to brain insults. BBB, blood-brain barrier; APC, antigen-presenting cell. Modified from reference 9

controlled responses and minimized collateral damage to neurons and processes which could be involved in responses by the immune system that signal injury, etc. The mechanism of this modulation is termed the immune-blood barrier (IBB). Because they are the most studied components of the IBB, this chapter focuses on the Fas-FasL and the CD40-CD40L systems.

Of course, all aspects of brain disease and protection are complicated by aging. In this regard, the immune system plays a dual role in responding to both the degenerative processes that accompany aging and normal brain stress, insults and injury. Since, in part, these responses underlie the development of dystrophies such as Alzheimer's disease, it is especially important to understand the mechanisms of the immune system's homeostatic and responsive actions and the role of estrogen in their regulation.

ACKNOWLEDGEMENT

We appreciate support from the Eli Lilly Company (AG15457 to F.N.).

References

1. Ramon y Cajal, S. Notas preventives sobre la degeneracion y regeneration de las vias nerviosas centrals. *Trab Labor Invest Biol* 1906;4:295-301
2. Naftolin F, Mor G, Horvath TL, *et al.* Synaptic remodeling in the arcuate nucleus during the estrous cycle is induced by estrogen and pre-

cedes the preovulatory gonadotrophin surge. *Endocrinology* 1996;137:1537–43
3. Silva I, Mor G, Naftolin F. Estrogen and the aging brain. *Maturitas* 2001;38:95–101
4. Steinman L, Martin R, Bernard C, Conlon P, Oksenberg JR. Multiple sclerosis: deeper understanding of its pathogenesis reveals new targets for therapy. *Annu Rev Neurosci* 2002;25:491–505
5. Baulieu EE, Schumacher M. Progesterone as a neuroactive neurosteroid, with special reference to the effect of progesterone on myelination. *Steroids* 2002;65:605–12
6. Hayden PG. Glia: listening and talking to the synapse. *Nature Rev Neurosci* 2001;2:185–92
7. Garcia-Ovejero D, Veiga S, Garcia-Segura M, Doncarlos LL. Glial expression of estrogen and androgen receptors after rat brain injury. *J Comp Neurol* 2002;450:256–71
8. Silva I, Nilsen J, Williams S, *et al.* Estrogen effects on microglia and immune checkpoint proteins in the brain. In Schneider HPG, ed. *Menopause: The State of the Art - in Research and Management, The Official Proceedings of the 10th World Congress on the Menopause.* London, UK: Parthenon Publishing, 2002:186–90
9. Bechmann I, Mor G, Nilsen J, *et al.* FasL (CD95L, Apo1L) is expressed in the normal rat and human brain - evidence for the existence of an immunological brain barrier. *Glia* 1999;27:62–74
10. Mor G, Nilsen J, Horvath T, *et al.* Estrogen and microglia: a regulatory system that affects the brain. *J Neurobiol* 1999;40:484–96
11. Flynn G, Maru S, Loughlin J, Romero IA, Male D. Regulation of chemokine receptor expression in human microglia and astrocytes. *J Immunol* 2003; 136:84–93
12. Mor G, Naftolin F. Oestrogen, menopause and the immune system. *J Br Menopause Soc* 1998; S1:4–8
13. Esch T, Stefano G. Proinflammation: a common denominator or initiator of different pathophysiological disease processes. *Med Sci Monit* 2002;8: HY1–9
14. Bechmann I, Nitsch R. Plasticity following lesion: help and harm from the immune system. *Restor Neurol Neurosci* 2001;19:189–98
15. Eyupoglu IY, Bechmann I, Nitsch R. Modification of microglia function protects from lesion-induced neuronal alterations and promotes sprouting in the hippocampus. *FASEB J* 2003;17:1110–11
16. Mor G, Yue W, Santen RJ, *et al.* Macrophages, estrogen and microenvironment of breast cancer. *J Steroid Biochem Mol Biol* 1998;67:403–11
17. Jakab RL, Horvath TL, Leranth C, Harada N, Naftolin F. Aromatase immunoreactivity in the rat brain: gonadectomy-sensitive hypothalamic neurons and an unresponsive 'limbic ring' of the lateral septum-bed nucleus–amygdala complex. *J Steroid Biochem Mol Biol* 1993;44:481–98
18. Garcia-Segura ML, Wozniak A, Azcoitia I, Rodriguez R, Hutchison RE, Hutchison JB. Aromatase expression by astrocytes after brain injury: implications for local estrogen formation in brain repair. *Neuroscience* 1999;89:567–78
19. Stoffel-Wagner B, Watzka M, Schramm J, Bidlingmaier F, Klingmuller D. Expression of CYP19 (aromatase) mRNA in different areas of the human brain. *J Steroid Biochem Mol Biol* 1999; 70:237–41
20. Adamson DC, Wildemann B, Sasaki M, *et al.* Immunologic NO synthase: elevation in severe AIDS dementia and induction by HIV-1 gp41. *Science* 1996;274:1917–21
21. Stalder A, Pagenstecher A, Yu NC, *et al.* Lipopolysaccharide-induced IL-12 expression in the central nervous system and cultured astrocytes and microglia. *J Immunol* 1997;159:1344–51
22. Garcia-Estrada J, Del Rio JA, Luquin S, Garcia-Segura LM. Gonadal hormones down-regulate reactive gliosis and astrocyte proliferation after a penetrating brain injury. *Brain Res* 1993;628:271–8
23. Klepper S, Naftolin F, Peipmeier JM. Verapamil treatment attenuates immunoreactive GFAP at cerebral cortical lesion site. *Brain Res* 1995;695: 245–9
24. Du S, Rubin A, Klepper S, *et al.* Calcium influx and activation of calpain I mediate acute reactive gliosis in injured spinal cord. *Exp Neurol* 1999;157:96–105
25. Bechmann I, Lossau S, Steiner B, Mor G, Gimsa U, Nitsch R. Reactive astrocytes upregulate Fas (CD95) and Fas ligand (CD95L) expression but do not undergo programmed cell death during the course of anterograde degeneration. *Glia* 2000; 32:25–41
26. Kamradt T, Mitchison NA. Tolerance and autoimmunity. *N Engl J Med* 2001;344:655–64
27. Bruce-Keller AJ. Microglia-neuronal interactions in synaptic damage and recovery. *J Neurosci Res* 1999;58:191–201
28. Dhandapani KM, Brann DW. Protective effects of estrogen and selective estrogen receptor modulators in the brain. *Biol Reprod* 2002;67: 1379–85
29. Mor G, Sapi E, Abrahams VM, *et al.* Interaction of the estrogen receptors with the Fas ligand promoter in human monocytes. *J Immunol* 2003;170:114–22
30. Hoffman GE, Le WW, Murphy AZ, Koski CL. Divergent effects of estrogen steroids on neuronal survival during experimental allergic encephalitis in Lewis rats. *Exp Neurol* 2001;171:272–84

Brain phenotype of the aromatase knock-out mouse 4

E. R. Simpson, R. A. Hill, M. van den Buuse, M. E. Jones and W. C. Boon

INTRODUCTION

Temporary retention of verbal or visual information and its active manipulation are intrinsically involved in working memory tasks. The importance of the frontal cortex in working memory has been demonstrated using a wide variety of techniques, including lesion studies in monkeys and patients[1,2] as well as functional neuroimaging in healthy human volunteers[3,4]. In addition, it has been reported that age-related degeneration of the frontal cortex is greater than the degeneration of other areas of the human brain[5], and Alzheimer's disease patients have less total prefrontal cortex gray matter than age-matched healthy subjects[6]. In one study, specifically examining the effect of estrogen on prefrontal cortex-dependent working memory, Duff and Hampson[7] found that healthy postmenopausal women taking estrogen exhibited significantly better performance on both verbal (Digit Ordering) and spatial (Spatial Working Memory) working memory tasks, but did not differ from healthy non-users on control tasks involving simple passive recall.

Similar results were reported in another study[8] which conducted neuropsychological tests on memory, verbal fluency, executive functions, attention and concentration and psychomotor function in healthy postmenopausal women aged over 60 years, with or without estrogen replacement therapy. Although no statistical significance was found for general demographic, intellectual and psychological measures, scores from both the Weschler Memory Scale Visual Reproduction (delayed recall) and the Digital Vigilance Test (attention) showed statistically significant better performance and fewer errors in the group of women taking estrogen replacement therapy.

These results are consistent with a more recent study[9] of the cognitive effects of 10 years of hormone replacement therapy with tibolone, a drug that exhibits estrogenic, progestogenic and androgenic activities, in women aged between 54 and 66 years. Results from this study revealed that women taking tibolone (when compared with placebo) felt significantly less clumsy. After exposure to a mildly stressful test, the control group felt more anxious, and the treatment group scored significantly higher on semantic memory tests. Carlson and Sherwin[10] also found that lifetime hormone replacement therapy use was associated with better baseline modified Mini-Mental State Examination scores and slower rates of decline.

AROMATASE EXPRESSION IN THE BRAIN

Aromatization of androgens to estrogens was first recognized in neural tissue from the non-human primate in 1973, by Flores and colleagues[11]. Several investigations followed, establishing the expression of aromatase in specific regions of the brain. One early report demonstrated that, in males, aromatization was present in the hypothalamus and limbic structures of the rat, rabbit, rhesus monkey and human fetus[12]. In a similar study of fetal brain aromatase expression in rabbits, significant rates of aromatase activity were expressed in the forebrain, with high rates occurring in the diencephelon of both male and female embryos between days 19 and 25 of gestation. More recently, the rate of aromatase activity in male rhesus monkeys has been measured throughout the brain, revealing the highest amount of activity occurring within specific regions of the hypothalamus and amygdala[13]. Specific regions of high aromatase activity include the medial preoptic area anterior hypothalamus (MPAH), ventromedial hypothalamus (VMH), bed nucleus of the stria terminalis (BMST), cortical amygdala (CA) and medial amygdala[13]. Levels of aromatase mRNA-containing cells were also observed to be highest in specific regions of the hypothalamus, including the medial preoptic nucleus and ventromedial hypothalamic nucleus[13]. Similar results were observed for rat brain[14,15].

Aromatase activity under normal conditions is believed to be centralized to neuronal cell bodies and neuronal processes (such as axon terminals) of the non-human primate, and other vertebrate species[3,16–18]. However, increased aromatase activity and induced expression of aromatase was recently observed to occur in reactive astroglia in rat brains after induced injury to the brain. After applying neurotoxins and mechanical lesions to specific areas of the brain, including the cortex, corpus callosum, striatum, hippocampus, thalamus and hypothalamus, all areas displayed aromatase expression in astroglia[19].

In summary, aromatase appears to be expressed in the frontal cortex, diencephelon, hippocampus, hypothalamus amygdala and pons regions, while aromatase activity is highest in the hypothalamus and amygdala. The activity of aromatase seems to be centralized to neurons and neuronal processes, but may occur in astroglia after injury.

THE *CYP19* GENE

The human P450arom enzyme is encoded by the *CYP19* gene. The *CYP19* gene was characterized over a decade ago[20–22], and it encodes a protein comprising approximately 500 amino acids[23]. The coding region of P450arom spans nine exons beginning with exon II[20]. The *CYP19* gene also displays tissue-specific expression, which is determined by the use of tissue-specific promoters, which give rise to transcripts with unique 5′-non-coding termini[24]. While placental transcripts contain at their 5′ end the distal untranslated exon I.1, transcripts in the ovary contain sequence at the 5′ end, which is immediately upstream of the start of translation. This is achieved by utilizing a proximal promoter, promoter II[25]. Adipose tissue contains transcripts with another distal exon, exon I.4, and a brain-specific 5′ untranslated transcript (exon If) has also been described[26]. This is a sequence that is present in rat amygdala and in the hypothalamus–preoptic area (HPOA). Promoter II-specific transcripts have also been detected in amygdala and HPOA regions[27]. More recently, different patterns of utilization of exon I in different areas of the brain have been discovered. Both males and females utilize promoter If or II in hypothalamic or limbic structures, while the pons and frontal lobe utilize I.4[27,28]. The coding region of the mouse *Cyp19* gene is similar to that of the human; however, the promoter regions are still being investigated.

THE AROMATASE KNOCK-OUT MOUSE

Aromatase knock-out (ArKO) mice (129_{SV}/J × c57BL/6J) were generated by disruption of the *Cyp19* gene by homologous recombination[29]. Homologous null or wild-type offspring were bred by crossing mice heterozygous for the disrupted gene. The pups were genotyped by polymerase chain reaction (PCR) as described elsewhere[30]. Animals had *ad libitum* access to water and soy-free mouse chow.

Brain phenotype of the female ArKO mouse

The results of histological studies (dUTP nick-end labelling (TUNEL) and immunostaining), RNase protection assay and 17β-estradiol replacement showed that a consequence of estrogen deficiency in female ArKO mice is apoptosis and cell loss in the frontal cortex of the brain. Our results demonstrated that estrogen probably exerts its survival effect on the neurons through up-regulation of antiapoptotic genes (*bcl-2*, *bfl-1*, *bcl-W* and *bcl-XL*) and down-regulation of at least one proapoptotic gene TRADD. Although there have been reports that cultured neurons undergo apoptosis in the absence of estrogen[31–33], this is the first *in vivo* study to show that neurons undergo spontaneous apoptosis in the absence of estrogen, in contrast to cell death caused by neurotoxins[34,35], ischemia[36,37] or impact-accelerated head injury[38]. Regional neuronal hypocellularity in the brain cortex[39] has been reported in the estrogen receptor β knockout mouse (ERβKO), but no apoptosis in the brain of these mice has been reported to date.

In addition, we have shown using the Y-maze test that the neuronal loss is associated with spatial working memory (short-term memory) deficit in these female ArKO mice. This is demonstrated by a lack of preference for the 'novel' arm during the second exploration session in the Y-maze test. The 'reluctance' to visit or spend more time in the 'novel' arm is not due to increased anxiety in ArKO mice. In fact, employing another test, namely the elevated plus maze test, female ArKO mice were more inclined to explore the open arms, compared with female wild-type mice, which did not enter the open arms at all. Hence, we may conclude that young female ArKO mice have a short-term memory deficit. Interestingly, Krezel and colleagues[40] have reported that the female ERβKO mouse displays increased anxiety, but not the female ERαKO. No report is available to date on the short-term memory of the ERβKO or ERαKO mouse.

A third test was employed, namely the Morris watermaze test. The results of this test showed that the spatial learning behavior of young female ArKO mice was not compromised. If anything, they exhibited evidence of improved spatial learning ability, compared with wild-type mice, in the free-swim trials. These results may be a consequence of increased transcript levels of the *N*-methyl-D-aspartate (NMDA) receptor NR2B in the ArKO mouse hippocampus. Previously, it has been demonstrated that over-expression of NR2B led to the superior ability of NR2B transgenic mice in learning and memory[41], including better performance in the Morris water-maze test. Thus, our data are consistent with the observation of Tang and colleagues[41] that higher transcript levels of NR2B correlate with improvement in watermaze performance. In addition, Rissman and associates[42], also using a Morris watermaze test, demonstrated that ovariectomized ERβKO mice on low doses of estrogen were delayed in learning acquisition, compared with their wild-type counterparts, while ovariectomized ERβKO mice administered a higher dose of estrogen failed to learn the task and, hence, were impaired in spatial learning. Therefore, the inference from these data is that estrogen influences various cognitive functions differently, depending on which estrogen receptors it is acting through.

ACKNOWLEDGEMENTS

This work was supported in part by National Health and Medical Research Council (NH&MRC) Project Grant no. 169010 and by US Public Health Service (PHS) Grant no. R37AG08174.

References

1. Petrides M. Impairments in working memory after frontal cortical excision. *Adv Neurol* 2000; 84:111–18
2. Petrides M. Impairments on nonspatial self-ordered and externally ordered working memory tasks after lesions of the mid-dorsal part of the lateral frontal cortex in the monkey. *J Neurosci* 1995;1:359–75
3. Postle BR, Berger JS, Taich AM, *et al.* Activity in human frontal cortex associated with spatial working memory and saccadic behavior. *J Cogn Neurosci* 2000;12(Suppl 2):2–14
4. Owen AM. The functional organization of working memory processes within human lateral frontal cortex: the contribution of functional neuroimaging. *Eur J Neurosci* 1997;9:1329–39
5. Raz N, Gunning FM, Head D, *et al.* Selective aging of the human cerebral cortex observed *in vivo* – differential vulnerability of the prefrontal gray matter. *Cereb Cortex* 1997;7:268–82
6. Salat DH, Kaye JA, Janowsky JS. Selective preservation and degeneration within the prefrontal cortex in aging and Alzheimer disease. *Arch Neurol* 2001;58:1403–8

7. Duff SJ, Hampson E. A beneficial effect of estrogen on working memory in postmenopausal women taking hormone replacement therapy. *Horm Behav* 2000;48:262-76
8. Smith YR, Giordani B, Lajiness-O'Neill R, *et al.* Long-term estrogen replacement is associated with improved nonverbal memory and attentional measures in postmenopausal women. *Fertil Steril* 2001;76:1101-7
9. Fluck E, File SE, Rymer J. Cognitive effects of 10 years of hormone-replacement therapy with tibolone. *J Clin Psychopharmacol* 2002;22:62-7
10. Carlson LE, Sherwin BB. Steroid hormones, memory and mood in a healthy elderly population. *Psychoneuroendocrinology* 1998;23:583-603
11. Flores F, Naftolin F, Ryan KJ. Aromatization of androstenedione and testosterone by rhesus monkey hypothalamus and limbic system. *Neuroendocrinology* 1973;11:177-82
12. Naftolin F, Ryan KJ, Davies IJ. The formation and metabolism of estrogens in brain tissues. *Adv Biosci* 1975;15:105-21
13. Roselli CE, Resko JA. Cytochrome P450 aromatase (CYP19) in the non-human primate brain: distribution, regulation and functional significance. *J Steroid Biochem Mol Biol* 2001;79: 247-53
14. Lauber ME, Lichtensteiger W. Pre- and postnatal ontogeny of aromatase cytochrome P450 in RNA expression in the male rat brain studied by *in situ* hybridisation. *Endocrinology* 1994;135:1661-8
15. Wagner CK, Morrell JI. Neuroanatomical distribution of aromatase mRNA in the rat brain: indicators of regional regulation. *J Steroid Biochem Mol Biol* 1997;61:307-14
16. MacLusky NJ, Naftolin F. Sexual differentiation of the central nervous system. *Science* 1981;211: 1294-302
17. Hutchison JB, Beyer C, Hutchison RE, *et al.* Sexual dimorphism in the developmental regulation of brain aromatase. *J Steroid Biochem Mol Biol* 1995;53:307-13
18. Lephart ED. A review of brain aromatase cytochrome P450. *Brain Res Rev* 1996;22:1-26
19. Garcia-Segura LM, Wozniak A, Azcoitia I. Aromatase expression by astrocytes after brain injury: implications for local estrogen formation in brain repair. *Neuroscience* 1999;89:567-78
20. Means GD, Mahendroo MS, Corbin CJ, *et al.* Structural analysis of the gene encoding human aromatase cytochrome P450, the enzyme responsible for estrogen biosynthesis. *J Biol Chem* 1989; 264:19385-91
21. Harada N, Yamada K, Saito K, *et al* Structural characterization of the human estrogen synthetase (aromatase) gene. *Biochem Biophys Res Commun* 1990;166:365-72
22. Toda K, Terashima M, Kawamoto T, *et al.* Structural and functional characterization of human aromatase P450 gene. *Eur J Biochem* 1990; 193:559-65
23. Simpson ER, Zhao Y, Agarwal VR, *et al.* Aromatase expression in health and disease. *Recent Prog Horm Res* 1997;52:185-213
24. Mahendroo MS, Mendelson CR, Simpson ER. Tissue-specific and hormonally controlled alternative promoters regulate aromatase cytochrome P450 gene expression in human adipose tissue. *J Biol Chem* 1993;268:19463-70
25. Jenkins C, Michael D, Mahendroo M, *et al.* Exon-specific Northern analysis and rapid amplification of cDNA ends (RACE) reveal that the proximal promoter II (PII) is responsible for aromatase cytochrome P450 (CYP19) expression in human ovary. *Mol Cell Endocrinol* 1993;97:R1-6
26. Harada N, Utsumi T, Takagi Y. Tissue-specific expression of the human aromatase cytochrome P450 gene by alternative use of multiple exons 1 and promoters, and switching of tissue-specific exons 1 in carcinogenesis. *Proc Natl Acad Sci USA* 1993;90:11312-16
27. Kato J, Yamada-Mouri N, Hirata S. Structure of aromatase mRNA in the rat brain. *J Steroid Biochem Mol Biol* 1997;61:381-5
28. Sasano H, Takashashi K, Satoh F, *et al.* Aromatase in the human central nervous system. *Clin Endocrinol (Oxf)* 1998;48:325-9
29. Fisher CR, Parlow GK, Simpson ER. Characterization of mice deficient in aromatase (ArKO) because of targeted disruption of the *cyp19* gene. *Proc Natl Acad Sci USA* 1998;95:6965-70
30. Jones ME, Thorburn AW, Britt KL, *et al.* Aromatase-deficient (ArKO) mice have a phenotype of increased adiposity. *Proc Natl Acad Sci USA* 2000,97.12735-40
31. Belcredito S, Brusadelli A, Maggi A. Estrogens, apoptosis and cells of neural origin. *J Neurocytol* 2000;29:359-65
32. Honda K, Shimohama S, Sawada H, *et al.* Non-genomic antiapoptotic signal transduction by estrogen in cultured cortical neurons. *J Neurosci Res* 2001;64:466-75
33. Kajta M, Budziszewska B, Marszal M, *et al.* Effects of 17-β estradiol and estriol on NMDA-induced toxicity and apoptosis in primary cultures of rat cortical neurons. *J Physiol Pharmacol* 2001;52: 437-46
34. Azcoitia I, Sierra A, Veiga S, *et al.* Brain aromatase is neuroprotective. *J Neurobiol* 2001;47:318-29
35. Hosoda T, Nakajima H, Honjo H. Estrogen protects neuronal cells from amyloid β-induced apoptotic cell death. *Neuroreport* 2001;12:1965-70
36. Fukuda K, Yao H, Ibayashi S, *et al.* Ovariectomy exacerbates and estrogen replacement attenuates photothrombotic focal ischemic brain injury in rats. *Stroke* 2000;31:155-60
37. Dubal DB, Zhu H, Yu J, *et al.* Estrogen receptor α, not β, is a critical link in estradiol-mediated

protection against brain injury. *Proc Natl Acad Sci USA* 2001;98:1952-7
38. Roof RL, Hall ED. Estrogen-related gender difference in survival rate and cortical blood flow after impact-acceleration head injury in rats. *J Neurotrauma* 2000;17:1155-69
39. Wang L, Andersson S, Warner M, *et al.* Morphological abnormalities in the brains of estrogen receptor β knockout mice. *Proc Natl Acad Sci USA* 2001;98:2792-6
40. Krezel W, Dupont S, Krust A, *et al.* Increased anxiety and synaptic plasticity in estrogen receptor β-deficient mice. *Proc Natl Acad Sci USA* 2001; 98:12278-82
41. Tang YP, Shimizu E, Dube GR, *et al.* Genetic enhancement of learning and memory in mice. *Nature (London)*1999:401:63-9
42. Rissman EF, Heck AL, Leonard JE, *et al.* Disruption of estrogen receptor β gene impairs spatial learning in female mice. *Proc Natl Acad Sci USA* 2003; 99:3996-4001

Neurosteroids and γ-aminobutyric acid type A receptor function and plasticity

5

E. Sanna, P. Follesa and G. Biggio

INTRODUCTION

γ-Aminobutyric acid (GABA) is the most important and widely distributed inhibitory neurotransmitter in the mammalian central nervous system, and mediates fast synaptic inhibition by activating type A ($GABA_A$) receptors[1,2]. $GABA_A$ receptors are ligand-gated chloride channels, and structurally they possess a pentameric structure composed of α(1-6), β(1-4), γ(1-4), δ, ε, π and θ subunits[3-5].

These receptors are the site of action of various pharmacologically and clinically important drugs, such as benzodiazepines, barbiturates, general anesthetics and convulsants[3,6]. In addition, a large body of experimental evidence has been provided in the past decade indicating that steroid hormones synthesized in the brain and periphery are among the most selective, potent and efficacious allosteric modulators of $GABA_A$ receptors identified to date. The term neurosteroids refers to steroid derivatives that are synthesized *de novo* from cholesterol in the central nervous system[7-11]. The action of some of these neurosteroids, such as 3α,5α-tetrahydroprogesterone (3α,5α-TH PROG or allopregnanolone) and 3α,5α-tetrahydrodeoxycorticosterone (3α,5α-TH DOC) at $GABA_A$ receptors results in a rapid onset and offset strong potentiation of GABA-evoked inhibitory postsynaptic Cl^- currents[12-15], with potency and efficacy similar to or greater than that of benzodiazepines and barbiturates[13,14,16]. Neurosteroids are thus considered the endogenous modulators of $GABA_A$ receptor-mediated neurotransmission. Modulation of synaptic activity through the interaction of neurosteroids with membrane-bound ionotropic neurotransmitter receptors[11-15,17,18] thus represents a mechanism of action of steroid hormones additional to the classic genomic action of these compounds[19].

The capability of neurosteroids to enhance $GABA_A$ receptor function is believed to form the basis for their pharmacological and behavioral properties, including the anxiolytic, analgesic, sedative, hypnotic, anticonvulsant and, at certain concentrations, anesthetic actions[13,20]. Therefore, the anxiolytic and anticonvulsant effects of progesterone are mostly attributable to its reduced metabolites[21-26].

It is proposed that such neurosteroids play an important physiological role to modulate locally neuronal excitability by 'fine-tuning' the action of GABA acting at $GABA_A$ receptors[18]. In addition, many molecular, neurochemical and neurophysiological studies have demonstrated that fluctuations of neurosteroid plasma or brain concentrations might have a profound influence on emotional and affective behaviors. Accordingly, changes in the peripheral as well as central synthesis of progesterone and 3α,5α-TH PROG have been measured during physiological conditions such as following the administration of a stressful stimulus, pregnancy, menstrual cycle and menopause. Such altered neurosteroid levels could be crucial in regulating the changes in $GABA_A$ receptor function and plasticity, as well as behaviors that are associated with these conditions[27-33]. In addition, alterations in neurosteroid brain levels might also be important in a variety of neurological and psychiatric disorders characterized by changes in sleep pattern and neuronal excitability. In fact, a decrease in plasma and cerebrospinal fluid concentrations of 3α,5α-TH PROG in depressed patients has been demonstrated[34].

Fluctuations of the secretion of neurosteroids are probably important neurochemical factors that may regulate $GABA_A$ receptor gene expression and function. Changes in the brain concentration of progesterone and 3α,5α-TH PROG have recently been proposed to represent a key factor in regulation of the expression of various subunits of the $GABA_A$ receptor. Long-term exposure to progesterone or 3α,5α-TH PROG induces a reduction in the level of expression of various $GABA_A$ receptor subunit genes, whereas abrupt discontinuation of such treatment causes an increase in the expression of the α_4 subunit, which is associated with a decreased modulatory efficacy of neurosteroids and benzodiazepines[35,36].

$GABA_A$ receptor responsiveness to its neurotransmitter and sensitivity to allosteric positive as well as negative modulators is markedly dependent on the type and stoichiometry of its component subunits. Recent experiments with knock-in mice carrying a point mutation in the α subunit revealed that $GABA_A$ receptors containing the α_1 subunit are responsible for mediating the sedative-hypnotic effects of benzodiazepines[37,38], whereas those containing the α_2 subunit mediate the anxiolytic action of these drugs[39]. In addition to α_1- and α_2-containing receptors, receptors with the α_3 and α_5 subunits possess high affinity to benzodiazepines, although their precise role is not currently known. These different $GABA_A$ receptor subtypes have been classified as benzodiazepine-sensitive, in contrast with those containing either the α_4 or α_6 subunit, which show virtual non-affinity to these drugs and have been classified as benzodiazepine-insensitive[3].

The γ_2 subunit is also an essential determinant for the optimal benzodiazepine and benzodiazepine-like ligand modulatory effects[40,41]. However, the γ_2 subunit does not appear to be important for the modulatory action of the neurosteroid 3α,5α-TH PROG or 3α,5α-TH DOC. Therefore, characterization of the functional roles of $GABA_A$ receptors requires an understanding of the mechanisms by which receptor subunit composition is regulated.

REGULATION OF $GABA_A$ RECEPTOR GENE EXPRESSION BY NEUROSTEROIDS

Rat cerebellar granule neurons

In this study, we used rat cerebellar granule cells in primary culture to evaluate the effects of the prolonged interaction of neurosteroids, synthesized by neurons from the precursor PROG, with $GABA_A$ receptors in modulating both gene expression and function of these receptors. Accordingly, cultured cerebellar granule cells synthesize mRNAs encoding for 5α-reductase and 3α-hydroxysteroid oxidoreductase[35,42], the enzymes required for the conversion of PROG into 3α,5α-TH PROG. In accordance with the expression of these enzymes, long-term (5 days) exposure of cultured granule cells to PROG resulted in a marked enhancement (~450%) in the concentration of 3α,5α-TH PROG[35]. This effect was completely prevented by blocking the conversion of PROG into 3α,5α-TH PROG with the 5α-reductase inhibitor finasteride, suggesting that cerebellar granule neurons can indeed form neuroactive steroids from exogenous PROG[43,44].

Long-term treatment of granule cells in culture with PROG induced a significant decrease (~25%) in the abundance of mRNA encoding for the γ_{2S} and γ_{2L} subunits of the $GABA_A$ receptor[35]. A similar result was obtained following prolonged exposure of these cells to 3α,5α-TH PROG. In addition, prolonged PROG treatment significantly reduced mRNA levels of the α_1, α_3 and α_5 subunits, but failed to alter those for the α_4, β_1, or β_2 subunits[35].

Co-treatment of granule cells with PROG and finasteride resulted in a blockade of both PROG conversion to 3α,5α-TH PROG and PROG-induced decrease in the amount of transcripts of α_1, γ_{2S} and γ_{2L} subunits[35]. These data suggest that a metabolite of PROG produced by cerebellar granule neurons, rather than PROG itself, regulates $GABA_A$ receptor subunit gene expression. In line with this hypothesis, 3α,5α-TH PROG, but not PROG, exerts a strong direct potentiation of $GABA_A$ receptor function[14,45,46]. Furthermore, these data support the general idea that chronic treatment with positive allosteric modulators of $GABA_A$ receptors causes a down-regulation of the receptor through mechanisms which may involve, at least in part, a reduction of the expression of specific subunit genes[47-57]. In turn, these alterations in $GABA_A$ receptor subunit gene expression are paralleled by changes in $GABA_A$ receptor function as well as pharmacological sensitivity, as determined by electrophysiological recording from *Xenopus* oocytes expressing $GABA_A$ receptors from cultured cerebellar granule cells. In fact, long-term exposure of the neurons to PROG induces a decreased efficacy of both diazepam and the anxiogenic and convulsant β-carboline DMCM[58,59] to potentiate and inhibit, respectively, GABA-evoked Cl^- currents[35]. Thus, the reduced ability of diazepam and DMCM to modulate $GABA_A$ receptor function following long-term exposure of granule cells to PROG is consistent with the decreased abundance of α_1, α_3, α_5 and γ_2 subunit transcripts elicited by such treatment[35]. In fact, both α and γ_2 subunits are necessary for the optimal sensitivity of $GABA_A$ receptors to benzodiazepines as well as benzodiazepine receptor inverse agonists[3,41].

From these data, it is thus conceivable that neuronal metabolism of peripheral PROG may contribute to set the brain concentration of 3α,5α-TH PROG and to the physiological modulatory tone of GABAergic synapses by this neurosteroid. Moreover, physiological as well as pharmacological conditions characterized by altered PROG synthesis from peripheral organs may therefore cause changes in brain neuroactive steroids and, in turn, may regulate the expression of specific $GABA_A$ receptor subunit genes in different regions of the brain.

Discontinuation of long-term exposure of granule cells in culture with PROG, and the consequent abrupt decrease of 3α,5α-TH PROG synthesis, induced an increased level of α_4 subunit transcription, together with a persistent decrease in that of the α_1 and γ_{2L} subunits[35]. $GABA_A$ receptors containing the α_4 subunit are characterized by a reduced sensitivity to classical benzodiazepine receptor agonists as well as an altered pattern of regulation by flumazenil, DMCM and other positive and negative modulators[3]. $GABA_A$ receptors from cultured granule cells undergoing PROG withdrawal expressed in *Xenopus* oocytes were markedly less sensitive to the potentiating action of diazepam with respect to untreated cells[35]. In addition, consistent with the increased expression of the α_4 subunit[3,60], the benzodiazepine receptor antagonist flumazenil, devoid of any effect on control cells, enhanced GABA-evoked Cl^- currents in oocytes expressing $GABA_A$ receptors from PROG withdrawal cells. These results suggest that, in this *in vitro* cellular model, the increased transcription of α_4 subunit mRNA during PROG withdrawal is followed by the synthesis of $GABA_A$ receptors containing this subunit, which are endowed with distinct pharmacological properties. In agreement with this idea, withdrawal following chronic PROG treatment was also associated with a restored sensitivity to the negative modulatory action of DMCM, sensitivity that was reduced after prolonged PROG exposure. In fact, recombinant α_4-containing $GABA_A$ receptors, like α_1-containing receptors, are negatively modulated by this β-carboline inverse agonist[60].

The increased level of α_4 subunit expression observed during PROG withdrawal may represent a crucial neurochemical event that could contribute to the development of PROG withdrawal syndrome. Such a notion would allow us to speculate that a putative endogenous compound endowed with a profile of inverse agonist may become active in association with an increased density of α_4-containing receptors. Accordingly, an increase in α_4 subunit mRNA levels observed during PROG withdrawal in a rat pseudopregnancy model is associated with changes in the kinetics of hippocampal $GABA_A$ receptor-mediated currents, with experimental anxiety and with increased susceptibility to pentylentetrazole-induced seizures[25,36]. Interestingly, such changes related to PROG withdrawal were prevented by the previous administration of α_4 subunit antisense RNA, demonstrating the strict correlation between enhancement of α_4 subunit gene expression and the different electrophysiological and behavioral effects induced by neurosteroid withdrawal[61]. Moreover, the observation that the effects of PROG withdrawal on cultured granule cells were prevented by finasteride suggests that the withdrawal-induced increase of α_4 subunit mRNA abundance results from the sudden decrease in $3\alpha,5\alpha$-TH PROG concentration. It should be considered, however, that because the inhibition of 5α-reductase by finasteride also results in a decreased level of 5α-dihydroprogesterone (5α-DH PROG), blockade of a direct genomic action activated by this metabolite and directed to the regulation of $GABA_A$ receptor subunit gene expression cannot be ruled out. However, because PROG itself has no effect on $GABA_A$ receptor gene expression in the presence of finasteride, the possibility of a genomic effect elicited by 5α-DH PROG appears unlikely. Finally, it should also be considered that 5α-DH PROG lacks any appreciable direct modulatory action on $GABA_A$ receptor function[62].

Rat cerebral cortical neurons

To establish whether the effects of long-term treatment with PROG and PROG withdrawal on $GABA_A$ receptor subunit gene expression investigated in cerebellar granule cells would also occur in neurons from different brain regions, we examined the effects of such treatment on rat cerebral cortical neurons in culture.

At variance with cerebellar granule cell cultures, which comprise an approximately 95% pure population of glutamatergic granule neurons, cultures obtained from embryonic rat cerebral cortices consist of a heterogeneous population of different neuronal cell types.

The prolonged (5 days) exposure of cortical neurons in culture with PROG (1 μmol/l) failed to change significantly the abundance of mRNA encoding the α_1, α_4 or γ_{2S} subunits of the $GABA_A$ receptor. In contrast, withdrawal from PROG for 6 h induced a marked increase (~45%) in the abundance of the α_4 subunit mRNA. This increase of α_4 subunit transcription was accompanied by a decrease (~25%) of γ_{2S} mRNA concentration, compared with control cells. Furthermore, PROG withdrawal was associated, at variance with cerebellar granule cells, with an increase (~17%) in the abundance of α_1 subunit mRNA. Prolonged co-exposure of cortical neurons in culture to PROG and finasteride completely prevented the changes in receptor subunit mRNA abundance elicited by PROG withdrawal. Treatment of cortical neurons with only finasteride failed to modify the levels of $GABA_A$ receptor subunit mRNA. The effects of PROG withdrawal were therefore due to a sudden decrease in the concentration of PROG-derived neuroactive steroids.

The results suggest that discontinuation of PROG treatment induced similar but not identical alterations in $GABA_A$ receptor subunit gene expression in cerebellar granule cells and in cerebral cortical neurons. On the other hand, the lack of effects of long-term exposure of cortical neurons to PROG on $GABA_A$ receptor subunit gene expression may be explained by a reduced sensitivity of cortical $GABA_A$ receptors to PROG-derived neurosteroids compared with that of $GABA_A$ receptors from cerebellar granule cells. Alternatively, heterogeneity of the cortical neuron population may mask changes in receptor subunit mRNA transcription that occur in opposite directions in different cell types. Indeed, the expression of $GABA_A$ receptor subunit genes has been shown to be modified in opposite manners in different subpopulations of neurons in the brain[63,64]. Finally, it is also possible that other mechanisms regulating the expression of $GABA_A$ receptor subunit genes, or of specific enzymes involved in PROG metabolism, differ between cerebral cortical neurons and cerebellar granule cells in culture.

CONCLUSIONS

Our *in vitro* cellular data presented in this chapter suggest that neuroactive steroids such as $3\alpha,5\alpha$-TH PROG play an important role in the physiological modulation of $GABA_A$ receptor gene expression and function. The long-term conversion of PROG to $3\alpha,5\alpha$-TH PROG, occurring in PROG-treated cultured cells, results in a sustained increased level of this neurosteroid, which in turn, by interacting directly with $GABA_A$ receptors, activates intracellular mechanisms that lead to a marked alteration in the expression of specific subunit genes. Such a change in subunit expression would also result in an altered pattern of $GABA_A$ receptor subtypes expressed on the neuronal membrane, receptors that may possess different functional as well as pharmacological properties.

Discontinuation of long-term exposure of cultured cells to PROG, and therefore 3α,5α-TH PROG, is associated with an increase in the abundance of α_4 subunit mRNA as well as receptors containing this subunit. Given that the presence of the α_4 subunit in recombinant GABA$_A$ receptors has been shown to be associated with a reduced sensitivity to various positive modulators, such as classic benzodiazepines, and an increased sensitivity to negative modulators, such as DMCM, an enhanced expression of α_4-containing receptors in neurons subjected to PROG withdrawal may contribute to the development of tolerance, dependence and withdrawal syndrome following long-term administration of anxiolytic and hypnotic drugs.

The marked fluctuations in plasma and brain concentrations of neurosteroids associated with physiological conditions such as pregnancy, estrus cycle, menopause, aging and stress also suggest that the extent of neurosteroid synthesis represents an important determinant for the regulation of GABA$_A$ receptor gene expression and function. Changes in neurosteroid levels may also contribute to the development of mental disorders that are often associated with these physiological conditions. Further studies of these various physiological conditions should help to clarify in more detail the role of neurosteroids in the regulation of GABA$_A$ receptor function and in behaviors associated with these conditions.

References

1. Mehta AK, Ticku MK. An update on GABA$_A$ receptors. *Brain Res Brain Res Rev* 1999; 29:196–217
2. Vicini S. New perspectives in the functional role of GABA(A) channel heterogeneity. *Mol Neurobiol* 1999;19:97–110
3. Barnard EA, Skolnick P, Olsen RW, *et al.* International Union of Pharmacology. XV. Subtypes of γ-aminobutyric acid$_A$ receptors: classification on the basis of subunit structure and receptor function. *Pharmacol Rev* 1998;50:291–313
4. Sieghart W. Unraveling the function of GABA(A) receptor subtypes. *Trends Pharmacol Sci* 2000;21: 411-13
5. Whiting PJ, Bonnert TP, McKernan RM, *et al.* Molecular and functional diversity of the expanding GABA-A receptor gene family. *Ann NY Acad Sci* 1999;868:645–53
6. Sieghart W. Structure and pharmacology of γ-aminobutyric acid$_A$ receptor subtypes. *Pharmacol Rev* 1995;47:181–234
7. Hu ZY, Bourreau E, Jung-Testas I, *et al.* Neurosteroids: oligodendrocyte mitochondria convert cholesterol to pregnenolone. *Proc Natl Acad Sci USA* 1987;84:8215–19
8. Le Goascogne C, Robel P, Gouezou M, *et al.* Neurosteroids: cytochrome P-450scc in rat brain. *Science* 1987;237:1212–15
9. Mathur C, Prasad VV, Raju VS, *et al.* Steroids and their conjugates in the mammalian brain. *Proc Natl Acad Sci USA* 1993;90:85–8
10. Mellon SH, Deschepper CF. Neurosteroid biosynthesis: genes for adrenal steroidogenic enzymes are expressed in the brain. *Brain Res* 1993; 629:283–92
11. Prasad VV, Vegesna SR, Welch M, Lieberman S. Precursors of the neurosteroids. *Proc Natl Acad Sci USA* 1994;91:3220–3
12. Lambert JJ, Harney SC, Belelli D, Peters JA. Neurosteroid modulation of recombinant and synaptic GABA$_A$ receptors. *Int Rev Neurobiol* 2001;46:177–205
13. Majewska MD. Neurosteroids: endogenous bimodal modulators of the GABA$_A$ receptor. Mechanism of action and physiological significance. *Prog Neurobiol* 1992;38:379–95
14. Majewska MD, Harrison NL, Schwartz RD, *et al.* Steroid hormone metabolites are barbiturate-like modulators of the GABA receptor. *Science* 1986; 232:1004–7
15. Rupprecht R, Holsboer F. Neuroactive steroids: mechanisms of action and neuropsychopharmacological perspectives. *Trends Neurosci* 1999;22:410–16
16. Harrison NL, Simmonds MA. Modulation of the GABA receptor complex by a steroid anaesthetic. *Brain Res* 1984;323:287–92

17. Mienville JM, Vicini S. Pregnenolone sulfate antagonizes $GABA_A$ receptor-mediated currents via a reduction of channel opening frequency. *Brain Res* 1989;489:190-4
18. Paul SM, Purdy RH. Neuroactive steroids. *FASEB J* 1992;6:2311-22
19. Evans RM. The steroid and thyroid hormone receptor superfamily. *Science* 1988;240:889-95
20. Lambert JJ, Belelli D, Hill-Venning C, Peters JA. Neurosteroids and $GABA_A$ receptor function. *Trends Pharmacol Sci* 1995;16:295-303
21. Bitran D, Shiekh M, McLeod M. Anxiolytic effect of progesterone is mediated by the neurosteroid allopregnanolone at brain $GABA_A$ receptors. *J Neuroendocrinol* 1995;7:171-7
22. Freeman EW, Purdy RH, Coutifaris C, *et al.* Anxiolytic metabolites of progesterone: correlation with mood and performance measures following oral progesterone administration to healthy female volunteers. *Neuroendocrinology* 1993;58:478-84
23. Picazo O, Fernandez-Guasti A. Anti-anxiety effects of progesterone and some of its reduced metabolites: an evaluation using the burying behavior test. *Brain Res* 1995;680:135-41
24. Kokate TG, Banks MK, Magee T, *et al.* Finasteride, a 5α-reductase inhibitor, blocks the anticonvulsant activity of progesterone in mice. *J Pharmacol Exp Ther* 1999;288:679-84
25. Reddy DS, Rogawski MA. Enhanced anticonvulsant activity of ganaxolone after neurosteroid withdrawal in a rat model of catamenial epilepsy. *J Pharmacol Exp Ther* 2000;294:909-15
26. Bitran D, Purdy RH, Kellogg CK. Anxiolytic effect of progesterone is associated with increases in cortical allopregnanolone and $GABA_A$ receptor function. *Pharmacol Biochem Behav* 1993;45:423-8
27. Barbaccia ML, Roscetti G, Trabucchi M, *et al.* Time-dependent changes in rat brain neuroactive steroid concentrations and $GABA_A$ receptor function after acute stress. *Neuroendocrinology* 1996;63:166-72
28. Barbaccia ML, Roscetti G, Trabucchi M, *et al.* The effects of inhibitors of GABAergic transmission and stress on brain and plasma allopregnanolone concentrations. *Br J Pharmacol* 1997;120:1582-8
29. Bicikova M, Dibbelt L, Hill M, *et al.* Allopregnanolone in women with premenstrual syndrome. *Horm Metab Res* 1998;30:227-30
30. Biggio G, Follesa P, Sanna E, *et al.* $GABA_A$-receptor plasticity during long-term exposure to and withdrawal from progesterone. *Int Rev Neurobiol* 2001;46:207-41
31. Concas A, Mostallino MC, Porcu P, *et al.* Role of brain allopregnanolone in the plasticity of γ-aminobutyric acid type A receptor in rat brain during pregnancy and after delivery. *Proc Natl Acad Sci USA* 1998;95:13284-9
32. Follesa P, Floris S, Tuligi G, *et al.* Molecular and functional adaptation of the GABA(A) receptor complex during pregnancy and after delivery in the rat brain. *Eur J Neurosci* 1998;10:2905-12
33. Serra M, Pisu MG, Littera M, *et al.* Social isolation-induced decreases in both the abundance of neuroactive steroids and GABA(A) receptor function in rat brain. *J Neurochem* 2000;75:732-40
34. Uzunova V, Sheline Y, Davis JM, *et al.* Increase in the cerebrospinal fluid content of neurosteroids in patients with unipolar major depression who are receiving fluoxetine or fluvoxamine. *Proc Natl Acad Sci USA* 1998;95:3239-44
35. Follesa P, Serra M, Cagetti E, *et al.* Allopregnanolone synthesis in cerebellar granule cells: roles in regulation of GABA(A) receptor expression and function during progesterone treatment and withdrawal. *Mol Pharmacol* 2000;57:1262-70
36. Smith SS, Gong QH, Li X, *et al.* Withdrawal from 3α-OH-5α-pregnan-20-one using a pseudopregnancy model alters the kinetics of hippocampal $GABA_A$-gated current and increases the $GABA_A$ receptor α_4 subunit in association with increased anxiety. *J Neurosci* 1998;18:5275-84
37. McKernan RM, Rosahl TW, Reynolds DS, *et al.* Sedative but not anxiolytic properties of benzodiazepines are mediated by the GABA(A) receptor α_1 subtype. *Nat Neurosci* 2000;3:587-92
38. Rudolph U, Crestani F, Benke D, *et al.* Benzodiazepine actions mediated by specific γ-aminobutyric acid(A) receptor subtypes. *Nature (London)* 1999;401:796-800
39. Low K, Crestani F, Keist R, *et al.* Molecular and neuronal substrate for the selective attenuation of anxiety. *Science* 2000;290:131-4
40. Gunther U, Benson J, Benke D, *et al.* Benzodiazepine-insensitive mice generated by targeted disruption of the γ_2 subunit gene of γ-aminobutyric acid type A receptors. *Proc Natl Acad Sci USA* 1995;92:7749-53
41. Pritchett DB, Sontheimer H, Shivers BD, *et al.* Importance of a novel $GABA_A$ receptor subunit for benzodiazepine pharmacology. *Nature (London)* 1989;338:582-5
42. Biggio G, Barbaccia ML, Follesa P, *et al.* *Neurosteroids and $GABA_A$ Receptor Plasticity*. New York: Lippincott Williams and Wilkins, 2000
43. Azzolina B, Ellsworth K, Andersson S, *et al.* Inhibition of rat α-reductases by finasteride: evidence for isozyme differences in the mechanism of inhibition. *J Steroid Biochem Mol Biol* 1997;61: 55-64
44. Rittmaster RS. Finasteride. *N Engl J Med* 1994; 330:120-5
45. Friedman L, Gibbs TT, Farb DH. γ-Aminobutyric $acid_A$ receptor regulation: chronic treatment with pregnanolone uncouples allosteric interactions

between steroid and benzodiazepine recognition sites. *Mol Pharmacol* 1993;44:191–7
46. Wu FS, Gibbs TT, Farb DH. Inverse modulation of γ-aminobutyric acid- and glycine-induced currents by progesterone. *Mol Pharmacol* 1990; 37:597–602
47. Holt RA, Bateson AN, Martin IL. Chronic treatment with diazepam or abecarnil differently affects the expression of $GABA_A$ receptor subunit mRNAs in the rat cortex. *Neuropharmacology* 1996;35: 1457–63
48. Holt RA, Martin IL, Bateson AN. Chronic diazepam exposure decreases transcription of the rat GABA(A) receptor γ_2-subunit gene. *Brain Res Mol Brain Res* 1997;48:164–6
49. Impagnatiello F, Pesold C, Longone P, *et al.* Modifications of γ-aminobutyric $acid_A$ receptor subunit expression in rat neocortex during tolerance to diazepam. *Mol Pharmacol* 1996;49:822–31
50. Mhatre MC, Pena G, Sieghart W, Ticku MK. Antibodies specific for $GABA_A$ receptor α subunits reveal that chronic alcohol treatment down-regulates α-subunit expression in rat brain regions. *J Neurochem* 1993;61:1620–5
51. Mhatre MC, Ticku MK. Chronic ethanol administration alters γ-aminobutyric $acid_A$ receptor gene expression. *Mol Pharmacol* 1992;42:415–22
52. Montpied P, Ginns EI, Martin BM, *et al.* γ-Aminobutyric acid (GABA) induces a receptor-mediated reduction in $GABA_A$ receptor α subunit messenger RNAs in embryonic chick neurons in culture. *J Biol Chem* 1991;266:6011–14
53. Morrow AL, Montpied P, Paul SM. $GABA_A$ receptor function and expression following chronic ethanol and barbiturate administration. *Ann NY Acad Sci* 1991;625:496–507
54. Roca DJ, Schiller GD, Friedman L, *et al.* γ-Aminobutyric $acid_A$ receptor regulation in culture: altered allosteric interactions following prolonged exposure to benzodiazepines, barbiturates, and methylxanthines. *Mol Pharmacol* 1990; 37:710–19
55. Roca DJ, Rozenberg I, Farrant M, Farb DH. Chronic agonist exposure induces down-regulation and allosteric uncoupling of the γ-aminobutyric acid/benzodiazepine receptor complex. *Mol Pharmacol* 1990;37:37–43
56. Yu R, Follesa P, Ticku MK. Down-regulation of the GABA receptor subunits mRNA levels in mammalian cultured cortical neurons following chronic neurosteroid treatment. *Brain Res Mol Brain Res* 1996;41:163–8
57. Follesa P, Mancuso L, Biggio F, *et al.* γ-Hydroxybutyric acid and diazepam antagonize a rapid increase in GABA(A) receptors α(4) subunit mRNA abundance induced by ethanol withdrawal in cerebellar granule cells. *Mol Pharmacol* 2003; 63:896–907
58. Braestrup C, Nielsen M, Honore T. Binding of [3H]DMCM, a convulsive benzodiazepine ligand, to rat brain membranes: preliminary studies. *J Neurochem* 1983;41:454–65
59. Braestrup C, Schmiechen R, Neef G, *et al.* Interaction of convulsive ligands with benzodiazepine receptors. *Science* 1982;216:1241–3
60. Whittemore ER, Yang W, Drewe JA, Woodward RM. Pharmacology of the human γ-aminobutyric $acid_A$ receptor α_4 subunit expressed in *Xenopus laevis* oocytes. *Mol Pharmacol* 1996;50:1364–75
61. Smith SS, Gong QH, Hsu FC, *et al.* GABA(A) receptor α_4 subunit suppression prevents withdrawal properties of an endogenous steroid. *Nature (London)* 1998;392:926–30
62. Rupprecht R, Reul JM, Trapp T, *et al.* Progesterone receptor-mediated effects of neuroactive steroids. *Neuron* 1993;11:523–30
63. Weiland NG, Orchinik M. Specific subunit mRNAs of the $GABA_A$ receptor are regulated by progesterone in subfields of the hippocampus. *Brain Res Mol Brain Res* 1995;32:271–8
64. Fenelon VS, Herbison AE. Plasticity in $GABA_A$ receptor subunit mRNA expression by hypothalamic magnocellular neurons in the adult rat. *J Neurosci* 1996;16:4872–80

Sex hormone receptors in the human hypothalamus in different stages of human life

6

D. F. Swaab, F. P. M. Kruijver and A. Hestiantoro

INTRODUCTION

The interaction between sex hormones and the brain, in development, may be the basis not only for sex differences in reproduction (menstrual cycle), gender identity (feeling of being male or female) and sexual orientation (heterosexuality, homosexuality), but later in life also for sex differences in the prevalence of psychiatric and neurological diseases in adulthood, changes in central functions in postmenopausal women and age-related neurodegeneration such as Alzheimer's disease. The proportions of cases are more than 75% women in Rett syndrome, lymphocytic hypophysitis, anorexia and bulimia nervosa and hypnic headache syndrome, and more than 75% men in dyslexia, attention deficit hyperactivity disorder (ADHD), autism, sleep apnea, Gilles de la Tourette syndrome, rabies, Kallman syndrome and Kleine-Levin syndrome (Table 1). Whether sex differences in the brain that arise in development ('organizing effect') are indeed the basis for the sex difference in neurological or psychiatric diseases has yet to be established. An alternative mechanism for sex differences in the prevalence of brain disorders is the immediate effect of circulating sex hormone levels ('activating effect') as shown in, for example, sleep apnea. Both effects may be mediated by sex hormone receptors. This chapter focuses on the hypothalamus.

Table 1 Ratios of women/men suffering from a selection of neurological and psychiatric diseases[1]

Disease	*Percentage women/ percentage men*
Rett syndrome	100/0
Postoperative hyponatremic encephalopathy with permanent damage or death	96/4
Anorexia nervosa	93/7
Lymphocytic hypophysitis	90/10
True (central) precocious puberty	90/10
Hypnic headache syndrome	84/16
Bulimia	75/25
Senile dementia of the Alzheimer type	74/26
Multiple sclerosis	67/33
Anxiety disorder	67/33
Post-traumatic stress disorders	66/34
Dementia	64/36
Unipolar depression, dysthymia	63/37
Whiplash	60/40
Severe learning disability	38/62
Substance abuse	34/66
Stuttering	29/71
Schizophrenia	27/73
REM sleep behavioral disorder	24/76
Male-to-female versus female-to-male transsexuals	28/72
Dyslexia	23/77
ADHD	20/80
Autism	20/80
Sleep apnea	18/82
Kallmann syndrome	17/83
Rabies	13/87
Gilles de la Tourette	10/90
Kleine-Levin	0/100

REM, rapid eye movement; ADHD, attention deficit hyperactivity disorder

SEX DIFFERENCES IN SEX HORMONE RECEPTOR DISTRIBUTION IN THE HYPOTHALAMUS

'The brain is our biggest sexual organ: a pity it is hidden in the skull'

Sex hormones act on the brain at least partly mediated by sex hormone receptors. In young adults there are many sex differences in receptor distribution in the brain, which vary in a complex, region-specific way according to area and receptor type.

In most hypothalamic areas that contain the androgen receptor, staining, nuclear staining in particular, is less intense in young adult women than in men (Figure 1). The strongest sex difference was found in the lateral and the medial mamillary nucleus[2]. The mamillary body complex is known to receive input from the hippocampus by the fornix, and to be involved in cognition. Moreover, this complex is also involved in several aspects of sexual behavior, such as penile erection (see below). In addition, a sex difference in androgen receptor staining is present in the horizontal diagonal band of Broca, the sexually dimorphic nucleus of the preoptic area (SDN-POA), medial preoptic area, the dorsal and ventral zone of the periventricular nucleus, paraventricular nucleus (PVN), supraoptic nucleus (SON), ventromedial hypothalamic nucleus (VMN) and the infundibular nucleus. No sex differences were observed in androgen receptor staining in the bed nucleus of the stria terminalis (BST), the nucleus basalis of Meynert (NBM) and the island of Calleja[2]. Nuclear androgen receptor activity in the mamillary complex of heterosexual men did not differ from that of homosexual men, but it was significantly stronger in men than in women. A female-like pattern was found in men with low testosterone levels, for example, in two castrated male-to-female transsexuals, in 26-year-old and 53-year-old castrated men and in intact elderly men. These data indicate that the amount of nuclear receptor staining in the mamillary complex is dependent on the circulating levels of androgens, rather than on gender identity or sexual orientation. This idea is supported by the finding that a male-like pattern of androgen receptor staining was found in a 36-year-old bisexual non-castrated male-to-female transsexual, and in a heterosexual virilized woman of 46 years of age[3].

Various sex differences were observed for estrogen receptor-α (ERα) staining in the hypothalamus and adjacent areas of young human subjects (Figure 2). More intense nuclear ERα immunoreactivity was found in young men, compared with young women, in neurons of the medial part of the bed nucleus of the stria terminalis (BSTm), the SDN-POA, the SON, the PVN, the dorsal periventricular zone (DPe) and the lateral hypothalamic area (LHA). Women revealed a stronger nuclear ERα-immunoreactivity in the diagonal band of Broca (DBB/Ch2), suprachiasmatic nucleus (SCN), VMN and medial mamillary nucleus (MMN). No sex differences in nuclear ERα staining were found in, for example, the lateral septum (LS), the central part of the BST (BSTc), the islands of Calleja (Cal) or in the infundibular nucleus (INF). Sex differences in cytoplasmic staining with a stronger staining in men were found in the BST, the SCN, the NBM, the INF, the tuberomamillary complex (TM) and the lateromamillary nucleus (LMN). An ovariectomized 46-year-old female subject, a castrated and estrogen-treated 50-year-old male-to-female transsexual and a 31-year-old male subject with high estrogen levels due to an estrogen-producing tumor revealed ERα distribution patterns according to their level of circulating estrogens in most areas, suggesting that the majority of the observed sex differences in ERα-immunoreactivity are 'activating' rather than 'organizing' in nature[4].

In general, ERβ-immunoreactivity was observed more frequently in the cytoplasm than in the nucleus, with a stronger staining in women in the NBM, horizontal diagonal band of Broca (hDBB) and TM and in men in the medial preoptic area (MPO). A more intense nuclear ERβ staining of a low to intermediate level was found, in men, in neurons of the BSTc, the BSTm, the islands of Calleja, the SDN-POA, the DBB/Ch2 and the VMN, as well as the paratenial nucleus (PT) and the paraventricular nucleus of the thalamus. Women revealed more nuclear ERβ of a low to intermediate level in the SCN, the SON, the PVN, the INF, the nucleus tuberalis lateralis and the

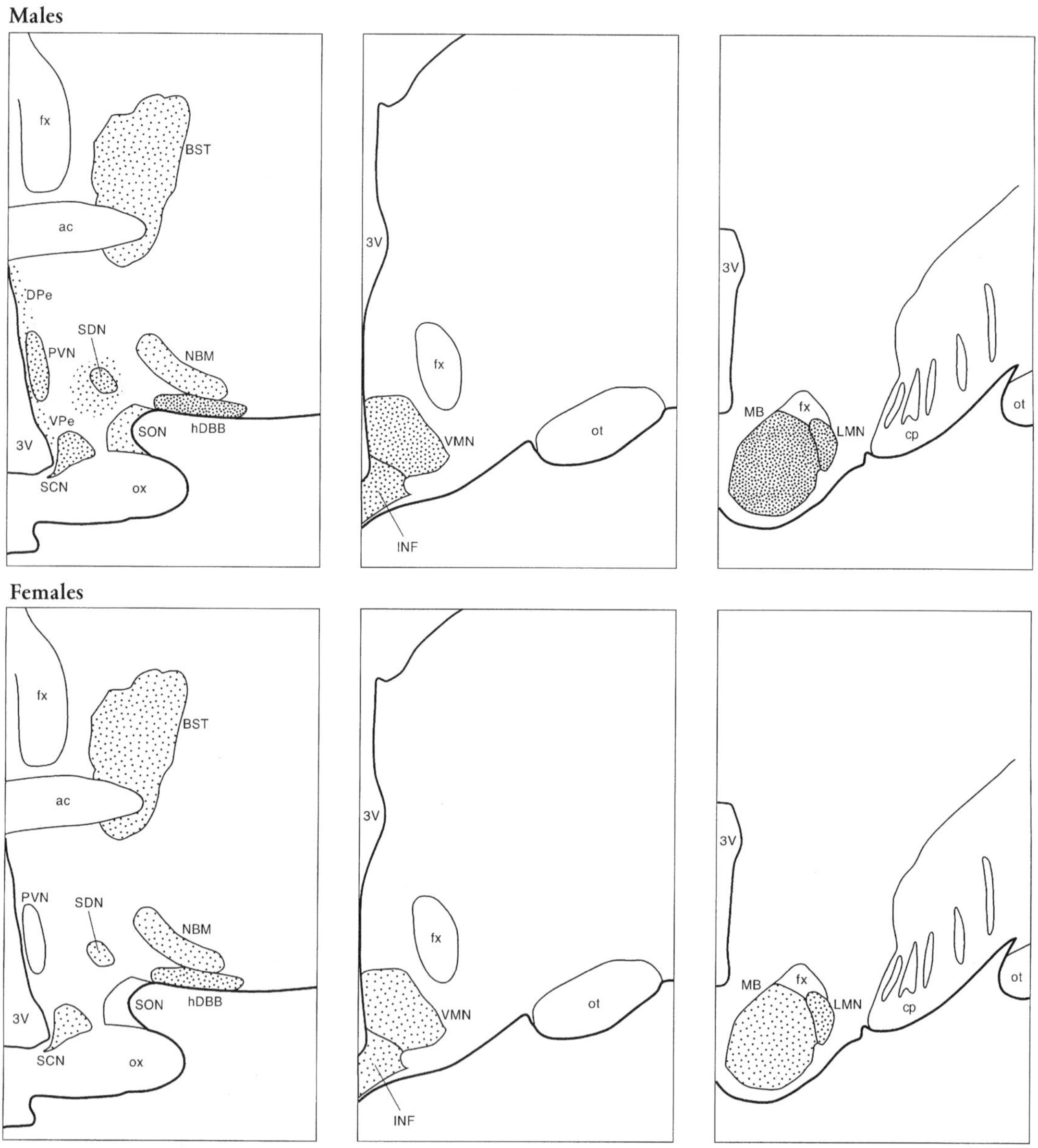

Figure 1 Schematic representation of sex differences in the intensity of androgen receptor immunoreactivity in the human hypothalamus. ox, optic chiasm; NBM, nucleus basalis of Meynert; hDBB, horizontal limb of diagonal band of Broca; SDN, sexually dimorphic nucleus of preoptic area; SCN, suprachiasmatic nucleus; BST, bed nucleus of stria terminalis; PVN, paraventricular nucleus; SON, supraoptic nucleus; DPe, periventricular nucleus dorsal zone; VPe, periventricular nucleus ventral zone; fx, fornix; 3V, third ventricle; ac, anterior commissure; VMN, ventromedial hypothalamic nucleus; INF, infundibular nucleus; OT, optic tract; MB, mamillary body, i.e. MMN, medial mamillary nucleus; LMN, lateromamillary nucleus; cp, cerebral peduncle. From reference 2

MMN. ERβ-immunoreactivity was observed not only in neurons but also in endothelial cells and perivascular smooth muscle cells. Interestingly, a striking ERβ-immunoreactivity was observed in fibers of the internal capsule and in the BSTc, while in the latter structure also a 'basket-like' neuronal staining pattern suggestive of nerve terminal appositions was observed.

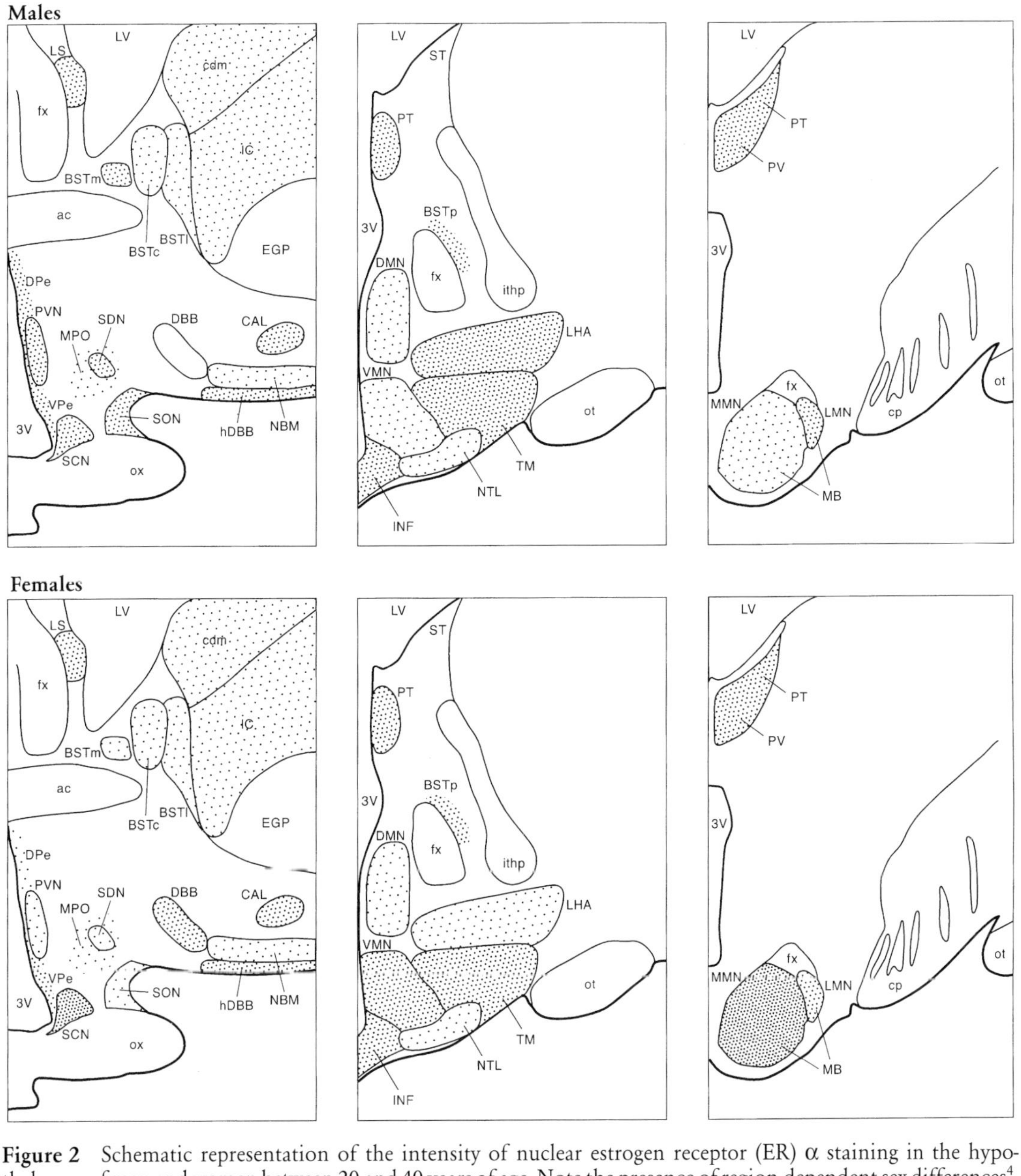

Figure 2 Schematic representation of the intensity of nuclear estrogen receptor (ER) α staining in the hypothalamus of men and women between 20 and 40 years of age. Note the presence of region-dependent sex differences[4]. For abbreviations see Figure 1, and: LS, lateral septum; LV, lateral ventricle; BSTm, medial part of bed nucleus of stria terminalis; BSTc, central part of BST; BSTl, lateral part of the BST; BSTp, posterior part of the BST; cdm, medial caudate nucleus; IC, internal capsule; EGP, external globus pallidus; MPO, medial preoptic area; CAL, islands of Callega; NTL, nucleus tuberculis lateralis; TM, tuberomamillary complex; LHA, lateral hypothalamic area; ithp, inferior thalamic peduncle; DMN, dorsomedial nucleus; PT, paratenial nucleus; ST, stria terminalis; PV, paraventricular nucleus of the thalamus

An ovariectomized 46-year-old female subject, a castrated and estrogen-treated 50-year-old male-to-female transsexual and a 31-year-old male subject with high estrogen levels owing to an estrogen-producing tumor revealed, in most areas, ERβ-immunoreactivity distribution patterns according to their level of circulating estrogens, suggesting again that the majority of the reported sex differences in ERβ-immunoreactivity are 'activational' rather than 'organizational' in nature (Kruijver and colleagues, *J Comp Neurol* 2003; in press).

The presence of ERα and -β in the hypothalamus at the mRNA level has been reported in the VMN, INF, SON and PVN, and generally agrees well with the protein levels we stained. In contrast to ERα mRNA, expression of the β subtype was generally very low in these areas[5].

HYPOTHALAMUS AND SEX HORMONES IN DEPRESSION

Depressive illness is presumed to result from an interaction between the effects of environmental stress and genetic/developmental predisposition. Sex hormones play a role in these complex interactions. The hypothalamic-pituitary-adrenal (HPA) axis, which is a key system in stress responses, is considered to be a final common pathway in depression. The set point of HPA axis activity is programmed by genotype, but can be changed to another level by early life events. Environmental stressors such as smoking by the mother during pregnancy may sensitize a person for depression. Stressful life events such as bereavement, child abuse or early maternal separation are also risk factors for depression. In addition there are genetic risk factors. Members of families with a high incidence of depression showed a primary functional defect in corticosteroid signal transduction, indicating the presence of a genetic factor. All the environmental and genetic factors seem ultimately to go together with increased HPA axis activity in adulthood (for review see reference 6). On the other hand, when patients are treated with antidepressants or electroconvulsive therapy, or show spontaneous remission, the HPA axis function returns to normal[7]. The corticotropin-releasing hormone (CRH) neurons of the PVN that regulate the HPA axis are indeed strongly activated in depression[8,9]. Depression is more common in women, specifically during times of changing sex hormone levels, such as premenstrual, antepartum and postpartum levels, and during transition to the postmenopausal period, pointing to an interaction of sex hormones with HPA axis activity.

Interestingly, M. Bleuer suggested, as early as 1919, that hormone treatment could be a potential antidepressant[10].

Unipolar depression and *dysthymia* are twice as common in women as in men[11,12], which may point to either an organizing or an activating effect of sex hormones in the pathogenesis of depression. The observation that adults with a history of prenatal exposure to diethylstilbestrol have an increased risk for depression argues in favor of an effect of prenatal estrogens in the organization of brain systems that are involved in affective disorders[13].

In untreated depressed female patients, significantly higher plasma concentrations of testosterone, androstenedione and dihydrotestosterone were found. These findings are best explained as a consequence of overstimulation of the adrenal glands in hypercortisolemic depressed patients. In contrast to women, depressed men seem to show decreased testosterone levels. In males, the activation of the HPA axis in depression may negatively affect gonadal function at every level of regulation[14–18]. In the infundibular nucleus, juxtapositions of CRH fibers were found, which formed multiple contacts with luteinizing hormone-releasing hormone (LHRH) neurons. This may be a substrate of such effects[19].

In severely depressed patients, testosterone levels are lower[20], and older men with lower bioavailable testosterone levels are more depressed[21]. In addition, low testosterone levels were found in men with dysthymic disorder[22]. Both testosterone level and androgen receptor polymorphism are related to the risk that middle-aged men run of becoming depressed. Men who have low total testosterone levels and a shorter CAG codon repeat length in the androgen receptor have a greater likelihood of becoming depressed[23]. In connection with the observed decreased sex hormone levels in depressed men, it is interesting that, in bodybuilders who took supraphysiological doses of testosterone, testosterone levels had a strong negative correlation with depression scores[24]. Studies in anabolic androgenic steroid users show that some of them develop manic or aggressive reactions to these drugs. Supraphysiological doses of testosterone indeed increased ratings of manic symptoms in normal men[25]. The sexual function and mood of hypogonadal men who received testosterone replacement improved[26,27]. However, there are not enough controlled studies at present to indicate that testosterone administration is effective in mood disorders[16].

In women with depression the blood levels of estradiol are significantly lower, which has been hypothesized to be due to the inhibiting effect of the HPA axis on the reproductive axis, in a way resembling that observed in stress and CRH administration[28]. Not only is estradiol lower in depressed women, but also the luteinizing hormone (LH) pulsatility frequency is slower and dysrhythmic[29]. The estrogen decrease in postmenopausal women may be a factor in both the pathogenesis of late-life depression and response to therapy. Estrogen replacement therapy may make women with Alzheimer's disease less vulnerable to depression[30], and may augment fluoxetine response in elderly depressed patients[31]. On the other hand, it should be noted that estrogen substitution in postmenopausal women with depressive symptoms was effective in some studies but not in others[32,33].

Premenstrual syndrome or *premenstrual dysphoric disorder* is characterized by depression, anxiety and mood swings during the last week of the luteal phase. Correlations have been reported between the premenstrual or menstrual phase and violent crimes, death as a result of accident or suicide, accidents, admission to hospital with psychiatric problems, taking a child to a medical clinic, and loss of control of aircraft and plane crashes in which the women pilots were said to be menstruating at the time of the crash[34]. Premenstrual dysphoric syndrome is characterized by disturbances in the timing and secretion patterns of circadian rhythms and their response to critically timed light administration, and interventions with bright light improve mood in these patients[35]. Although there is at present no conclusive evidence that premenstrual dysphoric disorder is indeed associated with abnormalities in the levels of sex hormones, both suppression of ovarian function by LHRH agonists and surgical oophorectomy are effective treatments for this type of mood disorder[32,36]. However, the observation that no differences were present in plasma levels of adrenocorticotropic hormone (ACTH), β-endorphin, cortisol or free testosterone does not support a primary endocrine abnormality in women with premenstrual syndrome[37]. Timing rather than quantitative measures of cortisol secretion were different in premenstrual dysphoric subjects, both during the menstrual cycle and in response to sleep-deprivation interventions[38]. Moreover, on the basis of animal experiments, neurosteroids have been proposed as potential etiological factors in this syndrome[39], and such effects would not be reflected in peripheral hormone changes.

Depression can also be associated with the use of oral contraceptives, pregnancy and the menopause[35].

Antepartum depression is found in 5% of pregnant women. This condition may be a risk factor for the development of pre-eclampsia, and is the strongest predictor of *postpartum depression*. Maternal depressive symptoms during pregnancy may lead to behavioral changes in the child[40]. The safety of pharmacological treatment of depression in pregnant women is controversial because of the possible behavioral-teratological effects[41]. It is therefore of great practical interest that an open trial showed that morning light therapy may be effective as an antidepressant during pregnancy[40]. A randomized controlled trial should confirm these promising data.

A characteristic hallmark of depression is elevated hypothalamic CRH production[6,8,9]. Because of all the evidence of a relationship between sex hormones and depression on the one hand, and depression and the HPA axis on the other, we recently used postmortem brain material to examine whether sex hormones might directly influence the CRH neurons in the hypothalamus of depressed patients and controls. We found that, in both populations of people, 40% of the CRH neurons contained ERα. Activation of the CRH neurons in depression is accompanied by a proportional rise of CRH neurons containing ERα, and sex hormones may thus affect these neurons directly (Bao and colleagues, unpublished data).

SEX DIFFERENCES IN RECEPTOR DISTRIBUTION MAY CHANGE DURING AGING AND IN MENOPAUSE

Males have higher vasopressin levels than females, even though the number of vasopressin neurons in the SON did not differ between men and women[42,43]. This sex difference is explained by the higher activity we found in vasopressin neurons in the SON of young males, compared with females, using the size of the Golgi apparatus and *in situ* hybridization for vasopressin mRNA as measures of neuronal activity. In the course of aging, probably triggered by the decrease in estrogen levels in postmenopausal women, the neuronal activity in the SON gradually increases in females, while it remains stable in males. The sex difference in neuronal activity in the SON thus disappears after the age of 50[44,45]. Consequently, this is an example of a hypothalamic system that shows no structural sex difference but a functional sex difference instead. It is also an example of a sex difference based on the 'activating' (or in this case 'inhibiting') effect of sex hormones. The activation of neurosecretory vasopressin neurons in postmenopausal women was confirmed by measurement of the cell size as a parameter for neuronal activity in immunocytochemically stained vasopressin neurons. Vasopressin neurons in the SON and PVN of the hypothalamus appeared to be larger in young men than in young women. In elderly women (> 50 years old), vasopressin cell size considerably exceeded that of young women. In addition, vasopressin cell size correlated positively with age in women, but not in men in both nuclei. Sex differences in the size of the PVN vasopressin neurons were pronounced on the left side and absent on the right, indicating the presence of functional lateralization of this nucleus. These data demonstrate sex differences in size of the vasopressin neurons, and thus in their function, that are age-dependent and probably also lateralized. No such changes were observed in oxytocin neurons in the PVN[45]. Sex- and age-related differences in the activity of vasopressin neurons in the human SON are probably mediated by differences in ERα and -β expression by these cells. Young women (≤ 50 years old) show 50 times more ERβ nuclear-positive vasopressin neurons than young men, and 250 times more than postmenopausal women. In contrast, ERα is present in a higher proportion of SON cells in young men and elderly women than in young women. The activation of vasopressin neurons in postmenopausal women is thus probably mediated by a decrease in nuclear ERβ as a possible mediator of inhibitory effects of estrogens, and an increase in nuclear ERα as a possible mediator of stimulatory effects of estrogens in these neurons[44] (Figure 3).

Another example of a sex difference based upon the activating effect of sex hormones was found in the mamillary body complex (MBC), which shows much stronger androgen receptor staining in males than in females[2]. Electrical stimulation of this area in monkeys induces penile erections[46,47]. In a follow-up study, we have shown that this sex difference depends on the

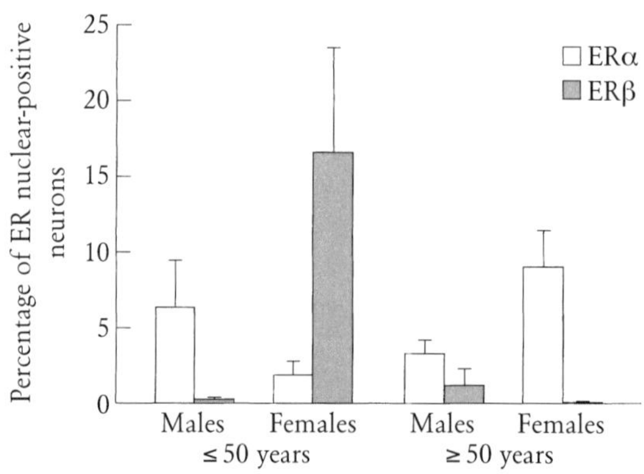

Figure 3 Graph depicting differential expression of nuclear estrogen receptors ERβ and ERα in vasopressin neurons in the dorsolateral supraoptic nucleus in relation to age and sex. In young women (39.5 ± 3.47 years old; six subjects), the percentage of nuclear ERβ-positive neurons is 50 times higher than that in young men (36.6 ± 3.6 years old; eight subjects) and 250 times higher than that in elderly women (70.9 ± 4.46 years old; ten subjects), whereas the proportion of ERα-positive cells in elderly women and in young and elderly men (68.9 ± 5.2 years old; eight subjects) exceeds that in young women by 4.5 and 3 times, respectively. From reference 44, with permission

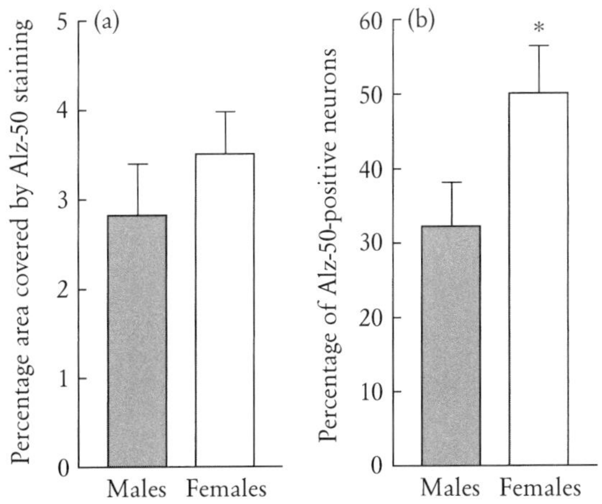

Figure 4 Graph depicting (a) mean of Alz-50 load and (b) mean percentage of Alz-50 stained neurons in males and females. Note that female subjects show a significant increase in mean percentage of Alz-50 stained neurons compared with males. $^*p = 0.039$. From reference 49, with permission

amount of circulating androgens in adulthood, while the sex difference in androgen receptors did not seem to be related to sexual orientation or gender identity[3]. Together, these data support the notion that a number of sex differences in the adult human hypothalamus are related to circulating levels of sex hormones. However, this is by no means a general phenomenon (see below).

SEX DIFFERENCES IN ALZHEIMER'S DISEASE AND SEX HORMONE RECEPTORS

A recent study indicated that, after the age of 90 years, the incidence of Alzheimer's disease (AD) is higher for women than for men, while the incidence of vascular dementia is higher in men than in women in all age groups[48]. Our observation of an increased number of neurons in the NBM, containing hyperphosphorylated tau in women, as compared with age-matched men[49] (Figure 4),

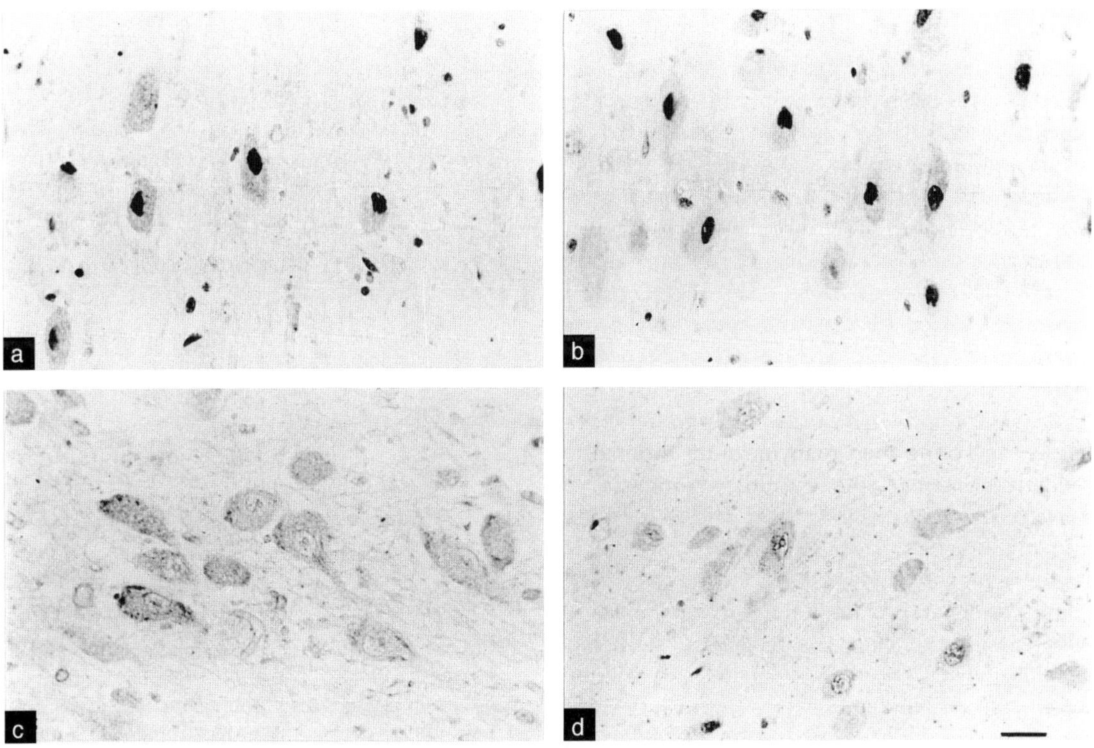

Figure 5 Immunocytochemical staining of estrogen receptor α (ERα) in the nucleus basalis of Meynert of Alzheimer's disease (AD) patients ((a) no. 91091, (b) no. 94029) and of their matched controls ((c) no. 98081, (d) no. 94074). Note intensive nuclear staining in AD patients compared with controls (scale bar = 25 μm). From reference 45, with permission

agrees with such a sex difference in AD. Unexpectedly, we found that in the NBM of AD patients, the proportion of neurons showing nuclear staining for ERα was markedly increased. In AD, the percentage of ERβ nuclear-positive neurons increased only in women and not in men[45] (Figure 5). In the vertical limb of the diagonal band of Broca an increased nuclear staining for ERα was also found (Ishunina and Swaab, *Exp Neurol* 2003;in press). These changes were unexpected, since in AD lower rather than higher sex hormone levels are reported. Whether the increased ERα staining is based upon local estrogen production by increased aromatase activity should be investigated.

The well-established Braak stages of both the neurofibrillary pathology and amyloid deposits indicate that the disease starts in the entorhinal cortex/hippocampal area, after which the neuropathological changes spread across the brain[50]. There is, however, one brain area that is an exception to this rule: the infundibular or arcuate nucleus of the hypothalamus. In this nucleus, AD pathology is already seen in non-demented control subjects without any AD pathology in the hippocampal area or neocortex. The pathology in the infundibular nucleus is characterized by neurofibrillary tangles, a network of neuropil threads and terminal-like vessel-associated processes (Figure 6). The AD pathology shows a striking sex difference[51-53] (Figure 7). From the age of 60 years onwards, the prevalence of neurofibrillary changes in the infundibular nucleus of non-demented male subjects rises from 20 to 90%, while in only 6–10% of the females such changes were observed[51-53].

The total number of neurons in the infundibular nucleus of pre- and postmenopausal women is not different, whereas the mean neuronal volume increases up to 40% in postmenopausal women, owing to an increase in neuronal size. Hypertrophy of neurons in this nucleus is thus not compensation for a loss of neurons, but rather the result of activation due to the loss of estrogen feedback in the menopause[54,55]. Some hypertrophy, although to a much lesser degree, also occurs in elderly men[56]. Sex steroid hormones influence gonadotropin secretion via negative feedback on the infundibular nucleus of the hypothalamus, and the removal of this inhibitory action of estrogens in postmenopausal women results in hyperactivity in this brain area, and increased gonadotropin-releasing hormone (GnRH) production[57]. A number of parameters indicate a strong increase of neuronal activity in the infundibular nucleus of postmenopausal women, such as increased cell size, an increase in nucleolar volume and number of nucleoli and an increase in expression of mRNAs of various peptides.

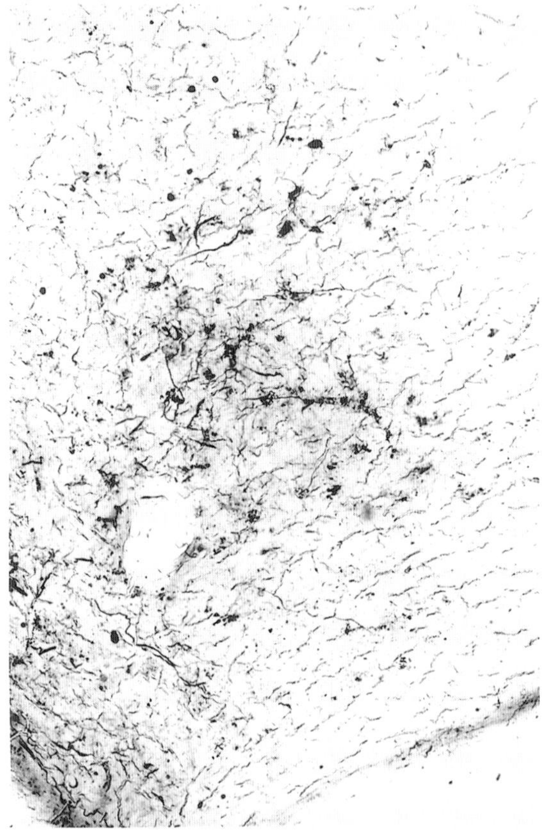

Figure 6 Mediobasal hypothalamus including the infundibular nucleus of a 66-year-old male with advanced cytoskeletal pathology stained by Alz-50 for hyperphosphorylated tau. Such pathology is rarely present in postmenopausal women, which suggests that hyperactivity of neurons protects them against Alzheimer changes

In the infundibular nucleus, a shift of ERα from the nucleus in young female controls to the cytoplasm in postmenopausal women was accompanied by a strong activation and a relative absence of AD neuropathology. In contrast, the

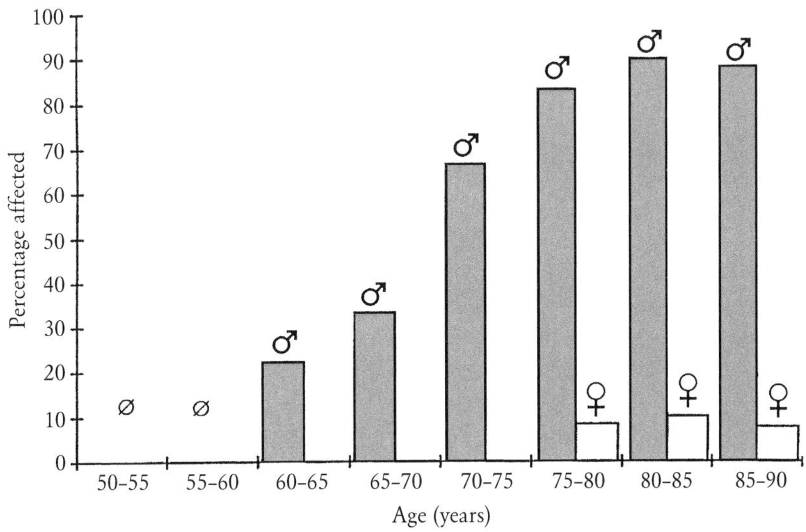

Figure 7 Percentage of male individuals affected by mediobasal hypothalamus (MBH) pathology increases markedly from age 60 to age 90 years. A marked or severe degree of MBH pathology was identified in 30% of all males at this age (not shown). In contrast, only a small percentage of elderly females is affected. From reference 52, with permission

expression of more nuclear ERα and basket-like nerve terminal ERβ in the infundibular nucleus of elderly non-demented men, compared with postmenopausal women was accompanied by less activation and a much stronger AD neuropathology (Hestiantoro and associates, unpublished data).

It is tempting to explain the sex difference in Alzheimer changes in the arcuate nucleus in relation to the strong activation of this structure in the menopause. Activation of neurons seems to protect them from Alzheimer changes, a phenomenon we paraphrased 'use it or lose it'[58,59].

Although the localization of ERα and ERβ in nearly all the brain areas, including hippocampus and neocortex, suggests that, in principle, all these brain areas may be a substrate for such replacement therapy, one may doubt the efficacy of estrogen replacement therapy in Alzheimer patients because there are so many different alterations in ERs in different systems in the brain, and some brain areas, such as the infundibular nucleus, may even be inhibited and subsequently develop Alzheimer changes. There is thus a need for the development of agonists that affect only selective brain areas.

CONCLUSION

Quite a number of structural and functional sex differences have been reported in the human hypothalamus and adjacent structures that may be related not only to reproduction, sexual orientation and gender identity, but also to the often pronounced sex differences in the prevalence of psychiatric and neurological diseases. A correlation between changing levels of sex hormones and depression has been documented extensively. Sex hormone receptors appear to be present in CRH neurons, the driving force of the HPA axis. Age- and menopause-related changes are observed in ER distribution in many brain areas, and may be related to activity changes, as is the case in, for example, the supraoptic nucleus. One of the recent focuses of interest in this respect is the possible beneficial effect of sex hormones on cognition in Alzheimer patients. The immunocytochemical localization of estrogen receptors α and β, and androgen receptors has shown that there are indeed numerous targets for sex hormones in the adult human brain. In the nucleus basalis of Meynert and diagonal band of Broca of Alzheimer patients, an unexpected up-regulation of nuclear

ERα and ERβ was found, suggesting increased local estrogen production. Observations in the infundibular nucleus have, however, indicated that in this area the hyperactivity resulting from a lack of estrogens in the menopause seems to protect females against Alzheimer changes, in contrast to males. It is thus quite possible that estrogen replacement therapy may, in such a brain area, lead to the inhibition of neuronal metabolism, and thus to the same proportion of Alzheimer changes as are observed in men. Knowledge about the functional sex differences in the brain and the effect of sex hormones on neuronal metabolism may thus provide clues, not only for the possible beneficial effects of estrogen replacement therapy, but also for the potential side-effects on the brain.

ACKNOWLEDGEMENTS

We would like to thank Ms W. T. P. Verweij for her excellent secretarial work. Brain material was obtained from the Netherlands Brain Bank (co-ordinator Dr R. Ravid). Financial support was obtained from the Hersenstichting Nederland, The International Stichting Alzheime Onderzach (ISAO), Alzheimer Nederland and The Netherlands Organization for Scientific Research (NWO).

References

1. Swaab DF. Gender issues in brain structures and functions and their relevance for psychopathology. In D'haenen H, Den Boer JA, Willner P, eds. *Biological Psychiatry*. New York: John Wiley and Sons Ltd, 2002:189-209
2. Fernández-Guasti A, Kruijver FPM, Fodor M, Swaab DF. Sex differences in the distribution of androgen receptors in the human hypothalamus. *J Comp Neurol* 2000;425:425-35
3. Kruijver FPM, Fernández-Guasti A, Fodor M, Kraan E, Swaab DF. Sex differences in androgen receptors of the human mamillary bodies are related to endocrine status rather than to sexual orientation or transsexuality. *J Clin Endocrinol Metab* 2001;86:818-27
4. Kruijver FPM, Balesar R, Espila AM, Unmehopa UA, Swaab DF. Estrogen receptor-α distribution in the human hypothalamus in relation to sex and endocrine status. *J Comp Neurol* 2002;454:115-39
5. Österlund MK, Hurd XL. Estrogen receptors in the human forebrain and the relation to neuropsychiatric disorders. *Prog Neurobiol* 2001;64: 252-67
6. Swaab DF, Fliers E, Hoogendijk WJG, Veltman DJ, Zhou JN. Interaction of prefrontal cortical and hypothalamic systems in the pathogenesis of depression. *Prog Brain Res* 2000;126:369-95
7. Nemeroff CB. The corticotropin-releasing factor (CRF) hypothesis of depression: new findings and new directions. *Mol Psychiatry* 1996;1:336-42
8. Raadsheer FC, Hoogendijk WJG, Stam FC, Tilders FJH, Swaab DF. Increased numbers of corticotropin-releasing hormone expressing neurons in the hypothalamic paraventricular nucleus of depressed patients. *Neuroendocrinology* 1994;60:436-44
9. Raadsheer FC, Van Heerikhuize JJ, Lucassen PJ, Hoogendijk WJG, Tilders FJH, Swaab DF. Corticotropin-releasing hormone mRNA levels in the paraventricular nucleus of patients with Alzheimer's disease and depression. *Am J Psychiatry* 1995;152:1372-6
10. Holsboer F. The corticosteroid receptor hypothesis of depression. *Neuropsychopharmacology* 2000;23: 477-501
11. Seeman, MV. Psychopathology in women and men: focus on female hormones. *Am J Psychiatry* 1997; 154:1641-7
12. Piccinelli M, Wilkinson G. Gender differences in depression. *Br J Psychiatry* 2000;177:486-92
13. Meyer-Bahlburg HFL, Ehrhardt AA. A prenatal-hormone hypothesis for depression in adults with a history of fetal DES exposure. In Halbreich U, ed. *Hormones and Depression*. New York: Raven Press, 1987:325-38
14. Baischer W, Koinig G, Hartmann B, Huber J, Langer G. Hypothalamic-pituitary-gonadal axis in depressed premenopausal women: elevated blood testosterone concentrations compared to normal controls. *Psychoneuroendocrinology* 1995;20:553-9

15. Albert DJ, Walsh ML, Jonk RH. Aggression in humans: what is its biological foundation? *Neurosci Biobehav Rev* 1993;17:405–25
16. Sternbach H. Age-associated testosterone decline in men: clinical issues for psychiatry. *Am J Psychiatry* 1998;155:1310–18
17. Schweiger U, Deuschle M, Weber B, *et al.* Testosterone, gonadotropin, and cortisol secretion in male patients with major depression. *Psychosom Med* 1999;61:292–6
18. Weber B, Lewicka S, Deuschle M, Colla M, Heuser I. Testosterone, androstenedione and dihydrotestosterone concentrations are elevated in female patients with major depression. *Psychoneuroendocrinology* 2000;25:765–71
19. Dudás B, Merchenthaler I. Close juxtapositions between luteinizing hormone-releasing hormone-immuno-immunoreactive neurons and corticotropin-releasing factor-immunoreactive axons in the human diencephalon. *J Clin Endocrinol Metab* 2002;87:5778–84
20. Heuser I. Depression, endocrinologically a syndrome of premature aging? *Maturitas* 2002;41 (Suppl 1):S19–23
21. Barrett-Connor E, Von Mühlen DG, Kritz-Silverstein D. Bioavailable testosterone and depressed mood in older men: the Rancho Bernardo study. *J Clin Endocrinol Metab* 1999;84: 573–7
22. Seidman SN, Araujo AB, Roose SP, *et al.* Low testosterone levels in elderly men with dysthymic disorder. *Am J Psychiatry* 2002;159:456–9
23. Seidman SN, Araujo AB, Roose SP, McKinlay JB. Testosterone level, androgen receptor polymorphism, and depressive symptoms in middle-aged men. *Biol Psychiatry* 2001;50:371–6
24. Dickerman RD, McCobathy WJ. Testosterone, vasopressin and depression. *Prog Neuro-Psychopharmacol Biol Psychiatry* 1997;21:247–8
25. Pope HG, Kouri EM, Hudson JI. Effects of supraphysiologic doses of testosterone on mood and aggression in normal men. *Arch Gen Psychiatry* 2000;57:133–40
26. Seidman SN, Walsh BT. Testosterone and depression in aging men. *Am J Geriatr Psychiatry* 1999; 7:18–33
27. Wong M-L, Kling MA, Munson PJ, *et al.* Pronounced and sustained central hypernoradrenergic function in major depression with melancholic features: relation to hypercortisolism and corticotropin-releasing hormone. *Proc Natl Acad Sci USA* 2000;97:325–30
28. Young EA, Midgley R, Carlson NE, Brown MB. Alteration in the hypothalamic-pituitary-ovarian axis in depressed women. *Arch Gen Psychiatry* 2000;57:1157–62
29. Meller WH, Grambsch PL, Bingham C, Tagatz GE. Hypothalamic pituitary gonadal axis dysregulation in depressed women. *Psychoneuroendocrinology* 2001;26:253–9
30. Carlson LE, Sherwin BB, Chertkow HM. Relationships between mood and estradiol (E_2) levels in Alzheimer's disease (AD) patients. *J Gerontol* 2000; B55:P47–53
31. Schneider LS, Small GW, Hamilton SH, Bystritsky A, Nemeroff CB, Meyers BS, Fluoxetine Collaborative Study Group. Estrogen replacement and response to fluoxetine in a multicenter geriatric depression trial. *Am J Geriatr Psychiatry* 1997;5: 97–106
32. Rubinow DR, Schmidt PJ, Roca CA. Estrogen-serotonin interactions: implications for affective regulation. *Biol Psychiatry* 1998;44:839–50
33. Rasgon NL, Altschuler LL, Fairbanks L. Estrogen-replacement therapy for depression. *Am J Psychiatry* 2001;158:1738
34. Parlee MB. The premenstrual syndrome. *Psychol Bull* 1973;80:454–65
35. Parry BL, Newton RP. Chronobiological basis of female-specific mood disorders. *Neuropsychopharmacology* 2001;25(Suppl 5):S102–8
36. Steiner M. Premenstrual dysphoric disorder. *Gen Hosp Psychiatry* 1996;18:244–50
37. Bloch M, Schmidt PJ, Su T-P, Tobin MB, Rubinow DR. Pituitary-adrenal hormones and testosterone across the menstrual cycle in women with premenstrual syndrome and controls. *Biol Psychiatry* 1998;43:897–903
38. Parry BL, Javeed S, Laughlin GA, Hauger R, Clopton P. Cortisol circadian rhythms during the menstrual cycle and sleep deprivation in premenstrual dysphoric disorder and normal control subjects. *Biol Psychiatry* 2000;48:920–31
39. Britton KT, Koob GF. Premenstrual steroids? *Nature (London)* 1998;392:869–70
40. Oren DA, Wisner KL, Spinelli M, *et al.* An open trial of morning light therapy for treatment of antepartum depression. *Am J Psychiatry* 2002;159: 666–9
41. Swaab DF, Boer K. Functional teratogenic effects of chemicals on the developing brain. In Levene MI, Chervenak FA, Whittle MJ, Bennett MJ, Punt J, eds. *Fetal and Neonatal Neurology and Neurosurgery*. London: Churchill Livingstone, 2001:1–26
42. Van Londen L, Goekoop JG, Van Kempen GMJ, *et al.* Plasma levels of arginine vasopressin elevated in patients with major depression. *Neuropsychopharmacology* 1997;17:284–92
43. Asplund R, Aberg H. Diurnal variation in the levels of antidiuretic hormone in the elderly. *J Int Med* 1991;229:131–4
44. Ishunina TA, Kruijver FP, Balesar R, Swaab DF. Differential expression of estrogen receptor α and β immunoreactivity in the human supraoptic nucleus in relation to sex and aging. *J Clin Endocrinol Metab* 2000;85:3283–91

45. Ishunina TA, Swaab DF. Increased expression of estrogen receptor α and β in the nucleus basalis of Meynert in Alzheimer's disease. *Neurobiol Aging* 2001;22:417-26
46. Poeck K, Pilleri G. Release of hypersexual behavior due to lesion in the limbic system. *Acta Neurol Scand* 1965;41:233-44
47. MacLean PD, Ploog DW. Cerebral representation of penile erection. *J Neurophysiol* 1962;25:29-55
48. Ruitenberg A, Ott A, Van Swieten JC, Hofman A, Breteler MMB. Incidence of dementia: does gender make a difference? *Neurobiol Aging* 2001;22: 575-80
49. Salehi A, Dubelaar EJG, Mulder M, Swaab DF. A sex difference and no effect of ApoE type on the amount of cytoskeletal alteration in the nucleus basalis of Meynert in Alzheimer's disease. *Neurobiol Aging* 1998;19:505-10
50. Braak H, Braak E. Neuropathological staging of Alzheimer-related changes. *Acta Neuropathol* 1991; 82:239-59
51. Schultz C, Braak H, Braak E. A sex difference in neurodegeneration of the human hypothalamus. *Neurosci Lett* 1996;212:103-6
52. Schultz C, Ghebremedhin E, Braak H, Braak E. Neurofibrillary pathology in the human paraventricular and supraoptic nuclei. *Acta Neuropathol* 1997;94:99-102
53. Schultz C, Ghebremedhin E, Braak E, Braak H. Sex-dependent cytoskeletal changes of the human hypothalamus develop independently of Alzheimer's disease. *Exp Neurol* 1999;160:186-93
54. Rance NE, McMullen NT, Smialek JE, Price DL, Scott Young W III. Postmenopausal hypertrophy of neurons expressing the estrogen receptor gene in the human hypothalamus. *J Clin Endocrinol Metab* 1990;71:79-85
55. Abel TW, Rance NE. Stereologic study of the hypothalamic infundibular nucleus in young and older women. *J Comp Neurol* 2000;424:679-88
56. Rance NE. Hormonal influences on morphology and neuropeptide gene expression in the infundibular nucleus of postmenopausal women. *Prog Brain Res* 1992;93:221-36
57. Rance NE, Uswandi SV. Gonadotropin-releasing hormone gene expression is increased in the medial basal hypothalamus of postmenopausal women. *J Clin Endocrinol Metab* 1996;81:3540-6
58. Swaab DF. Brain aging and Alzheimer's disease: 'wear and tear' versus 'use it or lose it'. *Neurobiol Aging* 1991;12:317-24
59. Swaab DF, Dubelaar EJG, Hofman MA, Scherder EJA, Van Someren EJW, Verwer RWH. Brain aging and Alzheimer's disease: use it or lose it. *Prog Brain Res* 2002;138:343-73

Progesterone in the nervous system: an old player in new roles

7

R. Guennoun, A. F. De Nicola, M. Schumacher and E. E. Baulieu

NEUROSTEROID CONCEPT

Concerning the origin of steroids in the nervous system, two possibilities have to be considered:

(1) Diffusion of steroids synthesized in peripheral steroidogenic tissues, such as the gonads and adrenals, across the blood-brain barrier; and

(2) *De novo* steroid biosynthesis within the nervous system itself.

Steroids synthesized in the nervous system by neurons and glial cells are called neurosteroids[1,2]. We have demonstrated that the levels of steroids in the rat brain persist up to 2 weeks after the removal of peripheral steroidogenic organs (Table 1). Furthermore, the enzymes and enzymatic activities of steroid biosynthesis have been demonstrated in the nervous system[3].

Among neurosteroids, we will focus on progesterone, its precursor pregnenolone, and its reduced metabolites 5α-dihydroprogesterone and 3α,5α-tetrahydroprogesterone (allopregnanolone). We will summarize in this review some new findings concerning their synthesis and effects in the peripheral and central nervous systems.

ORIGINS OF PROGESTERONE IN THE NERVOUS SYSTEM

Progesterone can originate from peripheral tissues or be locally synthesized in specific areas of the nervous system. As a hormone, progesterone is synthesized by ovaries, placenta and adrenal glands, and can then reach the target tissues via the blood circulation. It is generally admitted that circulating progesterone easily crosses the blood-brain barrier and diffuses throughout nervous tissues because of its lipid solubility. As a neurosteroid, progesterone is synthesized locally in the nervous system, i.e. in the brain, spinal cord, dorsal root ganglia and peripheral nerves, either *de novo* from cholesterol or from blood-derived pregnenolone. Progesterone accumulates in the nervous system, as indicated by a brain/plasma concentration ratio greater than 1[4,5].

Table 1 Neurosteroids in the male rat brain. Concentrations of pregnenolone, dehydroepiandrosterone (DHEA), their sulfates, their fatty acid esters and progesterone, in the intact and orchidectomized and adrenalectomized (ORX/ADX) male rat brain

	Pregnenolone	*Pregnenolone sulfate*	*Pregnenolone fatty ester*	*DHEA*	*DHEA sulfate*	*DHEA fatty ester*	*Progesterone*
Brain (ng/g)							
Intact	8.9 ± 2.4	14.2 ± 2.5	9.4 ± 2.9	0.24 ± 0.33	1.70 ± 0.32	0.45 ± 0.13	2.2 ± 1.1
ORX/ADX	2.6 ± 0.8	16.9 ± 4.6	4.9 ± 1.3	0.14 ± 0.13	1.64 ± 0.43	0.29 ± 0.12	3.2 ± 1.6
Plasma (ng/ml)							
Intact	1.2 ± 0.6	2.1	2.4 ± 0.9	0.06 ± 0.06	0.20 ± 0.08	0.18 ± 0.05	1.9 ± 0.7
ORX/ADX	0.3 ± 0.1	nd	1.3 ± 0.3	nm	nm	nm	0.1 ± 0.1

nm, not measured; nd, non-detectable

MECHANISMS OF ACTION OF PROGESTERONE IN THE NERVOUS SYSTEM

Genomic action

According to the common theory of steroid action, progesterone modulates gene transcription by interaction with intracellular nuclear receptors, which act as ligand-dependent transcription factors[6–8]. These receptors regulate gene expression by recognizing palindromic hormone response elements (HRE) at the DNA after homo- or heterodimerization of the ligand-receptor complex. Subsequently, transcription is initiated in conjunction with the basal transcription complex, different coactivators, repressors, and transcription regulators[8].

Membrane actions

Specific binding sites
The existence of progesterone membrane-binding sites in several regions of the brain has been demonstrated by the use of iodinated progesterone-bovine serum albumin (BSA) exhibiting K_d values in the nanomolar range[9–11]. In mouse brain membranes, photoaffinity labelling with a progesterone analog detected four protein bands with apparent molecular masses ranging from 29 to 64 kDa[12]. Wehling's group was able to characterize two membrane progesterone-binding sites (mPR) from porcine liver microsomes with apparent K_d values of 11 and 286 nmol/l, respectively[13]. After purification, the maximum capacity of binding corresponds to the enrichment of polypeptides with relative molecular masses of 28 and 56 kDa. The 56-kDa protein possibly represents a dimer of the 28-kDa protein[13]. Under native conditions, only one membrane-binding protein complex of 200 kDa, displaying progesterone-binding activity, was detected. These observations have led to the hypothesis that the native mPR may be an oligomeric protein complex, composed at least in part of the 28- and 56-kDa proteins[14].

Interestingly, the rat analog of mPR, the protein (25-Dx)[15], was suggested to be behaviorally relevant and expressed in the brain[16] and spinal cord[17]. Indeed, using differential display polymerase chain reaction (PCR), the mRNA of 25-Dx was found to be present and to be repressed by progesterone in the ventromedial hypothalamus after estradiol priming of ovariectomized rats. The expression of 25-Dx was found to be sexually dimorphic, and higher levels were seen in female PR knockout mice compared to their wild-type littermates. A GFP fusion construct transfected into the neuronal cell line GT-7 showed its membrane localization[16].

Interaction with receptors of neurotransmitters
Pregnenolone sulfate, progesterone and its metabolite 3α,5α-tetrahydroprogesterone can modulate the neurotransmission via interaction with neurotransmitter receptors.

γ-Aminobutyric acid type A ($GABA_A$) receptors 3α,5α-Tetrahydroprogesterone is a potent positive modulator of $GABA_A$ receptors, whereas pregnenolone sulfate has inhibitory effects[18]. 3α,5α-Tetrahydroprogesterone can mimic or enhance the effects of GABA and these actions may explain some of the psychopharmacological effects of progestins[18,19].

Sigma receptors The endogenous ligands of sigma receptors are not known, but it has been proposed that progesterone may be one of them[20,21]. Progesterone can bind to the sigma receptor *in vitro*[21,22]. Progesterone acts as a competitive inhibitor of 3H SKF-10,047 binding a selective sigma 1 agonist. In addition, progesterone inhibits, via sigma 1 receptors, the NMDA-evoked release of 3H norepinephrine from preloaded hippocampal slices[20].

Glycine receptors Progesterone modulates glycine receptors[23,24]. Pregnenolone sulfate rapidly and reversibly exerts its inhibitory effects on the glycine receptor-mediated response to glycine-induced currents[25].

Glutamate receptors Pregnenolone sulfate acts as a positive allosteric modulator of the NMDA receptor[26,27]. Progesterone rapidly attenuates excitatory amino acid responses of cerebellar Purkinje cells[28].

5-Hydroxytryptamine type 3 receptors ($5\text{-}HT_3$ receptors) Progesterone has been described as a functional antagonist of the $5\text{-}HT_3$ receptor in whole-cell voltage clamp recordings of HEK293 cells stably expressing 5-HT_3 receptors[29]. Progesterone also non-competitively inhibited the 5-HT_3 response by a voltage- and agonist-independent mechanism distinct from that of open-channel blockers[30]. Functional antagonistic properties at this ligand-gated ion channel have been shown for 3α,5α-tetrahydroprogesterone[29].

Action on microtubule-associated protein type 2 (MAP-2)

Fetal or adult rat-brain cytosol and fetal rat-brain microtubules contain a high-affinity, low-capacity pregnenolone-binding protein. The best competitors are pregnenolone sulfate, progesterone, Δ^5-pregnene-3β,20α-diol, and 3β-hydroxy-5α-pregnan-20-one. It was hypothesized that the pregnenolone-binding protein was related to microtubule-associated proteins. Because many proteins are associated with microtubules, binding assays were performed with purified calf-brain tubulin, MAP-2 and Tau protein. Only the MAP-2 fraction showed saturable [^{3}H]pregnenolone binding with an affinity close to that of rat-brain microtubules. Pregnenolone induced a dose-related increase in the rate and extent of MAP-2-induced tubulin assembly, whereas progesterone, which is inactive *per se*, counteracted the stimulatory effect of pregnenolone. The stimulatory effect on MAP-2-tubulin interaction was also observed in fetal rat-brain neuron cultures. Therefore, a potential effect of neurosteroids on microtubule assembly or, more generally, on neural cytoskeleton dynamics can be suggested[31].

PROGESTERONE AND ITS 5A-REDUCED METABOLITES

Synthesis of progesterone: the 3β-hydroxysteroid dehydrogenase enzyme

The synthesis of progesterone from pregnenolone is catalyzed by the 3β-hydroxysteroid dehydrogenase/Δ^5–Δ^4 isomerase (3β-HSD) enzyme (Figure 1). This enzymatic complex, which catalyzes the conversion of Δ^5-3β-hydroxysteroids into Δ^4-3-ketosteroids, plays a crucial role in the biosynthesis of all classes of steroid hormones. 3β-HSD has two distinct enzymatic activities: 3β-dehydrogenation and isomerization of the double bond from C5,6 in the B ring (Δ^5 steroids) to C4,5 in the A ring (Δ^4 steroids)[32-34]. This enzyme is encoded by multiple distinct genes, which are expressed in a tissue-specific manner[35]. Molecular cloning of the cDNAs encoding 3β-HSD has revealed the existence of two human isoforms of the enzyme: type I 3β-HSD which is mainly expressed in the placenta[33] and type II 3β-HSD which is predominantly expressed in the adrenal gland and gonads[36]. Four types of 3β-HSD cDNAs (types I–IV) have been characterized in the rat[35,37,38] and six types (types I–VI) in the mouse[39,40]. The rodent type III 3β-HSD isoform possesses the structural features common to all 3β-HSD but does not display the expected classical 3β-HSD activity.

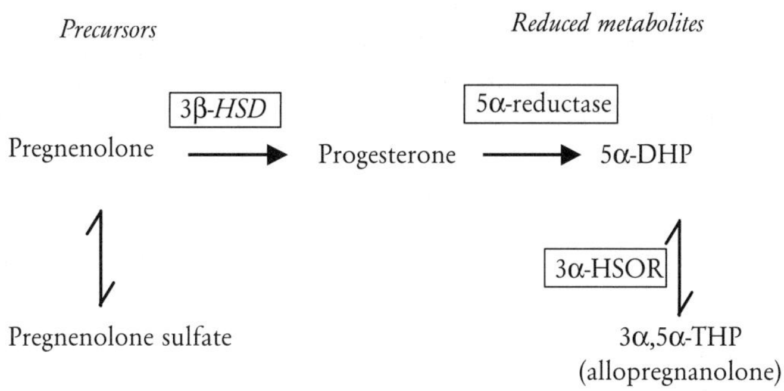

Figure 1 Progesterone biosynthesis and metabolism in the nervous system. Both progesterone and 5α-dihydroprogesterone (5α-DHP) can bind to the intracellular progesterone receptor. 3α,5α-Tetrahydroprogesterone (3α,5α-THP) is a positive allosteric modulator of γ-aminobutyric acid activating type A ($GABA_A$) receptors. 3β-HSD, 3β-hydroxysteroid dehydrogenase; 3α-HSOR, 5α-reductase and 3α-oxidoreductase

3β-HSD in brain

The first data suggesting the existence of 3β-HSD in the central nervous system have been provided by Weidenfield and colleagues[41] who showed that homogenates of rat amygdala and septum are capable of converting pregnenolone into

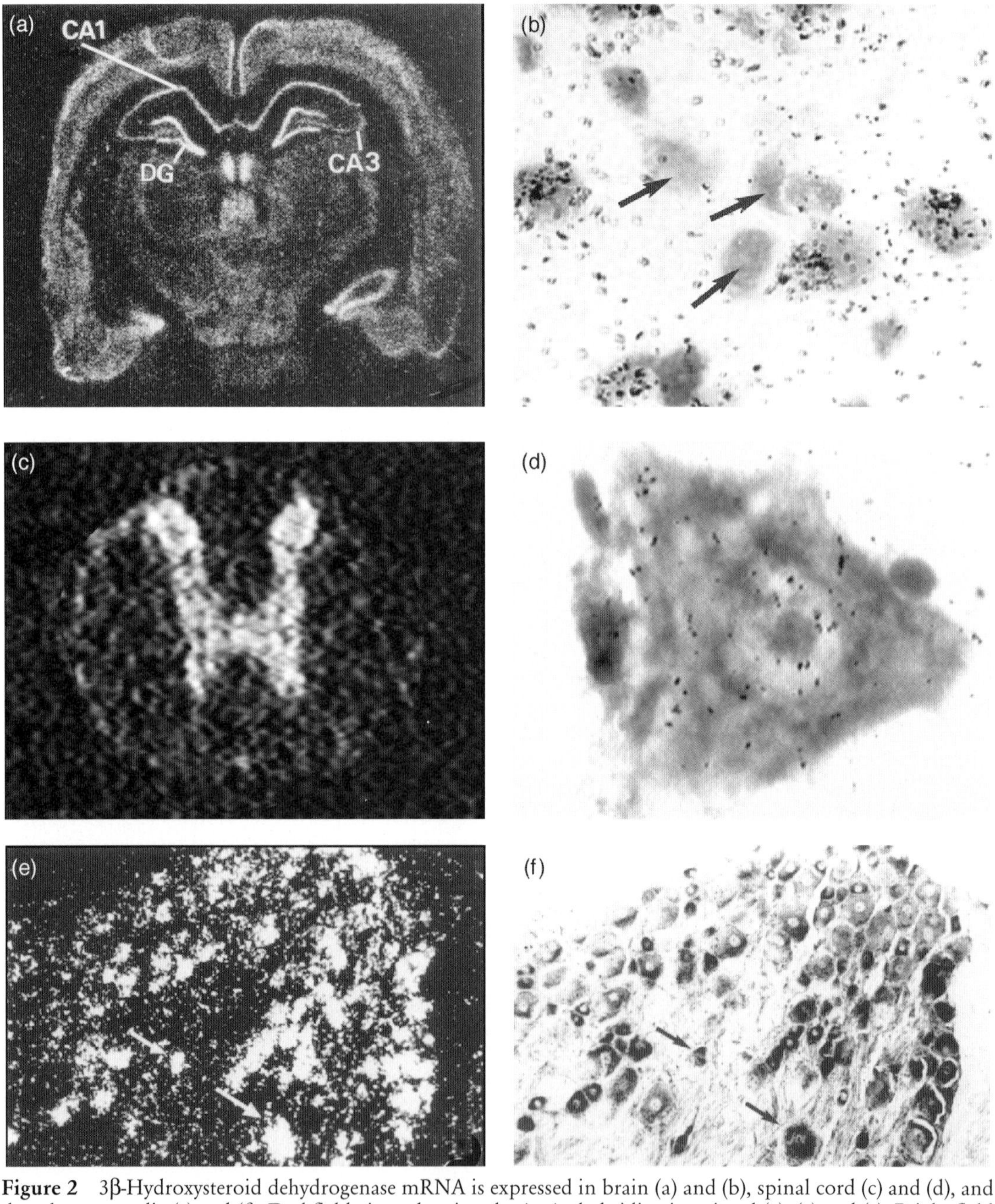

Figure 2 3β-Hydroxysteroid dehydrogenase mRNA is expressed in brain (a) and (b), spinal cord (c) and (d), and dorsal root ganglia (e) and (f). Darkfield views showing the *in situ* hybridization signal (a), (c) and (e). Bright-field microscopic views showing silver grains over neurons (b), (d) and (f). Small neurons in the striatum (b), large motoneuron in the spinal cord (d) and sensory neurons in dorsal root ganglia (f). Arrows in (b), unlabelled neurons; arrows in (e) and (f), large and small labelled sensory neurons. CA1–CA3, fields 1–3 of Hammon's horn; DG, dendate gyrus

progesterone. The biological activity of 3β-HSD has also been detected in primary cultures of rodent oligodendrocytes[42], astrocytes[43], and neurons[44]. Our *in situ* hybridization studies have revealed that the mRNAs encoding for 3β-HSD in the rat brain are localized in the olfactory bulb, nucleus accumbens, hippocampus, thalamus, hypothalamus, and cerebellum. 3β-HSD mRNAs were only detected in neuronal cell bodies[45] (Figure 2). The cerebellum showed the highest level of expression of 3β-HSD mRNAs, corresponding to a transcript of 1.8 kb. Nucleotide sequencing of the cloned PCR-amplified cDNA fragments from cerebellar mRNA indicated that the four known rat 3β-HSD isoforms are expressed in the cerebellum (Guennoun, unpublished results). These findings do not exclude the possibility of the expression of another isoform(s) in the cerebellum or in other brain regions not studied. Different studies have shown the expression of the 3β-HSD protein in rat brain[45,46]. Our recent ontogenetic study[47] showed that both the expression of the 3β-HSD gene and the concentrations of progesterone and pregnenolone in the hippocampus are maximum at birth, a period of intense cerebral maturation, suggesting that this enzyme could be implicated in several important neurotrophic events during postnatal development.

In human brain, Yu and colleagues[48] have quantified 3β-HSD mRNA by real-time reverse transcriptase-polymerase chain reaction (RT-PCR) in the human amygdala, caudate nucleus, cerebellum, corpus callosum, hippocampus, thalamus, and spinal cord. The 3β-HSD mRNA was present in all brain regions examined, and highest levels were found in the myelin-rich corpus callosum[48]. Both 3β-HSD and progesterone receptor mRNA were found to be present within distinct regions, suggesting local synthesis and autocrine/paracrine actions of progesterone in the human brain[49]. Cultured human oligodendroglial, astroglial and neuronal cell lines expressed the 3β-HSD[50]. The observation that human glioma cells with an oligodendroglial phenotype (expressing the myelin basic protein) express both P450scc and 3β-HSD suggests that human oligodendrocytes may have the capacity to synthesize progesterone *de novo* from cholesterol[50].

3β-HSD in spinal cord

Using *in situ* hybridization analysis, we have shown that 3β-HSD mRNA is widely expressed at all the levels from the cervical to the sacral segment. There is a higher expression in the gray matter than in the white matter (Figure 2). 3β-HSD is expressed by both motoneurons (Figure 2) and small neurons of the dorsal horn, but the grain densities per cell were similar. Further evidence for the expression of 3β-HSD in the spinal cord was obtained by Western blot analysis, which revealed an immunoreactive protein of 45 kDa. Castration and adrenalectomy did not influence the expression of 3β-HSD mRNA and protein. Gas chromatography/mass spectrometry measurements showed higher levels of pregnenolone and progesterone in the spinal cord than in the plasma. After castration and adrenalectomy, their levels remained elevated in the spinal cord, suggesting that these steroids may be synthesized locally. The wide distribution of 3β-HSD, and the high levels of pregnenolone and progesterone in the spinal cord even after castration and adrenalectomy, strongly suggest a potential endogenous production of progesterone and an important signalling function of this steroid in the spinal cord[51].

3β-HSD in sciatic nerve and dorsal root ganglia

In the peripheral nervous system, 3β-HSD is expressed and is functional in both sciatic nerve[52–54] and dorsal root ganglia (Figure 2e, f)[55]. Progesterone formation in the sciatic nerve is regulated by cellular interactions between Schwann cells and sensory neurons[54] and by some steroids, in particular by estradiol and by progesterone[52].

The regulation of progesterone synthesis in Schwann cells may be important for the normal functioning and regeneration of peripheral nerves. Several Schwann cell genes and functions have been shown to be under the control of neuronal signals, requiring either direct contact between cells or involving diffusible molecules[56–58]. The possibility that progesterone synthesis in Schwann cells may also be under neuronal control has been investigated. We have shown that mRNA expression and activity of 3β-HSD are induced in Schwann cells by sensory neurons. This was demonstrated *in vitro*, using different co-culture paradigms of dorsal root ganglia neurons and Schwann cells, and in the regenerating rat sciatic nerve after different types of lesions (cryolesion, nerve transection). Thus, progesterone synthesis in the peripheral nervous system is regulated by cellular interactions[54].

Metabolism of progesterone: 5α-reductases and 3α-oxidoreductase enzymes

The main metabolic pathway of progesterone in the nervous system is achieved through a 5α-reductase, which converts progesterone into 5α-dihydroprogesterone (Figure 1). Two 5α-reductase isoforms have been cloned[59] that share only 44% homology. The 5α-reductase type 1 is the main isoform expressed in the rat brain, type 2 having only transient expression during the perinatal period[60]. 5α-Dihydroprogesterone is susceptible to 3α- reduction by the enzyme 3α-oxidoreductase and can be converted into 3α,5α-tetrahydroprogesterone (allopregnanolone). The enzymatic activity of the 5α-reductase was first demonstrated in human brain tissues by using either progesterone or testosterone as substrates[61,62]. The enzymatic activities of the 5α-reductase and the 3α-oxidoreductase were found to co-localize at all life stages in the cerebral cortex and subcortical white matter of both men and women, but no sex-specific differences in enzyme activities were observed[63].

STIMULATORY EFFECT OF PROGESTERONE ON MYELINATION

Progesterone effect on myelination in sciatic nerve

The stimulatory effect of progesterone on myelination was first demonstrated in the peripheral nervous system[64]. The presence and activity of the 3β-HSD enzyme have been demonstrated in Schwann cells isolated from embryonic rat dorsal root ganglia[55], and its functional implication in myelination has been demonstrated in the regenerating mouse sciatic nerve by using the 3β-HSD inhibitor trilostane after cryolesion of the sciatic nerve[64]. Blocking the local synthesis of progesterone by trilostane impaired remyelination (Figure 3). In addition, blocking progesterone activity by mifepristone (RU486), its potent competitive antagonist, also impaired remyelination, indicating that the classical intracellular progesterone receptor (PR) is involved in this progesterone effect. The stimulatory effect of progesterone on myelination has also been demonstrated in both the aging rodent sciatic nerve and in dorsal root ganglia explant cultures[64–67].

One mechanism by which progesterone may promote myelination is by activating the expression of genes coding for specific myelin proteins[68]. Its actions in peripheral nerves may be autocrine, as Schwann cells not only synthesize progesterone, but also express an intracellular receptor for the steroid, as has been demonstrated by RT-PCR, immunocytochemistry and ligand binding studies[69]. It has been shown that, in sciatic nerves, progestins promote myelination through the classical intracellular progesterone receptor and through membrane $GABA_A$ receptors[70]. These two receptor systems were found to activate the expression of distinct peripheral myelin proteins. Progesterone and 5α-dihydroprogesterone, which both bind with high affinity to the intracellular progesterone receptor, increased P0 expression. 3α,5α-Tetrahydroprogesterone, a positive allosteric modulator of $GABA_A$ receptors which does not bind to the progesterone receptor, increased PMP22 expression[70,71].

Progesterone effect on myelination in brain

We have recently shown that the stimulatory effect of progesterone on myelination can be extended to the central nervous system. Indeed, progesterone stimulates myelination in organotypic slice cultures of 7-day-old (P7) rat and mouse cerebellum. Myelination was evaluated by immunofluorescence analysis of the myelin basic protein (MBP) expression. This *in vitro* system closely reproduces developmental *in vivo* events and thus provides a unique model for examining the process of myelin formation and its regulation in detail[72]. It has already been used to study the effects of progesterone on dendritic growth and synaptogenesis of developing Purkinje neurons[73].

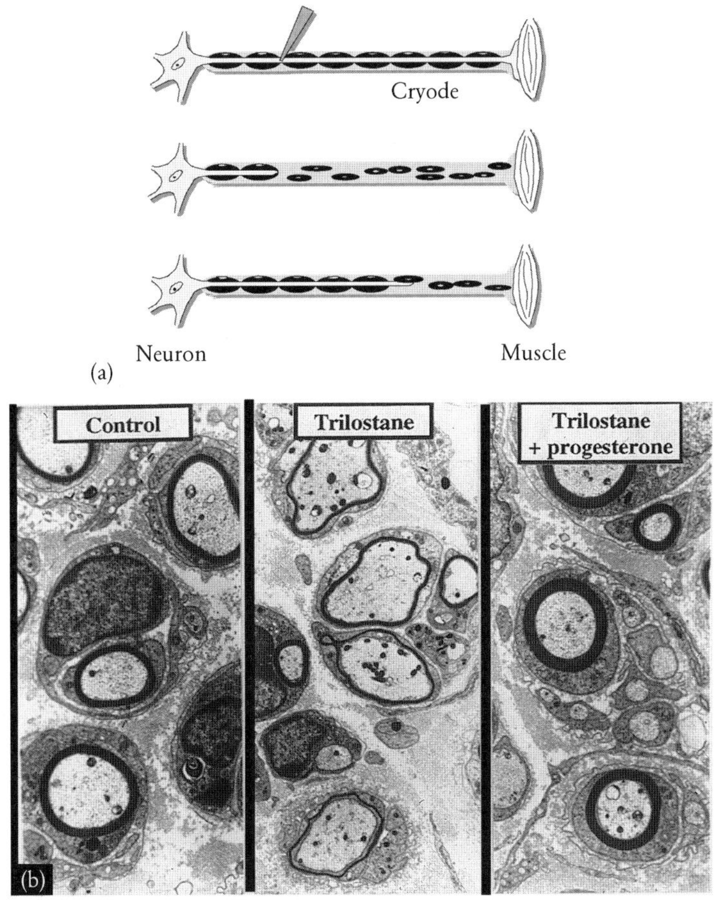

Figure 3 Role of local progesterone biosynthesis in the formation of myelin sheaths. (a) Cryolesion model of the sciatic nerve. The sciatic nerve was exposed and lesioned with a copper cryode (diameter, 0.5 mm) that had been dipped in liquid nitrogen and was repeatedly applied to the upper part of the nerve. The extent of the lesion was 1 mm. In this model, axons can regenerate and Schwann cells surround them with new myelin sheaths. (b) Effect of trilostane in the absence (center panel) or presence (right panel) of progesterone on the thickness of myelin sheaths. Adapted from reference 64

We evaluated the rate of myelination by measuring MBP accumulation, as the quantification of MBP-immunostaining provides a reliable and sensitive method for assessing the progress of myelination in the brain[74,75].

After 7 days in culture (7DIV), adding progesterone (2–5×10^{-5} mol/l) to the culture medium caused a 4-fold increase in MBP expression when compared to control slices (Figure 4). This effect involves both the classical intracellular progesterone receptor and $GABA_A$ receptors. Indeed, the selective progesterone receptor agonist R5020 significantly increased MBP expression and the progesterone receptor antagonist RU486 completely abolished the effect of progesterone (Figure 5). Moreover, treatment of P7-cerebellar slice cultures from progesterone receptor knockout mice with progesterone had no significant effect on MBP expression. In rat cerebellum slices, progesterone was metabolized into 5α-dihydroprogesterone and then to 3α,5α-tetrahydroprogesterone. The 5α-reductase inhibitor L685-273 partially inhibited the effect of progesterone, and 3α,5α-tetrahydroprogesterone significantly stimulated the MBP expression, although to a lesser extent than progesterone. The increase in MBP expression by 3α,5α-tetrahydroprogesterone involved $GABA_A$ receptors, as it could be inhibited

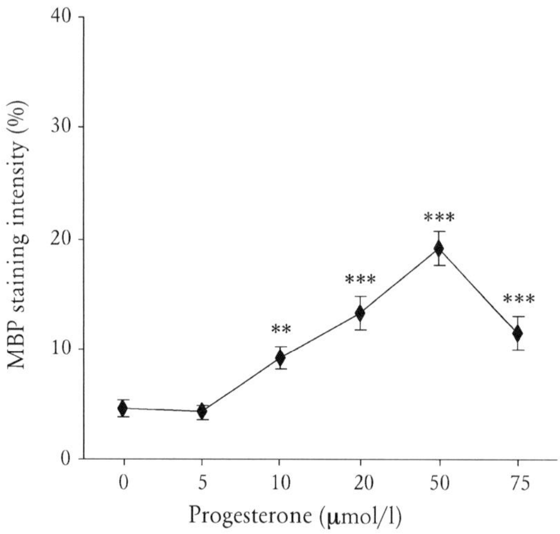

Figure 4 Progesterone stimulates myelination in organotypic slice cultures of rat cerebellum. Stimulatory effect of progesterone on myelination: dose-response curve. Organotypic slice cultures of rat cerebellum were treated with different concentrations of progesterone (5–75 μmol/l). The intensity of MBP staining was measured by quantifying MBP immunostaining using the National Institutes of Health image software and expressed as a percentage of light pixels (mean ± SEM). $^{***}p \leq 0.001$; $^{**}p \leq 0.01$ as indicated by Newman-Keuls tests after one-way ANOVA. Adapted from reference 76

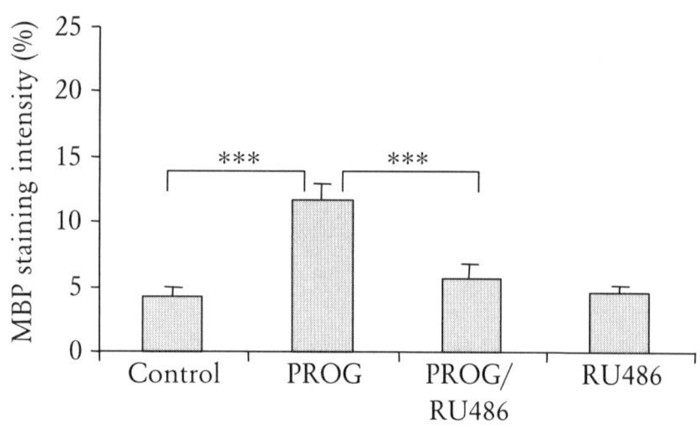

Figure 5 The intracellular progesterone (PROG) receptor is necessary for the progesterone effect on myelination in organotypic cerebellar slice cultures. Cerebellar slices from P7-rats were treated for 7 days with progesterone (20 μmol/l), and/or the progesterone receptor antagonist mifepristone (RU486) (10 μmol/l). Control cultures were treated with vehicle (dimethylsulfoxide) alone. $^{***}p \leq 0.001$ when compared to the control group or as indicated by Newman-Keuls tests after one-way ANOVA. MBP, myelin basic protein. Adapted from reference 92

by the selective $GABA_A$ receptor antagonist bicuculline. These findings demonstrated that progestins stimulate MBP expression in the central nervous system via two signalling systems, the intracellular progesterone receptors and membrane $GABA_A$ receptors, and suggested a new role of $GABA_A$ receptors in myelination. Immunostaining of two other myelin-specific markers, O4 and galactocerebroside (GalC), was also increased by progesterone to the same extent as that of MBP. The stimulatory effect of progesterone on MBP expression is clearly mediated by the classical intracellular progesterone receptor, while the increase of MBP expression by its metabolite 3α,5α-tetrahydroprogesterone involves membrane $GABA_A$ receptors[76].

The finding that progestins regulate myelination in a concerted manner through the intracellular progesterone receptor and through membrane $GABA_A$ receptors in both the central and peripheral nervous systems is a new concept and is notable, because it shows that steroids can regulate slow processes such as myelination by acting on a membrane neurotransmitter receptor.

Progesterone and remyelination in the central nervous system

In the central nervous system, systemic progesterone administration results in a partial reversal of the age-associated decline in the remyelination process following toxin-induced demyelination in old male rats. Indeed, administration of progesterone for 5 weeks promoted the slow remyelination of axons by oligodendrocytes after ethidium bromide-induced demyelination[77].

Progesterone in the oligodendroglial lineage

Studying the biology of oligodendroglial cells is essential for understanding the myelination process and may also provide some keys for a better comprehension of remyelination. We investigated the capacities of synthesis and metabolism of progesterone at three stages of the oligodendroglial lineage (Figure 6), with a special interest in the early stages, which are likely to be the source of remyelinating cells in the brain. This study was conducted *in vitro* using primary cell cultures prepared either from newborn rat brains for the early stages of the lineage, oligodendrocyte pre-progenitors (OPP) and oligodendrocyte progenitors (OP), or from 4-week-old rat brains for oligodendrocytes (OL). Our results showed that only OPP and OP, but not OL, expressed 3β-HSD mRNA and were able to synthesize progesterone from pregnenolone. In the three cell types studied, progesterone was metabolized by the type 1 isoform of 5α-reductase into 5α-dihydroprogesterone. 5α-Reductase activity was 5-fold higher in OL than in OPP and OP. 5α-Dihydroprogesterone was transformed into 3α,5α-tetrahydroprogesterone. This activity was 10-fold higher in OPP than in the other cells studied[78]. These results revealed dramatic changes of progesterone biosynthesis and metabolism during oligodendrocyte differentiation, suggesting the existence of different requirements for progesterone and its metabolites at different stages of the oligodendroglial lineage.

Progestins may promote myelination in the CNS by acting directly on the myelinating glial cells. Indeed, oligodendrocytes in culture have been shown to express a functional progesterone receptor[69] and cells of the oligodendroglial lineage express different $GABA_A$ receptor subunits (N. Gago and M. El-Etr, unpublished observations). Whether progestins stimulate the maturation of oligodendrocytes or whether they promote the elaboration of the myelin sheaths remains to be studied.

NEUROPROTECTIVE EFFECTS OF PROGESTERONE IN BRAIN AND SPINAL CORD

Progesterone neuroprotection in traumatic brain injury

Female rats with high levels of progesterone at the time of injury recover better than males. Progesterone is effective in post-injury treatment of both males and females. The effects of progesterone are pleotropic: progesterone reduces the necrotic damage, edema formation, cell loss, and restores the cognitive performances[79,80]. The mechanisms by which progesterone exerts its neuroprotective effects in this model are not well known.

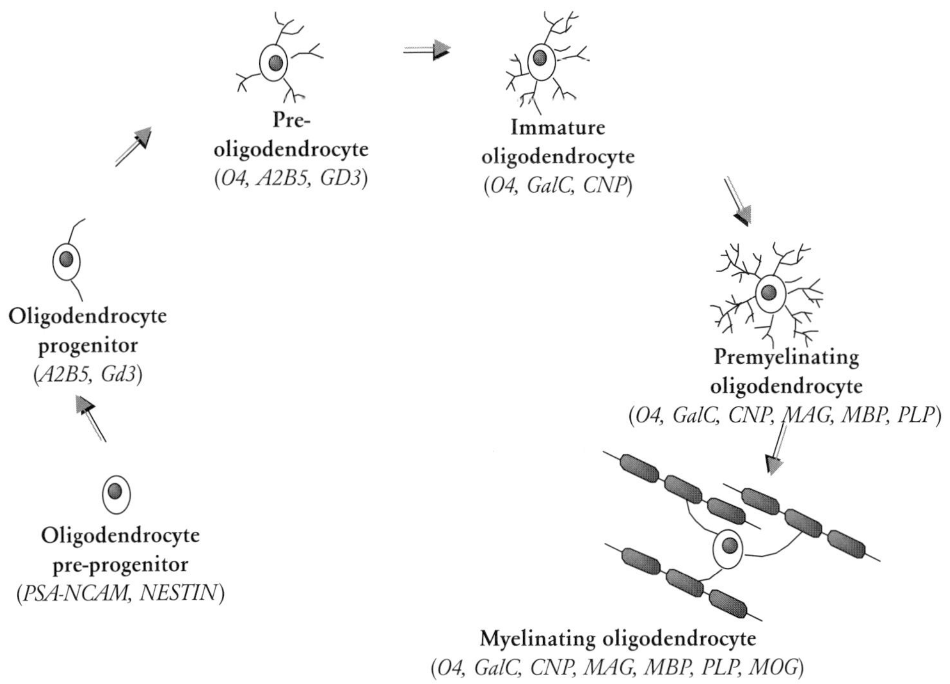

Figure 6 Oligodendroglial lineage. Specific markers of each stage are indicated in italic

Progesterone neuroprotection in spinal cord

Injury model

Reports from different groups demonstrated that progesterone can be added to the growing list of neuroprotective steroids in this model. Indeed, rats receiving progesterone had a better functional and histological recovery compared to untreated injured rats[81]. The progesterone precursor, pregnenolone, also facilitates recovery[82]. This effect may be due to increased local synthesis of progesterone from pregnenolone, a step enhanced after spinal cord injury[83].

After spinal cord transection, treatment with progesterone induced an up-regulation of glial cell parameters, including astrocyte NADPH-diaphorase, an accepted histochemical marker for nitric oxid synthase (NOS)[84], MBP, and the chondriotin sulfate proteoglycan NG2[85]. These effects can be supportive of neuronal recuperation. Motoneurons from spinal cord-transected animals presented several biochemical abnormalities, as the acetylcholine-synthesizing enzyme (ChAT), the sodium pump and GAP-43. These parameters were reverted to normal after progesterone treatment, with the exception of GAP-43 mRNA which was further enhanced[86].

The mechanisms by which progesterone exerts these protective effects in the spinal cord are not well known and may involve protection against excitotoxicity[87], inhibition of free radical-induced lipid membrane peroxidation[88], and selective regulation of gene expression. Both motoneurons and glial cells express the classical progesterone receptor[89], while the progesterone membrane binding site 25-Dx is expressed only in neurons. The two binding systems differed in their localization, response to lesion and hormone treatment[17]. Their function may differ under normal and pathological functions. Since only progesterone receptor was detected in glial cells, genomic mechanisms may play some role on progesterone effects in astrocytes and oligodendrocytes. Nevertheless, the fact that progesterone receptor declined after spinal cord transection and progesterone treatment, while 25-Dx expression increased, suggested that alternative mechanisms may also take place in the injured spinal cord. These observations point to a novel and potential important role of the progesterone binding protein 25-Dx after injury of the nervous system and suggest that the neuroprotective effects of progesterone may not necessarily be mediated exclusively by the classical progesterone receptor but may involve distinct membrane binding sites including 25-Dx and $GABA_A$ receptors.

Model of neurodegenerative diseases

In the Wobbler mouse, a model for degenerative motoneuron diseases such as amytropic lateral sclerosis (ALS)[90,91], progesterone has recently been shown to rescue motoneurons from degeneration, based on histological abnormalities and on $\alpha 3$ and $\beta 1$ subunit Na,K-ATPase mRNA levels[92,93].

EFFECTS OF SYNTHETIC PROGESTINS IN THE NERVOUS SYSTEM

In the nervous system, estradiol, progesterone or 19-norprogesterone, alone or in combination, protect hippocampal neurons against glutamate cytotoxicity. Medroxyprogesterone acetate (MPA) is not only ineffective in protecting the neurons, but this compound also inhibited the neuroprotective effects of estradiol when co-administered. In agreement with this observation, estradiol, progesterone or 19-norprogesterone increased expression of the antiapoptotic protein B-cell leukemia/lymphoma (Bcl-2), whereas MPA blocked estrogen-induced Bcl-2 expression[94]. Continuous MPA users reported depressive symptoms more than controls[95,96]. MPA also opposes the beneficial association between estrogen and cognitive changes[97]. However, a recent study has reported beneficial effects of MPA on mood in postmenopausal women, and in particular in those with a history of premenstrual syndrome[98].

Steroid enantiomers offer interesting perspectives for the treatment of age-dependent cognitive impairment or neurodegenerative diseases. These are mirror-symmetric, non-superimposable images of the molecules, with identical physical properties (except for the different rotation of polarized light[99]). The synthetic (-) enantiomer of pregnenolone sulfate was ten times more potent in activating memory functions than natural (+) pregnenolone sulfate. This effect showed enantiomeric selectivity: in contrast to (+) pregnenolone sulfate, the promnesic effects of (-) pregnenolone sulfate could not be blocked by a selective NMDA receptor antagonist[100].

HORMONE REPLACEMENT THERAPY

In contrast to the preclinical findings reporting beneficial effects of steroids on the nervous system, the results of clinical studies are not conclusive. There is still no clear evidence for beneficial effects of hormone replacement therapy (HRT) on mood and cognitive functions in the elderly. After the initial euphoria prompted by studies suggesting that estradiol replacement therapy in postmenopausal women may protect against the onset of Alzheimer's disease and even improve cognitive functions in women who already suffer from the disease, a series of studies have questioned these beneficial effects of estrogen. Moreover, recent results from a very large trial conducted by the Women's Health Initiative have not only questioned the benefits of estrogen plus progestin therapy in postmenopausal women, but they have also pointed to the risks. One reason for the outcome of this trial may be related to the conditions of the treatment, and in particular to the use of the synthetic progestin MPA, which has androgenic properties and which antagonizes beneficial effects of estrogens on the cardiovascular and nervous systems. Whether 'pure' progestins, which do not interfere with other steroid receptor systems, may exert beneficial effects on the aging nervous system, as strongly suggested by animal studies, is so far unknown (for review, see reference 101).

Hormone replacement therapy may become an important component of preventive strategies against age-dependent cognitive dysfunctions, ranging from mild cognitive impairment to dementing diseases such as Alzheimer's disease. The success of this strategy will depend on the development of safer and more selective steroid receptor ligands, targeting of alternative steroid signalling pathways and/or stimulation of neurosteroid synthesis.

CONCLUSIONS

Progesterone, originating either from peripheral glands or synthesized locally in the nervous system, has positive effects on myelination and neuroprotection. Progesterone effects are pleotropic and can be achieved via different mechanisms involving different receptors.

ACKNOWLEDGEMENTS

We thank our colleagues and collaborators who contributed to the work summarized in this review, particularly Drs N. Gago, A. Ghoumari, C. Ibanez, K. Murakami from INSERM U488, France and Drs F. Labombarda, H. Coirini, M. C. Gonzalez-Deniselle from Instituto de Biologia y Medicina Experimental, University of Buenos Aires, Buenos Aires, Argentina.

References

1. Baulieu EE. Neurosteroids: a new function in the brain. *Biol Cell* 1991;71:3-10
2. Baulieu EE. Neurosteroids: of the nervous system, by the nervous system, for the nervous system. *Recent Prog Horm Res* 1997;52:1-32
3. Robel P, Schumacher M, Baulieu EE. Neurosteroids: from definition and biochemistry to physiological function. In Baulieu EE, Robel P, Schumacher M, eds. *Neurosteroids. A New Regulatory Function in the Nervous System*. Totowa, NJ: Humana Press, 1999:1-25
4. Marynick SP, Smith GB, Ebert MH, Loriaux DL. Studies on the transfer of steroid hormones across the blood-cerebrospinal fluid barrier in

the rhesus monkey. II. *Endocrinology* 1977;101: 562–7
5. Pardridge WM, Moeller TL, Mietus LJ, Oldendorf WH. Blood-brain barrier transport and brain sequestration of steroid hormones. *Am J Physiol* 1980;239:96–102
6. Evans RM. The steroid and thyroid hormone receptor superfamily. *Science* 1988;240:889–95
7. Beato M, Chavez S, Truss M. Transcriptional regulation by steroid hormones. *Steroids* 1996; 61:240–51
8. Beato M, Klug J. Steroid hormone receptors: an update. *Hum Reprod Update* 2000;6:225–36
9. Ke FC, Ramirez VD. Binding of progesterone to nerve cell membranes of rat brain using progesterone conjugated to ^{125}I-bovine serum albumin as a ligand. *J Neurochem* 1990;54:467–72
10. Caldwell JD, Walker CH, Faggin BM, Carr RB, Pedersen CA, Mason GA. Characterization of progesterone-3-[^{125}I-BSA] binding sites in the medial preoptic area and anterior hypothalamus. *Brain Res* 1995;693:225–32
11. Ramirez VD, Zheng J, Siddique K. Membrane receptors for estrogen, progesterone, and testosterone in the rat brain: fantasy or reality. *Cell Mol Neurobiol* 1996;16:175–98
12. Bukusoglu C, Krieger NR. Photoaffinity labelling with progesterone-11α-hemisuccinate-(2-[^{125}I] iodohistamine) identifies four protein bands in mouse brain membranes. *J Neurochem* 1994;63: 1434–8
13. Meyer C, Schmid R, Scriba PC, Wehling M. Purification and partial sequencing of high affinity progesterone-binding site(s) from porcine liver membranes. *Eur J Biochem* 1996;239:726–31
14. Meyer C, Schmid R, Schmieding K, Falkenstein E, Wehling M. Characterization of high affinity progesterone-binding membrane proteins by antipeptide antiserum. *Steroids* 1998;63:111–16
15. Selmin O, Lucier GW, Clark GC, *et al.* Isolation and characterization of a novel gene induced by 2,3,7,8-tetrachlorodibenzo-*p*-dioxin in rat liver. *Carcinogenesis* 1996;17:2609–15
16. Krebs CJ, Jarvis ED, Chan J, *et al.* A membrane-associated progesterone-binding protein, 25-Dx, is regulated by progesterone in brain regions involved in female reproductive behaviors. *Proc Natl Acad Sci USA* 2000;97:12816–21
17. Labombarda F, Gonzalez SL, Gonzalez Deniselle MC, *et al.* Effects of injury and progesterone treatment on progesterone receptor and progesterone binding protein 25-Dx expression in the rat spinal cord. *J Neurochem* 2003;in press
18. Majewska MD, Harrison NL, Schwartz RD, Barker JL, Paul SM. Steroid hormone metabolites are barbiturate-like modulators of the GABA receptor. *Science* 1986;232:1004–7
19. Paul SM, Purdy RH. Neuroactive steroids. *FASEB J* 1992;6:2311–22
20. Monnet FP, Mahé V, Robel P, Baulieu EE. Neurosteroids, via σ receptors, modulate the [^{3}H]norepinephrine release evoked by *N*-methyl-D-aspartate in the rat hippocampus. *Proc Natl Acad Sci USA* 1995;92:3774–8
21. Meyer C, Schmieding K, Falkenstein E, Wehling M. Are high-affinity progesterone binding site(s) from porcine liver microsomes members of the sigma receptor family? *Eur J Pharmacol* 1998; 347:293–9
22. McCann DJ, Su TP. Solubilization and characterization of haloperidolsensitive (1)- [3H]SKF-10,047 binding sites (sigma sites) from rat liver membranes. *J Pharmacol Exp Ther* 1991;257:547–54
23. Wu FS, Gibbs TT, Farb DH. Inverse modulation of γ-aminobutyric acid and glycine-induced currents by progesterone. *Mol Pharmacol* 1990; 37:597–602
24. Prince RJ, Simmonds MA. Steroid modulation of the strychnine-sensitive glycine receptor. *Neuropharmacology* 1992;31:201–5
25. Wu FS, Chen SC, Tsai JJ. Competitive inhibition of the glycine-induced current by pregnenolone sulfate in cultured chick spinal cord neurons. *Brain Res* 1997;750:318–20
26. Wu FS, Gibbs TT, Farb DH. Pregnenolone sulfate: a positive allosteric modulator at the *N*-methyl-D-aspartate receptor. *Mol Pharmacol* 1991;40: 333–6
27. Park-Chung M, Wu F, Farb DH. 3α-Hydroxy-5β-pregnan-20-one sulfate: a negative modulator of the NMDA-induced current in cultured neurons. *Mol Pharmacol* 1994;46:146–50
28. Smith SS. Progesterone administration attenuates excitatory amino acid responses of cerebellar Purkinje cells. *Neuroscience* 1991;42:309–20
29. Wetzel CH, Hermann B, Behl C, *et al.* Functional antagonism of gonadal steroids at the 5-hydroxytryptamine type 3 receptor. *Mol Endocrinol* 1998; 12:1441–51
30. Wu FS, Lai CP, Liu BC. Noncompetitive inhibition of 5-HT3 receptor-mediated currents by progesterone in rat nodose ganglion neurons. *Neurosci Lett* 2000;278:37–40
31. Murakami K, Fellous A, Baulieu EE, Robel P. Pregnenolone binds to microtubule-associated protein 2 and stimulates microtubule assembly. *Proc Natl Acad Sci USA* 2000;97:3579–84
32. Lorence MC, Murry BA, Trant JM, Mason JI. Human 3 beta-hydroxysteroid dehydrogenase/ delta 5-4isomerase from placenta: expression in nonsteroidogenic cells of a protein that catalyzes the dehydrogenation/isomerization of C21 and C19 steroids. *Endocrinology* 1990;126:2493–8
33. Luu-The V, Lachance Y, Labrie C, *et al.* Full length cDNA structure and deduced amino acid sequence of human 3 beta-hydroxy-5-ene steroid dehydrogenase. *Mol Endocrinol* 1989;3: 1310–12

34. Thomas JL, Myers RP, Strickler RC. Human placental 3 beta-hydroxy-5-ene-steroid dehydrogenase and steroid 5-4-ene-isomerase: purification from mitochondria and kinetic profiles, biophysical characterization of the purified mitochondrial and microsomal enzymes. *J Steroid Biochem* 1989;33:209–17
35. Mason JI. The 3β-hydroxysteroid dehydrogenase gene family of enzymes. *Trends Endocrinol Metab* 1993;78:1003–8
36. Rhe´aume E, Lachance Y, Zhao HF, *et al.* Structure and expression of a new cDNA encoding the almost exclusive 3β-hydroxysteroid dehydrogenase/Δ5-Δ4 isomerase in human adrenals and gonads. *Mol Endocrinol* 1991;5:1147–57
37. Zhao HF, Rhe´aume E, Trudel C, Couet J, Labrie F, Simard J. Structure and sexual dimorphic expression of a liver-specific rat 3β-hydroxysteroid dehydrogenase/isomerase. *Endocrinology* 1990;127:3237–9
38. Zhao HF, Labrie C, Simard J, *et al.* Characterization of 3β-hydroxysteroid dehydrogenase Δ5-Δ4 isomerase cDNA and differential tissue specific expression of the corresponding mRNAs in steroidogenic and peripheral tissues. *J Biol Chem* 1991;266:583–93
39. Simard J, Durocher F, Mebarki F, *et al.* Molecular biology and genetics of the 3β-hydroxysteroid dehydrogenase/Δ5-Δ4 isomerase gene family. *J Endocrinol* 1996;150:S189–207
40. Abbaszade IG, Arensburg J, Park CH, Kasa-Vubu JZ, Orly J, Payne AH. Isolation of a new mouse 3β-hydroxysteroid dehydrogenase isoform, 3β-HSD VI, expressed during early pregnancy. *Endocrinology* 1997;138:1392–9
41. Weidenfield J, Sziegel RA, Chowers I. *In vitro* conversion of pregnenolone to progesterone by discrete brain areas of the male rat. *J Steroid Biochem* 1980;13:961–3
42. Jung-Testas I, Hu ZY, Baulieu EE, Robel P. Neurosteroids: biosynthesis of pregnenolone and progesterone in primary cultures of rat glial cells. *Endocrinology* 1989;125:2083–91
43. Akwa Y, Sananès N, Gouézou M, Robel P, Baulieu EE, Le Goascogne C. Astrocytes and neurosteroids: metabolism of pregnenolone and dehydroepiandrosterone. Regulation by cell density. *J Cell Biol* 1993;121:135–43
44. Bauer HC, Bauer H. Micromethod for the determination of 3β-HSD activity in cultured cells. *J Steroid Biochem* 1989;33:643–6
45. Guennoun R, Fiddes RJ, Gouézou M, Lombes M, Baulieu EE. A key enzyme in the biosynthesis of neurosteroids, 3 beta-hydroxysteroid dehydrogenase/delta 5-delta 4-isomerase (3 beta-HSD), is expressed in rat brain. *Mol Brain Res* 1995;30:287–300
46. Ukena K, Kohchi C, Tsutsui K. Expression and activity of 3beta-hydroxysteroid dehydrogenase/delta5-delta4-isomerase in the rat Purkinje neuron during neonatal life. *Endocrinology* 1999;140:805–13
47. Ibanez C, Guennoun R, Liere P, *et al.* Developmental expression of genes involved in neurosteroidogenesis: 3beta-hydroxysteroid dehydrogenase/delta(5)-delta(4) isomerase in the rat brain. *Endocrinology* 2003;144:2902–11
48. Yu L, Romero DG, Gomez-Sanchez CE, Gomez-Sanchez EP. Steroidogenic enzyme gene expression in the human brain. *Mol Cell Endocrinol* 2002;190:9–17
49. Inoue T, Akahira J, Suzuki T, *et al.* Progesterone production and actions in the human central nervous system and neurogenic tumors. *J Clin Endocrinol Metab* 2002;87:5325–31
50. Brown RC, Cascio C, Papadopoulos V. Pathways of neurosteroid biosynthesis in cell lines from human brain: regulation of dehydroepiandrosterone formation by oxidative stress and beta-amyloid peptide. *J Neurochem* 2000;74:847–59
51. Coirini H, Gouézou M, Liere P, *et al.* 3β-hydroxysteroid dehydrogenase expression in the spinal cord. *Neuroscience* 2002;113:883–91
52. Coirini H, Gouézou M, Delespierre B, *et al.* Characterization and regulation of the 3beta-hydroxysteroid dehydrogenase isomerase enzyme in the rat sciatic nerve. *J Neurochem* 2003;84:119–26
53. Coirini H, Gouézou M, Delespierre B, Schumacher M, Guennoun R. 3 Beta-hydroxysteroid dehydrogenase isomerase (3β-HSD) activity in the rat sciatic nerve: kinetic analysis and regulation by steroids. *J Steroid Biochem Mol Biol* 2003;85:89–94
54. Robert F, Guennoun R, Désarnaud F, *et al.* Synthesis of progesterone in Schwann cells: regulation by sensory neurons. *Eur J Neurosci* 2001;13:916–24
55. Guennoun R, Schumacher M, Robert F, *et al.* Neurosteroids: expression of functional 3beta-hydroxysteroid dehydrogenase by rat sensory neurons and Schwann cells. *Eur J Neurosci* 1997;9:2236–47
56. Bolin LM, Shooter EM. Neurons regulate Schwann cell genes by diffusible molecules. *J Cell Biol* 1993;123:237–43
57. Reynolds ML, Woolf CJ. Reciprocal Schwann cell-axon interactions [Review]. *Curr Opin Neurobiol* 1993;3:683–93
58. Snipes GJ, Suter U. Signalling pathways mediating axon-Schwann cell interactions. *Trends Neurosci* 1994;17:399–401
59. Normington K, Russell DW. Tissue distribution and kinetic characteristics of rat steroid 5alpha-reductase isozymes. Evidence for distinct physiological functions. *J Biol Chem* 1992;267:19548–54
60. Poletti A, Coscarella A, Negri-Cesi P, Colciago A, Celotti F, Martini L. 5Alpha-reductase isozymes

in the central nervous system. *Steroids* 1998; 63:246–51
61. Jenkins JS, Hall CJ. Metabolism of [^{14}C]testosterone by human fetal and adult brain tissue. *J Endocrinol* 1977;74:425–9
62. Saitoh H, Hirato K, Yanaihara T, Nakayama T. A study of 5 alpha-reductase in human fetal brain. *Endocrinol Jpn* 1982;29:461–7
63. Steckelbroeck S, Watzka M, Reichelt R, *et al.* Characterization of the 5alpha-reductase-3alpha-hydroxysteroid dehydrogenase complex in the human brain. *J Clin Endocrinol Metab* 2001; 86:1324–31
64. Koenig H, Schumacher M, Ferzaz B, *et al.* Progesterone synthesis and myelin formation by Schwann cells. *Science* 1995;268:1500–3
65. Chan JR, Phillips LJ, Glaser M. Glucocorticoids and progestins signal the initiation and enhance the rate of myelin formation. *Proc Natl Acad Sci USA* 1998;95:10459–64
66. Melcangi RC, Magnaghi V, Cavarretta I, Martini L, Piva F. Age-induced decrease of glycoprotein Po and myelin basic protein gene expression in the rat sciatic nerve. Repair by steroid derivatives. *Neuroscience* 1998;85:569–78
67. Notterpek L, Snipes GJ, Shooter EM. Temporal expression pattern of peripheral myelin protein 22 during *in vivo* and *in vitro* myelination. *Glia* 1999;25:358–69
68. Désarnaud F, Do-Thi A, Brown AM, *et al.* Progesterone stimulates the activity of the promoters of peripheral myelin protein-22 and protein zero genes in Schwann cells. *J Neurochem* 1998;71: 1765–8
69. Jung-Testas I, Schumacher M, Robel P, Baulieu EE. Demonstration of progesterone receptors in rat Schwann cells. *J Steroid Biochem Mol Biol* 1996;58:77–82
70. Magnaghi V, Cavarretta I, Galbiati M, Martini L, Melcangi RC. Neuroactive steroids and peripheral myelin proteins. *Brain Res Brain Res Rev* 2001;37:360–71
71. Notterpek LM, Bullock PN, Malek H, Fisher R, Rome LH. Myelination in cerebellar slice cultures: development of a system amenable to biochemical analysis. *J Neurosci Res* 1993;36:621–34
72. Melcangi RC, Magnaghi V, Cavarretta I, *et al.* Progesterone derivatives are able to influence peripheral myelin protein 22 and P0 gene expression: possible mechanisms of action. *J Neurosci Res* 1999;56:349–57
73. Sakamoto H, Ukena K, Tsutsui K. Effects of progesterone synthesized *de novo* in the developing Purkinje cell on its dendritic growth and synaptogenesis. *J Neurosci* 2001;21:6221–32
74. Hamano K, Iwasaki N, Takeya T, Takita H. A quantitative analysis of rat central nervous system myelination using the immunohistochemical method for MBP. *Dev Brain Res* 1996;93:18–22
75. Muse ED, Jurevics H, Toews AD, Matsushima GK, Morell P. Parameters related to lipid metabolism as markers of myelination in mouse brain. *J Neurochem* 2001;76:77–86
76. Ghoumari AM, Ibanez C, El-Etr M, *et al.* Progesterone and its metabolites increase myelin basic protein expression in organotypic slice cultures of rat cerebellum. *J Neurochem* 2003;in press
77. Ibanez C, Shields SA, Liere P, *et al.* Systemic progesterone administration results in a partial reversal of the age-associated decline in CNS remyelination following toxin-induced demyelination in male rats. *Neuropathol Appl Neurobiol* 2003;in press
78. Gago N, Akwa Y, Sananès N, *et al.* Progesterone and the oligodendroglial lineage: stage-dependent biosynthesis and metabolism. *Glia* 2001;36: 295–308
79. Stein DG. Brain damage, sex hormones and recovery: a new role for progesterone and estrogen? *Trends Neurosci* 2001;24:386–91
80. Shear DA, Galani R, Hoffman SW, Stein DG. Progesterone protects against necrotic damage and behavioral abnormalities caused by traumatic brain injury. *Exp Neurol* 2002;178:59–67
81. Thomas AJ, Nockels RP, Pan HQ, Shaffrey CI, Chopp M. Progesterone is neuroprotective after acute experimental spinal cord trauma in rats. *Spine* 1999;24:2134–8
82. Guth L, Zhang Z, Roberts E. Key role for pregnenolone in combination therapy promotes recovery after spinal cord injury. *Proc Natl Acad Sci USA* 1994;91:12308–12
83. Di Michele F, Lekieffre D, Pasini A, Bernardi G, Benavides J, Romeo, E. Increased neurosteroids synthesis after brain and spinal cord injury in rats. *Neurosci Lett* 2000;284:65–8
84. Labombarda F, Gonzalez S, Roig P, *et al.* Modulation of NADPH-diaphorase and glial fibrillary acidic protein by progesterone in astrocytes from normal and injured spinal cord. *J Steroid Biochem Mol Biol* 2000;73:159–69
85. De Nicola AF, Labombarda F, Gonzalez SL, *et al.* Steroid effects on glial cells: detrimental or protective for spinal cord function? *Prog Neurobiol* 2003;in press
86. Labombarda F, Gonzalez S, Gonzalez Deniselle MC, Guennoun R, Schumacher M, De Nicola AF. Cellular basis for progesterone neuroprotection in the injured spinal cord. *J Neurotrauma* 2002; 19:343–55
87. Ogata T, Nakamura Y, Tsuji K, Shibata T, Kataoka K. Steroid hormones protect spinal cord neurons from glutamate toxicity. *Neuroscience* 1993;55: 445–9
88. Roof R, Hoffman S, Stein D. Progesterone protects against lipid peroxidation following traumatic brain injury in rats. *Mol Chem Neuropathol* 1997;31:1–11

89. Labombarda F, Guennoun R, Gonzalez S, *et al.* Immunocytochemical evidence for a progesterone receptor in neurons and glial cells of the rat spinal cord. *Neurosci Lett* 2000;288:29–32
90. Duchen LW, Strich SJ. An hereditary motor neurone disease with progressive denervation of muscle in the mouse: the mutant 'wobbler'. *J Neurol Neurosurg Psychiatry* 1968;31:535–42
91. Price DL, Cleveland DW Koliatsos VE. Motor neurone disease and animal models. *Neurobiol Dis* 1994;1:3–11
92. Gonzalez Deniselle MC, Lopez-Costa JJ, Saavedra JP, *et al.* Progesterone neuroprotection in the wobbler mouse, a genetic model of spinal cord motor disease. *Neurobiol Dis* 2002;11:457–68
93. Gonzalez Deniselle MC, Lopez-Costa JJ, Gonzalez SL, *et al.* Basis of progesterone protection in spinal cord neurodegeneration. *J Steroid Biochem Mol Biol* 2003;83:199–209
94. Nilsen J, Brinton RD. Impact of progestins on estrogen-induced neuroprotection: synergy by progesterone and 19-norprogesterone and antagonism by medroxyprogesterone acetate. *Endocrinology* 2002;143:205–12
95. Civic D, Scholes D, Ichikawa L, *et al.* Depressive symptoms in users and non-users of depot medroxyprogesterone acetate. *Contraception* 2000; 61:385–90
96. Saaresranta T, Irjala K, Polo K, Polo O. Medroxyprogesterone-induced endocrine alterations after menopause. *Menopause* 2002;9:288–92
97. Rice MM, Graves AB, McCurry SM, *et al.* Postmenopausal estrogen and estrogen-progestin use and 2-year rate of cognitive change in a cohort of older Japanese American women: the Kame Project. *Arch Intern Med* 2000;160:1641-9
98. Bjorn I, Bixo M, Nojd KS, *et al.* The impact of different doses of medroxyprogesterone acetate on mood symptoms in sequential hormonal therapy. *Gynecol Endocrinol* 2002;16:1-8
99. Covey DF, Nathan D, Kalkbrenner M, *et al.* Enantioselectivity of pregnanolone-induced gamma-aminobutyric acid (A) receptor modulation and anesthesia. *J Pharmacol Exp Ther* 2000; 293:1009–16
100. Akwa Y, Ladurelle N, Covey DF, Baulieu EE. The synthetic enantiomer of pregnenolone sulfate is very active on memory in rats and mice, even more so than its physiological neurosteroid counterpart: distinct mechanisms? *Proc Natl Acad Sci USA* 2001;98:14033-7
101. Schumacher M, Weill-Engerer S, Liere P, *et al.* Steroid hormones and neurosteroids in normal and pathological aging of the nervous system. *Prog Neurobiol* 2003;in press

Testosterone metabolism and its effects on glial cells of the central nervous system

8

R. C. Melcangi and M. Galbiati

INTRODUCTION

The concept that steroid hormones play an important role in the control of several functions of the nervous system is now well accepted. It is well known that steroid hormones regulate the development and function of the central nervous system (CNS) and affect mood, behavior and cognition. Moreover, this concept has recently been amplified, since further observations have indicated that the nervous system is also able to synthesize the steroid hormones itself, forming so-called neurosteroids. Hormonal steroids coming from the periphery and neurosteroids may then be converted to metabolites called neuroactive steroids. It is interesting to highlight that neuroactive steroids may occasionally be more effective than their corresponding parent compounds, or may have totally different biological actions. Furthermore, these neuroactive steroids may exert their actions through either classical or non-classical receptors, which are localized both in the neuronal and in the glial compartments. In particular, the importance of glial cells as a target for neuroactive steroids has recently been suggested by the demonstration, in astrocytes and oligodendrocytes, of classical intracellular receptors for many families of hormonal steroids (e.g. receptors for androgens (AR), estrogens (ER), progestogens (PR), etc.) (for review see references 1 and 2). Moreover, astrocytes also express γ-aminobutyric acid type A ($GABA_A$) receptor[3,4], and consequently may respond to those neuroactive steroids that are able to interact with this neurotransmitter receptor (for review see references 5 and 6).

This chapter briefly analyzes only one of the major pathways converting hormonal steroids, namely the 5α-reductase-3α-hydroxysteroid dehydrogenase (5α-R-3α-HSD) enzymatic system, with a particular focus on the metabolism of testosterone. In addition, the effects of testosterone and its neuroactive derivatives on the glial cells of the CNS are taken into consideration.

5α-REDUCTASE AND 3α-HYDROXYSTEROID DEHYDROGENASE SYSTEM

General considerations

The enzymatic complex formed by 5α-R and 3α-HSD is not only found in the classical peripheral steroid target structures (e.g. prostate, epididymis, etc.) which respond to androgens, but is also present in the CNS (for review see references 5 and 6). This enzymatic system is very versatile, since every steroid possessing the Δ^4-3-keto configuration may be first 5α-reduced and subsequently 3α-hydroxylated. For instance, testosterone can be converted into dihydrotestosterone (DHT) and subsequently into 5α-androstane-3α,17β-diol (3α-diol). Similarly, progesterone and corticosterone may be converted into their metabolites, dihydroprogesterone (DHP) and dihydrocorticosterone, respectively (for review see references 5 and 6). The existence, in peripheral structures, of more than one 5α-R isoenzyme was postulated years ago on the basis of studies utilizing various inhibitors[7,8], and different substrates[7]. More recently, two isoforms of 5α-R (called type 1 and type 2) have been cloned, in man, in rat and in monkey[9–14]. Despite the fact that the two major isoforms of 5α-R (type 1 and type 2) catalyze the same reaction (e.g. testosterone to DHT, progesterone to DHP, etc.), they possess different biochemical and possibly functional properties. In the rat, the affinity of testosterone for the type 1 isoform is about 15–20-fold lower than that determined for the type 2 isoform. The difference in affinity is evident also in the case of the human enzymes, even if this is less marked. Both in rat and in man, the capability of reducing the substrate is much higher in the case of the type 1 isoform. The two isoforms have a different pH optimum: the type 1 isoform is active in a wide range of pH (from 5 to 8), while the type 2 5α-R possesses a narrow pH optimum of around 5, with a very low activity at pH 7.5[15].

The enzyme 3α-HSD, also known as 3α-hydroxysteroid oxidoreductase, may be considered the second element of the 5α-R-3α-HSD system. At variance with the two isoforms of 5α-R, this enzyme appears able to catalyze the controlled reaction both in the oxidative and in the reductive directions (for review see references 5 and 6).

Cellular localization in the central nervous system

Even if the majority of the earlier studies of 5α-R activity in the brain were performed on the hypothalamus (for review see references 5 and 6), later analyses have indicated that the conversion of testosterone to DHT is not limited to this cerebral area, but also occurs in several others (for review see references 5 and 6). In particular, it has also been reported that the conversion of testosterone to DHT is several times higher in brain structures composed mainly of white matter (e.g. corpus callosum, midbrain tegumentum, etc.)[16–20]. Moreover, as demonstrated by further observations, 5α-R activity is associated with the myelin compartment[18,19,21]. The proposed physiological meaning of the presence of 5α-R in the myelin is that 5α-reduced steroids formed locally in the myelin might play a role in the process of myelination (for review see references 5 and 6).

The cellular distribution of 5α-R has been analyzed in our laboratory in primary cultures of neurons, of oligodendrocytes and of type 1 (A1) and type 2 astrocytes, obtained from the fetal or neonatal rat brain[22,23]. The results obtained indicate that the formation of DHT from testosterone takes place preferentially in neurons; however, type 2 astrocytes and oligodendrocytes also possess measurable 5α-R activity, while A1 shows a much lower enzymatic activity. A completely different localization was observed for 3α-HSD, since the formation of 3α-diol from DHT appears to be prevalently, if not exclusively, present in A1. The compartmentalization of two strictly correlated enzymes (5α-R and 3α-HSD) in separate CNS cell populations suggests the simultaneous participation of neurons and glial cells in the 5α-reductive metabolism of testosterone and possibly of other hormonal steroids (see below).

It is relevant to emphasize that not only differentiated CNS cells possess the 5α-R-3α-HSD system, but that considerable enzymatic activities converting steroid hormones are also present in undifferentiated cells, as shown in our studies performed on undifferentiated stem cells originating from the mouse striatum[24].

Regulation of 5α-R-3α-HSD system

The data obtained to date indicate that, in the brain, the enzymatic system formed by 5α-R-3α-HSD is not sexually dimorphic. Moreover, a large amount of data indicate that this system is not regulated by sex steroids, since castration or substitutive therapies are unable to influence its activity (for review see reference 6). This has been shown in the whole rat brain, as well as in specific CNS areas. However, a few studies appear to disagree with this conclusion, since an increase in 5α-R activity has been observed after orchidectomy in the basolateral amygdala of the rhesus monkey[25].

Also, neural inputs seem to be ineffective in regulating the activity of 5α-R at least at hypothalamic level. This was shown in the rat by abolishing, with appropriate pharmacological manipulations, inputs reaching the hypothalamus from other brain centers. The use of reserpine, atropine, *p*-chlorophenylalanine, morphine and naloxone has excluded, respectively, the participation of adrenergic, serotoninergic, cholinergic and opioid mediators. The final demonstration of the lack of participation of inputs transported from extrahypothalamic neurons in the control of hypothalamic levels of 5α-R was obtained by performing a total hypothalamic deafferentation. In this experimental model, 5α-R activity remained unchanged in the isolated hypothalamus[26].

Some experiments have also been directed to analyze the possible control of the 5α-R-3α-HSD enzymatic system in cultures of mixed glial cells[27]. The results obtained indicate that the formation of DHT is not modified by the addition of phorbol esters, implying that probably protein kinase C is not involved in the intracellular signalling system controlling the enzyme 5α-R in these cells. On the contrary, a statistically significant increase of 5α-R activity over control levels has been observed after incubation with 8-Br-cAMP[27]. The effect of the cyclic adenosine monophosphate (cAMP) analog appears to be specific for 5α-R, since the activity of 3α-HSD did not show any variation.

Another important aspect that has emerged in the past few years is that growth factors originating in the astroglial cells may influence the activity of the enzymes 5α-R and 3α-HSD present in neuronal cell populations. In particular, we have observed that transforming growth factor-β1 (TGF-β1) is able to decrease 5α-R activity converting testosterone into DHT in GT1-1 cells (a cell line derived from a hypothalamic luteinizing hormone-releasing hormone (LHRH)-producing tumor, induced by genetically targeted tumorigenesis)[28].

The possible androgenic control of the gene expression of the two isozymes of 5α-R so far cloned has been analyzed *in vitro* on cultured hypothalamic neurons, as well as *in vivo*, exposing animals *in utero* to the androgen antagonist flutamide (for review see reference 29). Testosterone treatment greatly induced the expression of the 5α-R type 2 gene in cultured hypothalamic neurons, which normally do not express this isoenzyme. *In vivo* treatment with flutamide counteracted the expression of the type 2 gene occurring, at time of birth, in the whole brains of male neonates (for review see reference 29). When the same phenomenon was analyzed in the neonatal female brain, the effect of flutamide was not present, suggesting, for the first time, a sexual dimorphism of the 5α-R system in the brain; these data also lead us to hypothesize that factors other than androgens might control expression of 5α-R type 2 in the female brain. There was no effect of testosterone or flutamide on expression of the type 1 gene in the brain of either sex.

GLIAL-NEURONAL INTERACTIONS: THEIR EFFECTS ON TESTOSTERONE METABOLISM

It is now well known that glial cells not only provide mechanical support to neurons, but also play an important role in neuronal migration, neurite outgrowth and axonal guidance during neural development[30]. Moreover, it has recently been demonstrated that glial cells synthesize, and possibly release, an array of bioactive agents, such as neurotransmitters, growth factors, prostaglandins, neurosteroids, etc. (for review see references 31 and 32), which are likely to exert specific influences on neuronal activity. On the other hand, glial-neuronal interactions are certainly not one-way, since neurons can interfere with the proliferation and maturation of glial elements[33]. Thus, the emerging concept is that neurons and glia form in the CNS a functional unit, in which each single element exerts effects on the others. On this basis, we have investigated whether neurons and glial cells might interact, via humoral messages, to control the 5α-R-3α-HSD enzymatic complex. Two different experimental approaches have been utilized: a co-culture system in which neurons and glial cells remain physically separated but which allows the free transfer of secretory products from one to the other type of co-cultured cells; and the addition of conditioned medium (CM) of neurons to cultures of A1, and vice versa. The results obtained indicate that co-culture with neurons, or exposure to the neuronal CM, stimulates 5α-R and 3α-HSD activities in A1. In contrast, there was no effect of A1 on the enzymatic activity of neurons[34]. A similar effect was also evident when rat glioma cells (C6) were utilized[35]. The formation of DHT is generally considered to be a mechanism to amplify testosterone actions, while the subsequent conversion to 3α-diol is considered to be a mechanism of steroid catabolism. Consequently, a possible interpretation of our observations is that neuronal influences on A1 cells may increase (by acting on 5α-R) or decrease (by acting on 3α-HSD) the androgenic potential. However, a word of caution regarding this hypothesis may come from very recent observations indicating that 3α-diol might interact with the $GABA_A$ receptor (for review see reference 36), and consequently might exert some so far unknown anabolic effect.

The situation seems to be different when we have analyzed in the co-culture system the effects of A1 on specialized neurons such as GT1-1 cells. In this experimental model we have observed that A1 induces in GT1 cells a significant decrease of the formation of DHT[28]. Moreover, it is also interesting to note that A1 alters in opposite directions 5α-R activity in GT1-1 cells, depending on the substrate utilized. In fact, when we utilized progesterone as substrate, and subsequently the formation of DHP was analyzed, a significant increase in the formation of DHP was observed[28]. These findings are intriguing, since they suggest that the substrate itself may influence 5α-R activity. The differential effects on the formation of DHT and DHP cannot be explained on the basis of an effect on either one of the two isoforms of 5α-R so far cloned. Consequently, we have hypothesized the existence of a third 5α-R isoform, which has not been cloned to date. Several other of our observations support such a hypothesis. For instance, pluripotential CNS stem cells derived from mice striatum, when induced in culture to differentiate into glial cells, start to form DHT and DHP at totally different times[24]. The formation of DHP peaks on day 10, while that of DHT increases only after 14 days of differentiation. The CM of C6 glioma and of 1321N1 human astrocytoma cell lines are unable to modify the formation of DHT from testosterone in A1, while inducing a statistically significant decrease in the formation of DHP in the same type of culture[35]. The exposure of C6 cells to CM of rat fetal neurons stimulates the formation of DHT but not that of DHP[35].

EFFECTS OF TESTOSTERONE AND ITS METABOLITE ON GLIAL CELLS OF THE CENTRAL NERVOUS SYSTEM

As mentioned in the 'Introduction', it is well known that glial cells are a target for the action of neuroactive steroids. As also mentioned in the 'Introduction', several observations indicate that they possess classical (e.g. AR, ER, PR, etc.) and non-classical (e.g. $GABA_A$ receptor) steroid receptors. Consequently, the attention of many laboratories has been focused on the possible effects exerted by testosterone and its derivatives on different parameters of glial cells.

For instance, it has been demonstrated that castration of male rats decreases, at hypothalamic level, glial fibrillary acidic protein (GFAP) immunoreactivity[37]; this phenomenon seems to be counteracted by testosterone and DHT, but not by estradiol[37]. Androgens are also able to increase GFAP immunoreactivity of hypothalamic astrocytes in androgen-insensitive testicular feminized mice[38], and that of hypothalamic and hippocampal astrocytes in hypogonadal mice (*hpg*)[39]. Surprisingly, *hpg* mice, which possess normal sex hormone receptors, estrogens and aromatizable androgens, but not DHT, are able to normalize hippocampal but not hypothalamic GFAP immunoreactivity[39]. After a penetrating brain injury, testosterone in males is able to decrease the processes of gliosis and of astrocytic proliferation, resulting in a decrease in the number of GFAP-positive astrocytes in the cerebral cortex and in the hippocampus[40]. Analyzing the extension of GFAP-immunoreactive astroglial cell processes in hippocampal slice cultures obtained from castrated male rats, a significant decrease of GFAP-immunoreactive processes has been shown; in the same experimental conditions, testosterone increases the extension of this parameter[41]. The effects of testosterone, DHT and 3α-diol have also been evaluated on GFAP mRNA levels in A1 cultures[42]. Among these androgens, only DHT is effective on GFAP gene expression, inducing a significant decrease of the mRNA levels of this protein.

It has also been observed that the levels of GFAP mRNA and immunoreactivity show sex differences in the arcuate nucleus of the rat, lower levels being found in females than in males[43]. Androgenization of neonatal females increases GFAP mRNA to male levels, while castration of newborn males (without testosterone substitution) reduces GFAP mRNA to the levels found in females[44].

Gonadal steroids may influence astrocytes also in non-endocrine cerebral structures[45]. It has been demonstrated that the immunoreactivity for GFAP is markedly decreased after castration in the interpeduncular nucleus of adult male rats, and that testosterone is able to counteract this effect.

The 5α-reduced metabolite of testosterone, DHT, is also able to affect the physiology of astrocytes influencing the expression of a growth factor such as basic fibroblast growth factor (bFGF) (for review see reference 43). This growth factor, which exerts several effects on differentiation, proliferation and functionality of oligodendrocytes, astrocytes and neurons (for review see reference 46), seems also to be actively involved in the neuroendocrine control of LHRH neurons located in the hypothalamus. For instance, it has been demonstrated that, in GT1 cells, bFGF induces neuronal differentiation, promoting both neurite outgrowth and cell survival[47,48]. Moreover, this growth factor also enhances the processing of the LHRH prohormone[49]. Utilizing culture of hypothalamic A1 we have demonstrated that DHT reduces the expression of bFGF (for review see reference 43). This effect may be due to an interaction with the AR, which is expressed in astrocytes *in vitro* (for review see reference 2). However, testosterone, which is also able to bind to this receptor, albeit with a lower affinity than DHT, does not affect bFGF expression (for review see reference 43).

Some interesting observations have also emerged from analyzing the effect of testosterone on some parameters of the oligodendrocyte. For instance, using a monoclonal antibody which is able to recognize an oligodendrocyte-specific cell surface antigen, it has been demonstrated that testosterone is able to accelerate oligodendrocyte maturation in several brain areas[50]. Furthermore, *in vivo* treatment with testosterone in juvenile male zebra finches is able to increase the degree of myelination in the forebrain and in the cerebellum[50].

CONCLUSIONS

This chapter summarizes available information, clearly showing the importance of the metabolism of testosterone by the 5α-reductase-3α-hydroxysteroid dehydrogenase enzymatic complex in the central nervous system. In particular, relationships between neuronal and glial cells seem to play a significant role in modulating testosterone metabolism. The importance of such metabolism is also underlined by the fact that not only testosterone itself but also its metabolites exert significant effects on morphological and biochemical parameters of glial cells.

ACKNOWLEDGEMENTS

The financial support of MURST, 'FIRST - Special Project' and of the European Community - RTD program (contract QLK6-CT-2000-00179) is gratefully acknowledged.

References

1. Garcia-Segura LM, Chowen JA, Naftolin F. Endocrine glia: roles of glial cells in the brain actions of steroid and thyroid hormone and in the regulation of hormone secretion. *Front Neuroendocrinol* 1996;17:180–211
2. Melcangi RC, Magnaghi V, Galbiati M, *et al.* Glial cells: a target for steroid hormones. *Prog Brain Res* 2001;132:31–40
3. Bovolin P, Santi MR, Puia G, *et al.* Expression patterns of γ-aminobutyric acid type A receptor subunit mRNAs in primary cultures of granule neurons and astrocytes from neonatal rat cerebella. *Proc Natl Acad Sci USA* 1992;89:9344–8
4. Hosli E, Otten U, Hosli L. Expression of $GABA_A$ receptors by reactive astrocytes in explant and primary cultures of rat CNS. *Int J Dev Neurosci* 1997;15:949–60

5. Melcangi RC, Magnaghi V, Martini L. Steroid metabolism and effects in central and peripheral glial cells. *J Neurobiol* 1999;40:471-83
6. Melcangi RC, Magnaghi V, Galbiati M, *et al.* Formation and effects of neuroactive steroids in the central and peripheral nervous system. *Int Rev Neurobiol* 2001;46:145-76
7. Zoppi S, Lechuga M, Motta M. Selective inhibition of the 5α-reductase of the rat epididymis. *J Steroid Biochem Mol Biol* 1992;42:509-14
8. Motta M, Zoppi S, Brodie AM, *et al.* Effect of 1,4,6-androstatriene-3,17-dione (ATD), 4-hydroxy-4-androstene-3,17-dione (4-OH-A) and 4-acetoxy-4-androstene-3,17-dione (4-Ac-A) on the 5α-reduction of androgens in the rat prostate. *J Steroid Biochem* 1986;25:593-600
9. Andersson S, Bishop RW, Russell DW. Expression and regulation of steroid 5α-reductase, an enzyme essential for male sexual differentiation. *J Biol Chem* 1989;264:16249-55
10. Andersson S, Berman DM, Jenkins EP, *et al.* Deletion of steroid 5α-reductase 2 gene in male pseudohermaphroditism. *Nature (London)* 1991; 354:159-61
11. Labrie F, Sugimoto Y, Luu-The V, *et al.* Structure of human type 2 5α-reductase gene. *Endocrinology* 1992;131:1571-3
12. Normington K, Russell DW. Tissue distribution and kinetic characteristics of rat steroid 5α-reductase isozymes. Evidence for distinct physiological functions. *J Biol Chem* 1992;267: 19548-54
13. Russell DW, Wilson JD. Steroid 5α-reductase: two genes/two enzymes. *Ann Rev Biochem* 1994;63: 25-61
14. Levy MA, Brandt M, Sheedy KM, *et al.* Cloning, expression and functional characterization of type 1 and type 2 steroid 5α-reductases from cynomolgus monkey: comparison with human and rat isoenzymes. *J Steroid Biochem Mol Biol* 1995; 52:307-19
15. Thigpen AE, Russell DW. Four-amino acid segment in steroid 5α-reductase 1 confers sensitivity to finasteride, a competitive inhibitor. *J Biol Chem* 1992;267:8577-83
16. Krieger NR, Scott RG, Jurman ME. Testosterone 5α-reductase in rat brain. *J Neurochem* 1983;40: 1460-4
17. Krieger NR, Scott RG. 3α-Hydroxysteroid dehydrogenase in rat brain. *J Neurochem* 1984;42: 887-90
18. Melcangi RC, Celotti F, Ballabio M, *et al.* Testosterone 5α-reductase activity in the rat brain is highly concentrated in white matter structures and in purified myelin sheaths of axons. *J Steroid Biochem* 1988;31:173-9
19. Melcangi RC, Celotti F, Ballabio M, *et al.* Ontogenetic development of the 5α-reductase in the rat brain: cerebral cortex, hypothalamus, purified myelin and isolated oligodendrocytes. *Dev Brain Res* 1988;44:181-8
20. Sholl SA, Goy RW, Kim K. 5α-Reductase, aromatase, and androgen receptor levels in the monkey brain during fetal development. *Endocrinology* 1989;124:627-34
21. Melcangi RC, Celotti F, Ballabio M, *et al.* Effect of postnatal starvation on the 5α-reductase activity of the brain and of the isolated myelin membranes. *Exp Clin Endocrinol* 1989;94:253-61
22. Melcangi RC, Celotti F, Ballabio M, *et al.* 5α-Reductase activity in isolated and cultured neuronal and glial cells of the rat. *Brain Res* 1990; 516:229-36
23. Melcangi RC, Celotti F, Castano P, *et al.* Differential localization of the 5α-reductase and the 3α-hydroxysteroid dehydrogenase in neuronal and glial cultures. *Endocrinology* 1993;132:1252-9
24. Melcangi RC, Froelichsthal P, Martini, L, *et al.* Steroid metabolizing enzymes in pluripotential progenitor CNS cells: effect of differentiation and maturation. *Neuroscience* 1996;72:467-75
25. Roselli CE, Stadelman H, Horton LE, *et al.* Regulation of androgen metabolism and luteinizing hormone-releasing hormone content in discrete hypothalamic and limbic areas of male rhesus macaques. *Endocrinology* 1987;120:97-106
26. Celotti F, Negri-Cesi P, Limonta P, *et al.* Is the 5α-reductase of the hypothalamus and of the anterior pituitary neurally regulated? Effects of hypothalamic deafferentations and of centrally acting drugs. *J Steroid Biochem* 1983;19:229-34
27. Melcangi RC, Celotti F, Castano P, *et al.* Intracellular signalling systems controlling the 5α-reductase in glial cell cultures. *Brain Res* 1992; 585:411-15
28. Cavarretta I, Magnaghi V, Ferraboschi P, *et al.* Interactions between type 1 astrocytes and LHRH-secreting neurons (GT1-1 cells): modification of steroid metabolism and possible role of TGFβ1. *J Steroid Biochem Mol Biol* 1999;71:41-7
29. Melcangi RC, Poletti A, Cavarretta I, *et al.* The 5α-reductase in the central nervous system: expression and modes of control. *J Steroid Biochem Mol Brain Res* 1998;65:295-9
30. Fields RD, Stevens-Graham B. New insights into neuron-glia communication. *Science* 2002;298: 556-62
31. LoPachin RM Jr, Aschner M. Glial-neuronal interactions: relevance to neurotoxic mechanisms. *Toxicol Appl Pharmacol* 1993;118:141-58
32. Vernadakis A. Glia-neuron intercommunications and synaptic plasticity. *Prog Neurobiol* 1996;49: 185-214
33. Steward O, Torre ER, Tomasulo R, *et al.* Neuronal activity up-regulates astroglial gene expression. *Proc Natl Acad Sci USA* 1991;88:6819-23
34. Melcangi RC, Celotti F, Martini L. Neurons influence the metabolism of testosterone in cultured

astrocytes via humoral signals. *Endocrine* 1994; 2:709–13
35. Melcangi RC, Cavarretta I, Magnaghi V, *et al.* Crosstalk between normal and tumoral brain cells. Effect on sex steroid metabolism. *Endocrine* 1998; 8:65–71
36. Frye CA. The role of neurosteroids and non-genomic effects of progestins and androgens in mediating sexual receptivity of rodents. *Brain Res Rev* 2001;37:201–22
37. Day JR, Laping NJ, Lampert-Etchells M, *et al.* Gonadal steroids regulate the expression of glial fibrillary acidic protein in the adult male rat hippocampus. *Neuroscience* 1993;55:435–43
38. McQueen JK, Wright AK, Arbuthnott GW, *et al.* Glial fibrillary acidic protein (GFAP)-immunoreactive astrocytes are increased in the hypothalamus of androgen-insensitive testicular feminized *(Tfm)* mice. *Neurosci Lett* 1990;118:77–81
39. McQueen JK. Glial cells and neuroendocrine function. *J Endocrinol* 1994;143:411–15
40. Garcia-Estrada J, Del Rio JA, Luquin S, *et al.* Gonadal hormones down-regulate reactive gliosis and astrocyte proliferation after a penetrating brain injury. *Brain Res* 1993;628:271–8
41. Del Cerro S, Garcia-Estrada J, Garcia-Segura LM. Neuroactive steroids regulate astroglia morphology in hippocampal cultures from adult rats. *Glia* 1995;14:65–71
42. Melcangi RC, Riva MA, Fumagalli F, *et al.* Effect of progesterone, testosterone and their 5α-reduced metabolites on GFAP gene expression in type 1 astrocytes. *Brain Res* 1996;711:10–15
43. Melcangi RC, Cavarretta I, Magnaghi V, *et al.* Interactions between growth factors and steroids in the control of LHRH-secreting neurons. *Brain Res Rev* 2001;37:223–34
44. Chowen JA, Busiguina S, Garcia-Segura LM. Sexual dimorphism and sex steroid modulation of glial fibrillary acidic protein (GFAP) mRNA and immunoreactive levels in the rat hypothalamus. *Neuroscience* 1995;69:519–32
45. Hajos F, Halasy K, Gerics B, *et al.* Glial fibrillary acidic protein (GFAP)-immunoreactivity is reduced by castration in the interpeduncular nucleus of male rats. *Neuroreport* 1999;10:2229–33
46. Melcangi RC, Martini L, Galbiati M. Growth factors and steroid hormones: a complex interplay in the hypothalamic control of reproductive functions. *Prog Neurobiol* 2002;67:421–49
47. Tsai PS, Werner S, Weiner RI. Basic fibroblast growth factor is a neurotropic factor in GT1 gonadotropin-releasing hormone neuronal cell lines. *Endocrinology* 1995;136:3831–8
48. Ochoa A, Domenzain C, Clapp C, *et al.* Differential effects of basic fibroblast growth factor, epidermal growth factor, transforming growth factor-α, and insulin-like growth factor-I on a hypothalamic gonadotropin-releasing hormone neuronal cell line. *J Neurosci Res* 1997;49:739–49
49. Wetsel WC, Hill DF, Ojeda SR. Basic fibroblast growth factor regulates the conversion of pro-luteinizing hormone releasing hormone (pro-LHRH) to LHRH in immortalized hypothalamic neurons. *Endocrinology* 1996;137:2606–16
50. Kafitz KW, Herth G, Bartsch U, *et al.* Application of testosterone accelerates oligodendrocyte maturation in brain of zebra finches. *Neuroreport* 1992;3:315–18

Physiological mechanisms of menopausal hot flushes

9

R. R. Freedman

INTRODUCTION

Hot flushes are the most common symptom of the climacteric, and occur in the vast majority of postmenopausal women. Their prevalence in naturally menopausal women is estimated to be 68–82% in the USA[1,2], with an average age of onset of 51 years[3]. In ovariectomized women the prevalence is about 90%[2].

Hot flushes are reported as sudden sensations of intense heat, superior to the sternum, accompanied by sweating and flushing, and followed by chills and shivering. They typically last from 1 to 5 min and their occurrence persists for 1–5 years.

PHYSIOLOGY OF HOT FLUSHES

Peripheral vasodilatation, as evidenced by increased skin temperature and blood flow, occurs over virtually the entire body surface (Figure 1)[4–6]. The whole-body sweat rate during hot flushes has been measured to be about 1.3 g/min, with more sweat occurring in the upper half of the body[7]. Skin conductance, an electrical measure of sweating, also increases during hot flushes, and can be used objectively to indicate them[8,9]. It has been shown that an increase in skin conductance of 2 μmho/30 s, measured over the sternum, corresponds with patient self-reports in 95% of hot flushes recorded in the laboratory and 77–86% of those recorded during ambulatory monitoring[8,9].

Homeotherms regulate core body temperature (T_c) between upper thresholds, where sweating and peripheral vasodilatation occur, and a lower threshold, where shivering occurs. If T_c were elevated in women with hot flushes, their symptoms of sweating and peripheral vasodilatation could be explained. However, measurements of esophageal[10], rectal[11] and tympanic[12] temperatures were not found to be elevated prior to hot flushes. These studies all found declines of about 0.3°C following hot flushes, probably due to increased heat loss (peripheral vasodilatation) and evaporative cooling (sweating). However, esophageal and rectal temperatures have long thermal lag times, and respond too slowly to appear along with the rapid peripheral events of the hot flush[13]. Additionally, it has been shown that tympanic temperature does not reliably measure T_c because it is affected by peripheral vasodilatation and sweating[14].

Several studies were then conducted in which T_c was recorded with an ingested radiotelemetry pill, which responds more rapidly than esophageal and rectal temperature. We found that small but significant increases in core body temperature preceded 65–76% of hot flushes recorded in the laboratory, whereas rectal temperature did not change[4,11]. Small elevations in T_c may, therefore, be the triggering event for the majority of hot flushes.

Elevations in T_c can be caused by increased metabolic rate (heat production) and by peripheral vasoconstriction (decreased heat loss). We sought to determine whether either of these factors accounted for the core body temperature elevations preceding hot flushes. Significant elevations in metabolic rate (about 15%) occurred, but were simultaneous with sweating and peripheral vasodilatation and did not precede the T_c elevations (Figure 1). Peripheral vasoconstriction did not occur. Thus, increased metabolic rate and peripheral vasoconstriction did not account for the core body temperature elevations in these women.

CIRCADIAN RHYTHMS

The circadian rhythm of T_c is well known, and similar variations in other thermoregulatory

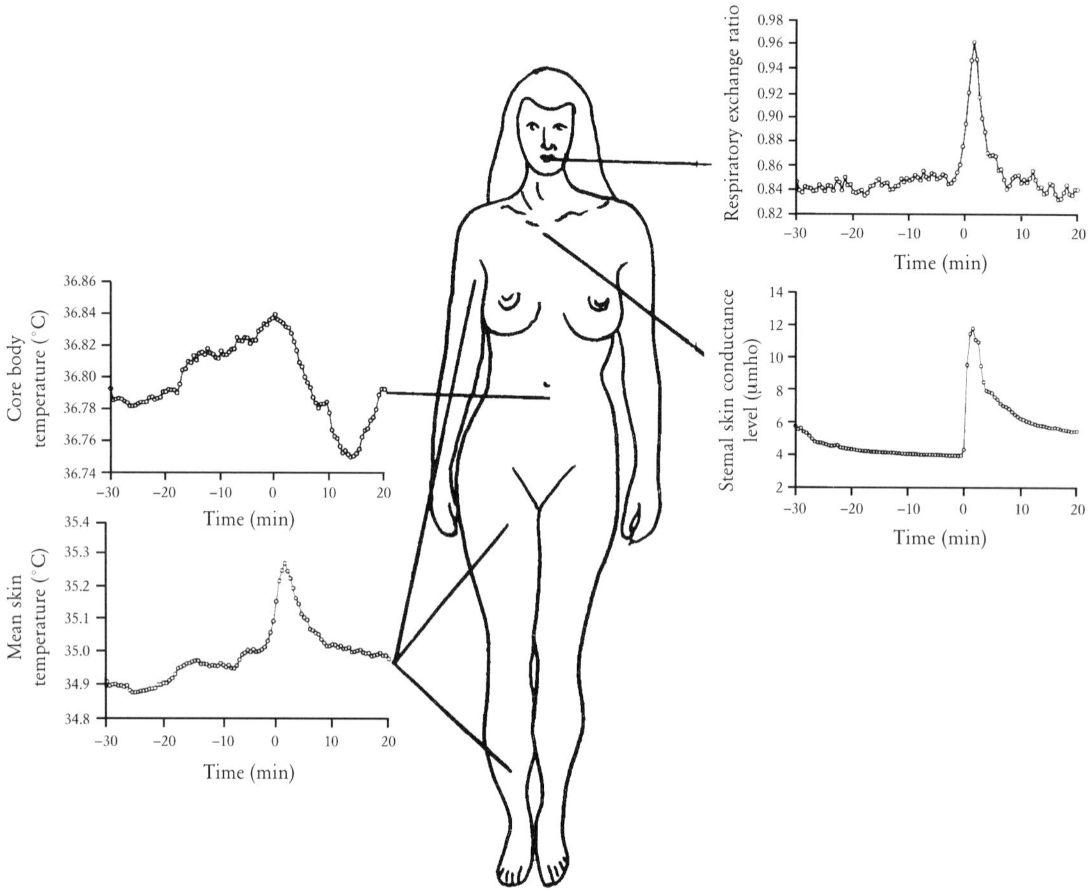

Figure 1 Peripheral physiological events of the hot flush. Data from reference 4. Drawing by Jeri Pajor

parameters, such as heat conductance and sweating, have also been demonstrated. These patterns suggest that the thermoregulatory effector responses of hot flushes might also demonstrate temporal variations. A previous study showed circadian rhythmicity of self-reported hot flushes in some menopausal women, but no physiological data were collected[15]. We therefore recorded sternal skin conductance level and T_c (with the telemetry pill) in symptomatic and asymptomatic postmenopausal women using 24-h ambulatory monitoring[16]. Cosinor analysis demonstrated a circadian rhythm ($p < 0.02$) of hot flushes with a peak around 18.25 (Figure 2). This rhythm lagged the circadian rhythm of T_c in symptomatic women by about 3 h. T_c values of the symptomatic women were lower than those of the asymptomatic women ($p < 0.05$) from 00.00 to 04.00, and at 15.00 and 22.00. The majority of hot flushes were preceded by elevations in T_c, a statistically significant effect ($p < 0.05$). Hot flushes began at significantly ($p < 0.02$) higher levels of T_c (36.82 ± 0.04°C) compared with all non-flush periods (36.70 ± 0.005°C). These data are consistent with the hypothesis that elevated T_c serves as part of the hot flush triggering mechanism.

ETIOLOGY

Estrogens

Because hot flushes accompany the decline of estrogens in the vast majority of naturally and surgically menopausal women, there is little doubt

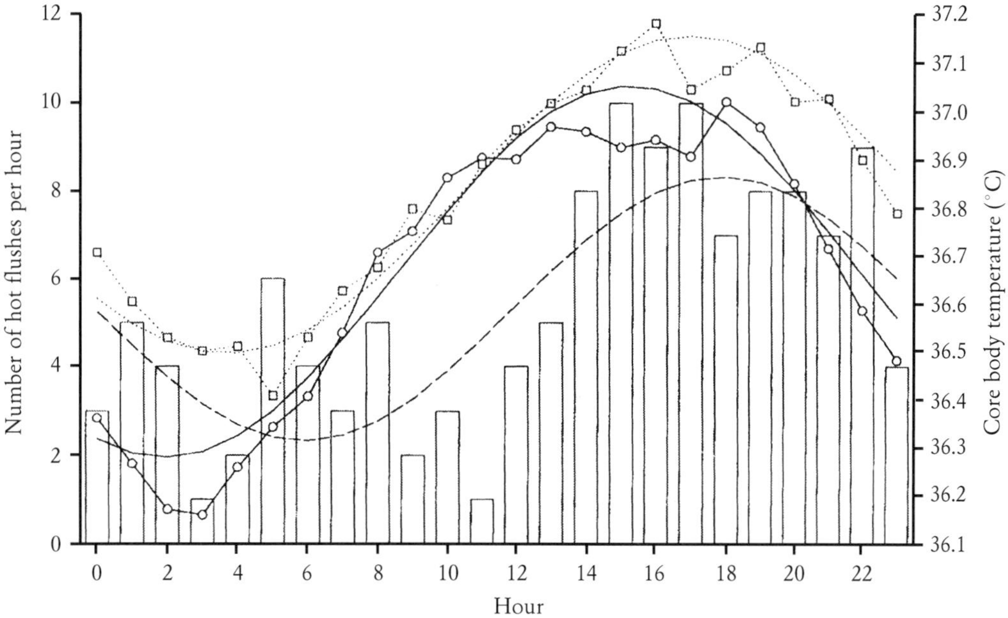

Figure 2 Hot flush (HF) frequency and core body temperature over 24 h. Hot flush frequency in ten symptomatic women shown as bars. Curves: best-fit cosine curve for hot flush frequency (- - -); 24-h core temperature data for ten symptomatic women (—○—) with best-fit cosine curve (——); 24-h core temperature data in six asymptomatic women (···□···) with best-fit cosine curve (. . . .)

that estrogens play a role in the genesis of hot flushes. However, estrogens alone do not appear to be responsible for hot flushes because there is no correlation between the presence of this symptom and plasma[17], urinary[18] or vaginal concentrations[19]. No differences in unconjugated plasma estrogen concentrations were found in symptomatic versus asymptomatic women[3-5]. Additionally, clonidine significantly reduces hot flush frequency without altering circulating estrogen values[20].

Gonadotropins

Because gonadotropins become elevated at the menopause, their possible role in the initiation of hot flushes has been investigated. Although no differences in luteinizing hormone (LH) concentrations were found between women with and without hot flushes[21], a temporal association was found between LH pulses and hot flush occurrence[22,23]. However, subsequent investigation revealed that women with a defect of gonadotropin-releasing hormone (GnRH) secretion (isolated gonadotropin deficiency) had hot flushes but no LH pulses, and women with abnormal input to GnRH neurons (hypothalamic amenorrhea) had some LH pulses but no hot flushes[24]. Additionally, hot flushes occur in hypophysectomized women, who have no LH release[25], in women with pituitary insufficiency and hypoestrogenism[26], and in women with LH release suppressed by GnRH analog treatment[27,28]. Thus, LH cannot be the basis for hot flushes.

Opiates

It was observed that alcohol-induced flushing in subjects taking chlorpropamide, a drug that stimulates insulin release and lowers blood glucose, was related to opiate receptor activation[29]. Lightman and colleagues[30] subsequently found that naloxone infusion significantly reduced hot flush and LH pulse frequencies in six postmenopausal women. However, DeFazio and associates[31] attempted to replicate this study and found no effects. Tepper and co-workers[32] found that plasma β-endorphin concentration decreased significantly before the occurrence of menopausal hot flushes, whereas Genazzani and colleagues[33] found significantly increased values preceding hot flushes. Thus, there is no consistent evidence of the involvement of an opioidergic system in menopausal hot flushes.

Catecholamines

There is considerable evidence that norepinephrine plays an important role in thermoregulation mediated, in part, through α_2-adrenergic receptors[34]. Injection of norepinephrine into the preoptic hypothalamus causes peripheral vasodilatation, heat loss and a subsequent decline in T_c[34]. Additionally, there is considerable evidence that gonadal steroids modulate central noradrenergic activity[35].

3-Methoxy-4-hydroxyphenylglycol (MHPG) is the main metabolite of norepinephrine and reflects whole-body sympathetic activation[36]. Basal levels of plasma MHPG are significantly higher in symptomatic than in asymptomatic postmenopausal women, and increase significantly further with the occurrence of each hot flush[37]. It was subsequently shown that plasma vanillymandelic acid (VMA), the peripheral metabolite of norepinephrine, does not change with hot flushes[4], lending support to the hypothesis that central norepinephrine levels are elevated in symptomatic women.

Clonidine, an α_2-adrenergic agonist, reduces central noradrenergic activation and hot flush frequency[38-40]. Conversely, yohimbine, an α_2-adrenergic antagonist, increases central noradrenergic activation and triggers hot flushes[41]. These data support the hypothesis that α_2-adrenergic receptors within the central noradrenergic system are involved in the initiation of hot flushes and that brain norepinephrine is elevated in this process.

THERMOREGULATION AND HOT FLUSHES

Increased thermosensitivity at the menopause has been noted in the literature for many years, and is reflected in reports of increased hot flush frequency and duration during warm weather[42,43]. Peripheral heating has been demonstrated to provoke hot flushes in most symptomatic subjects[8,44]. As noted above, T_c in homeotherms is regulated by hypothalamic centers between the thresholds of T_c for sweating and peripheral vasodilatation and for shivering. According to this mechanism, the heat dissipation responses of hot flushes (sweating, peripheral vasodilatation) would be triggered if body temperature were elevated or the sweating threshold lowered.

Three separate investigations have found that small elevations in T_c precede the majority of menopausal hot flushes[4,11,16]. Since these elevations also occur in asymptomatic women, they do not explain the entire triggering mechanism[45]. However, if the thermoneutral zone were sufficiently narrowed in symptomatic women, the T_c elevations would be a likely trigger.

This appears to be the case. A study was conducted in which the thermoneutral zone was measured to be 0.0°C in symptomatic postmenopausal women and 0.4°C in asymptomatic postmenopausal women[46]. Sweating rates were significantly higher in the symptomatic women, and hot flushes were triggered by T_c elevations produced by body heating and by exercise.

Animal studies have shown that increased brain norepinephrine narrows the width of the thermoneutral zone[34]. Conversely, clonidine reduces norepinephrine release, raises the sweating threshold and reduces hot flushes in symptomatic women[47]. Estrogen ameliorates hot flushes by raising the sweating threshold in symptomatic women[48].

Thus, it is proposed that elevated brain norepinephrine narrows the thermoregulatory interthreshold zone in symptomatic postmenopausal women, and that small elevations in core body temperature trigger hot flushes when the sweating threshold is crossed.

References

1. Neugarten BL, Kraines RJ. 'Menopausal symptoms' in women of various ages. *Psychosom Med* 1965;27:266–73
2. Feldman BM, Voda A, Grenseth E. The prevalence of hot flash and associated variables among perimenopausal women. *Res Nurs Health* 1985; 8:261–8
3. Hagstad A, Janson PO. The epidemiology of climacteric symptoms. *Acta Obstet Gynecol Scand Suppl* 1986;134:59–65
4. Freedman RR. Biochemical, metabolic, and vascular mechanisms in menopausal hot flashes. *Fertil Steril* 1998;70:1–6
5. Ginsburg J, Swinhoe J, O'Reilly B. Cardiovascular responses during the menopausal hot flush. *Br J Obstet Gynaecol* 1981;88:925–30
6. Sturdee DW, Reece BL. Thermography of menopausal hot flushes. *Maturitas* 1979;1:201–5
7. Molnar GW. Body temperature during menopausal hot flashes. *J Appl Physiol Respir Environ Exercise Physiol* 1975;38:499–503
8. Freedman RR. Laboratory and ambulatory monitoring of menopausal hot flashes. *Psychophysiology* 1989;26:573–9
9. Freedman RR, Woodward S, Norton D. Laboratory and ambulatory monitoring of menopausal hot flushes: comparison of symptomatic and asymptomatic women. *J Psychophysiol* 1992;6: 162–6
10. Kronenberg F, Cote LJ, Linkie DM, Dyrenfurth I, Downey JA. Menopausal hot flashes: thermoregulatory, cardiovascular, and circulating catecholamine and LH changes. *Maturitas* 1984;6:31–43
11. Freedman RR, Woodward S. Core body temperature during menopausal hot flushes. *Fertil Steril* 1996;65:1141–4
12. Tataryn IV, Lomax P, Bajorek JG, Chesarek W, Meldrum DR, Judd HL. Postmenopausal hot flushes: a disorder of thermoregulation. *Maturitas* 1980;2:101–7
13. Molnar GW, Read RC. Studies during open heart surgery on the special characteristics of rectal temperature. *J Appl Physiol* 1974;36:333–6
14. Skiraki K, Nobuhide K, Sagawa S. Esophageal and tympanic temperature responses to core blood temperature changes during hyperthermia. *J Appl Physiol* 1986;61:98–102
15. Albright DL, Voda AM, Smolensky MH, His B, Decker M. Circadian rhythms in hot flashes in natural and surgically-induced menopause. *Chronobiol Int* 1989;6:279–84
16. Freedman RR, Norton D, Woodward S, Cornelissen G. Core body temperature and circadian rhythm of hot flashes in menopausal women. *J Clin Endocrinol Metab* 1995;80:2354–8
17. Askel S, Schomberg DW, Tyrey L, Hammond CB. Vasomotor symptoms, serum estrogens, and gonadotropin levels in surgical menopause. *Am J Obstet Gynecol* 1976;126:165–9
18. Stone SC, Mickal A, Rye F, Rye PH. Postmenopausal symptomatology, maturation index, and plasma estrogen levels. *Obstet Gynecol* 1975;45:625–7
19. Hutton JD, Jacobs HS, Murray MAF, James VHT. Relation between plasma estrone and estradiol and climacteric symptoms. *Lancet* 1978;1:671–81
20. Schindler AE, Muller D, Keller E, Goser R, Runkel F. Studies with clonidine (Dixarit) in menopausal women. *Arch Gynecol* 1979;227:341–7
21. Campbell S. Intensive steroid and protein hormonal profiles on postmenopausal women experiencing hot flashes and a group of controls. In Campbell S, ed. *Management of the Menopause and Post-Menopause Years*. London: MTP Press, 1976
22. Casper RF, Yen SSC, Wilkes MM. Menopausal flushes: a neuroendocrine link with pulsatile luteinizing hormone secretion. *Science* 1979;205: 823–5
23. Tataryn IV, Meldrum DR, Lu KH, Frumar AM, Judd HL. LH, FSH, and skin temperature during menopausal hot flush. *J Clin Endocrinol Metab* 1979;49:152–4
24. Gambone J, Meldrum DR, Laufer L, Chang RJ, Lu JKH, Judd, HL. Further delineation of hypothalamic dysfunction responsible for menopausal hot flashes. *J Clin Endocrinol* 1984;59:1092–102
25. Mulley G, Mitchell RA, Tattersall RB. Hot flushes after hypophysectomy. *Br Med J* 1977;2:1062
26. Meldrum DR, Erlik Y, Lu JKH, Judd HL. Objectively recorded hot flushes in patients with pituitary insufficiency. *J Clin Endocrinol Metab* 1981;52:684–7
27. Casper RF, Yen SSC. Menopausal flushes: effect of pituitary gonadotropin desensitization by a potent luteinizing hormone releasing factor agonist. *J Clin Endocrinol Metab* 1981;53:1056–8
28. DeFazio J, Meldrum DR, Laufer L, *et al.* Induction of hot flashes in premenopausal women treated with a long-acting GnRH agonist. *J Clin Endocrinol Metab* 1983;56:445–8
29. Leslie RDG, Pyke DA, Stubbs WA. Sensitivity to enkephalin as a cause of non-insulin dependent diabetes. *Lancet* 1979;1:341–3
30. Lightman SL, Jacobs HS, Maquire AK, McGarrick G, Jeffcoate SL. Climacteric flushing: clinical and endocrine response to infusion of naloxone. *Br J Obstet Gynaecol* 1981;88:919–24
31. DeFazio J, Vorheugen C, Chetkowski R, Nass T, Judd HL, Meldrum DR. The effects of naloxone on hot flashes and gonadotropin secretion in

postmenopausal women. *J Clin Endocrinol Metab* 1984;58:578–81
32. Tepper R, Neri A, Kaufman H, Schoenfield A, Ovadia J. Menopausal hot flushes and plasma β-endorphins. *Obstet Gynecol* 1987;70:150–2
33. Genazzani AR, Petraglia F, Facchinetti F, Facchini V, Volpe A, Alessandrini G. Increase of proopiomelanocortin-related peptides during subjective menopausal flushes. *Am J Obstet Gynecol* 1984; 149:775–9
34. Brück K, Zeisberger E. Adaptive changes in thermoregulation and their neuropharmacological basis. In Schönbaum E, Lomax P, eds. *Thermoregulation: Physiology and Biochemistry*. New York: Pergamon, 1990:255–307
35. Insel PA, Motulskey HJ. Physiologic and pharmacologic regulation of adrenergic receptors. In Insel PA, ed. *Adrenergic Receptors in Man*. New York: Dekker, 1987:201–36
36. Lambert GW, Kaye DM, Vaz M, *et al.* Regional origins of 3-methoxy-4-hydroxyphenylglycol in plasma: effects of chronic sympathetic nervous activation and denervation, and acute reflex sympathetic stimulation. *J Autom Nerv Syst* 1995;55: 169–78
37. Freedman RR, Woodward S. Elevated α_2-adrenergic responsiveness in menopausal hot flushes: pharmacologic and biochemical studies. In Schönbaum E, Lomax P, eds. *Thermoregulation: The Pathophysiological Basis of Clinical Disorders*. Basel: Karger, 1992:6–9
38. Clayden JR, Bell JW, Pollard P. Menopausal flushing: double blind trial of a non-hormonal medication. *Br Med J* 1974;1:409–12
39. Laufer LR, Erlik Y, Meldrum DR, Judd HL. Effect of clonidine on hot flushes in postmenopausal women. *Obstet Gynecol* 1982;60:583–9
40. Schmitt H. The pharmacology of clonidine and related products. *Handb Exp Pharmacol* 1977;39: 299–396
41. Freedman RR, Woodward S, Sabharwal SC. α_2-Adrenergic mechanism in menopausal hot flushes. *Obstet Gynecol* 1990;76:573–8
42. Molnar GW. Menopausal hot flashes: their cycles and relation to air temperature. *Obstet Gynecol* 1981;57(Suppl 6):52–5
43. Kronenberg F, Barnard RM. Modulation of menopausal hot flashes by ambient temperature. *J Therm Biol* 1992;17:43–9
44. Sturdee DW, Wilson KA, Pipili E, Crocker D. Physiological aspects of menopausal hot flush. *Br Med J* 1978;2:79–80
45. Freedman RR. Core body temperature variation in symptomatic and asymptomatic postmenopausal women: brief report. *Menopause* 2002;9: 399–401
46. Freedman RR, Krell W. Reduced thermoregulatory null zone in postmenopausal women with hot flashes. *Am J Obstet Gynecol* 1999;181:66–70
47. Freedman RR, Dinsay MD. Clonidine raises the sweating threshold in symptomatic but not in asymptomatic postmenopausal women. *Fertil Steril* 2000;74:20–3
48. Freedman RR, Blacker CM. Estrogen raises the sweating threshold in postmenopausal women with hot flashes. *Fertil Steril* 2002;77:487–90

Menopause, hormone replacement therapy and sleep disturbance 10

E. O. Bixler, A. N. Vgontzas, H.-M. Lin and A. Vela-Bueno

INTRODUCTION

A complaint of sleep disturbance is commonly reported for women who are menopausal[1]. In order to understand the extent of and the factors associated with this complaint, we need to first address several closely associated dimensions. These dimensions include the effects of aging, gender, menopause, and hormone replacement therapy (HRT) on sleep as well as on complaints of sleep disturbance. Finally, we will address the issue of sleep-disordered breathing in terms of age, gender, menopause, and HRT.

NORMAL SLEEP

Age

It is well accepted that, as we age, we tend to sleep less soundly[2,3]. We recently evaluated this question in our Penn State Cohort, which is a random sample of the general public (n = 1741), aged from 20 to 100 years and recorded polysomnographically in the sleep laboratory[4,5]. We selected a subsample of normal sleepers from this cohort, excluding those with insomnia, excessive daytime sleepiness and sleep apnea (apnea/hypopnea index (A/HI) ≥ 5)[6]. In this subsample of 1324, we observed that the ability to sleep worsened with increasing age. Specifically, the amount of sleep (sleep efficiency) decreased with age and the time to fall asleep (sleep latency) and duration of light or drowsy sleep (stage 1) increased with age. In addition, decreases were observed in both deep sleep (slow wave sleep) and, to a lesser degree, dreaming sleep (REM). Recently, Vgontzas and colleagues reported a possible mechanism for this decline in ability to sleep soundly with increasing age[7]. In this study, a bolus of corticotropin releasing hormone (CRH) was injected 10 min after sleep onset in a sample of young and middle-aged men. The anticipated increased levels of cortisol in response to this stimulus of CRH were observed and the increased levels of cortisol were similar in the two age groups. However, the two age groups differed dramatically in terms of their response to this physiological stimulus. The middle-aged group responded with increased wakefulness levels that were significantly higher than in the young group. This supports the hypothesis that, as one ages, the overall sleep mechanism is weakening and is more vulnerable to physiological and psychological stimuli.

Gender

We have recently evaluated the effects of gender on sleep in the subsample of men and women without sleep disorders recorded polysomnographically within our Penn State Cohort[6]. We observed that the women compared to the men tended to sleep better. Specifically, they slept more (sleep efficiency), had less drowsy sleep (stage 1), more deep sleep (slow wave) and dreaming sleep (REM) than men. However, the times taken by men and women to fall asleep (sleep latency) were similar across all ages.

Menopause

There are only a few studies that have assessed the association between objectively recorded sleep and menopause. Data reported to date would suggest that, in population studies, there is little support for a general sleep deterioration associated with menopause. In a recent report from the Wisconsin Sleep Cohort Study of 539 women aged 30–60 years, the sleep recorded polysomnographically in menopausal women was similar to the sleep recorded in premenopausal women[8]. As mentioned above, in our Penn State Cohort subsample without sleep disorders, we observed that women slept better than men in terms of both quantity and quality[6]. This increased amount of sleep in women compared to men occurred primarily between the ages of 45 and 70 years. Thus, objective data do not support the assumed increase of sleep deterioration associated with menopause. There are, however, data that would support the conclusion that the presence of hot flushes is associated with objective sleep disturbance[9–11].

Hormone replacement therapy

Assessment of the influence of HRT on sleep patterns using polysomnographic data is not clear, mainly due to the lack of well-designed studies. In those studies using only estrogen, the majority of the studies have studied women with symptoms and have shown improved sleep[12]. In one study, estrogen HRT was evaluated in postmenopausal women without symptoms. In this sample, those women with HRT were shown to have less sleep disturbance associated with an external stimulus of nocturnal blood sampling[13]. Thus, the general conclusion is that estrogen used as HRT is associated with improved sleep. High levels of progesterone have a marked sedative effect[14]. We are aware of only one study that evaluated progesterone alone in order to evaluate its effects on sleep-disordered breathing[12]. This study reported that sleep efficiencies as well as sleep-disordered breathing were not changed. Finally, in the studies that have evaluated estrogen plus progesterone, the results are mixed[12]. It appears from these data that, in the doses employed for HRT, estrogen has sleep-enhancing properties while progesterone may not. The timing of administration in relation to onset of menopause, as well as the duration of administration, may be important variables to be considered in the design of future studies.

SLEEP DISTURBANCE

Association with mental and physical disorders

Estimates of the prevalence of insomnia range from about 10 to 35%, depending upon the definition employed[15]. The class of variables most consistently reported to be associated with insomnia has been psychopathology. Insomnia is a common symptom associated with psychiatric disorders[16]. In fact, it is commonly employed as a diagnostic criterion with many psychiatric disorders, especially mood disorders. In contrast, it is also well established that psychopathology is commonly present in patients with a complaint of chronic insomnia[3,17]. The strong interaction between insomnia and psychopathology has been further demonstrated in association with treatment. For example, it has been shown that successful treatment of psychiatric disorders will improve the sleep disorder[18,19], and the degree of success of treating the psychiatric disorder is associated with the severity of the sleep disorder[20,21]. In addition, it has been demonstrated that the successful treatment of the sleep disorder may also improve the psychiatric disorder[22,23]. Finally, there are data derived from large longitudinal epidemiological studies that indicate that the presence of insomnia at baseline is associated with an increased risk for new-onset major depression at follow-up[24,25]. There are also considerable data that support the model that the complaint of insomnia is associated with various physical health problems[15,16,26]. In the Penn State Cohort, we evaluated the association between chronic insomnia and various physical and mental health symptoms, as well as objective measures of sleep disturbance[15]. Multivariate analysis indicated that depression was the single most strong factor followed by gender (Figure 1). Minority status, and a history of colitis, hypertension, and anemia were also associated. The final model did not include age, body mass index or any of the sleep laboratory findings.

Gender

There is strong consensus that women are at a greater risk for the complaint of insomnia than

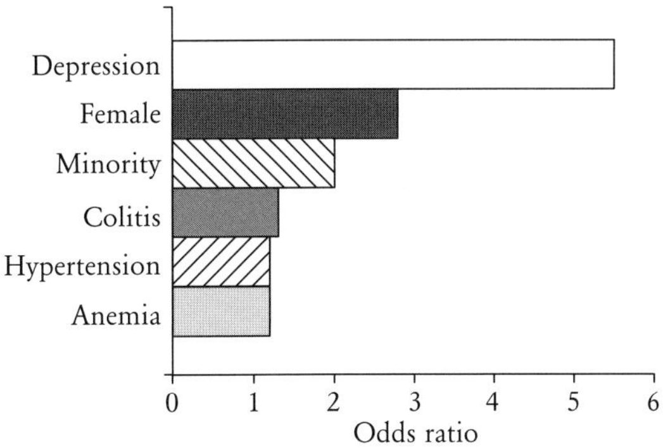

Figure 1 Odds ratios of the variables included in the final model of logistic regression predicting chronic insomnia in the Penn State Cohort controlling for age, body mass index and gender

men[3]. In our Penn State Cohort, female gender made an independent contribution to the presence of chronic insomnia[15]. Given that women tend to sleep better than men, it appears that an increased prevalence of a complaint of chronic insomnia in women might be unexpected[6]. However, this apparent inconsistency can at least partially be understood in terms of the strong relationship between chronic insomnia and depression. In patients with a primary complaint of chronic insomnia, the most common depressive disorder observed is dysthymic depression[3]. Women have an increased prevalence of depression, including dysthymic depression, compared to men[27]. Thus, the complaint of insomnia may be more strongly associated with mood than with actual sleep time.

Menopause

Sleep disturbance is a common complaint of women entering menopause. An early study reported by Lugaresi and colleagues appeared to support this finding[28]. In a large sample of the general public, they demonstrated that the complaint of insomnia increased with age. Men and women reported about the same prevalence until age 40, when the prevalence of insomnia demonstrated a dramatic increase in women compared to men. It was hypothesized that this increase was associated with the onset of menopause. In a subsample of women selected from a large volunteer cohort established by the American Cancer Society, a significant association between insomnia and menopause was observed[29]. More recently, it has been shown, in a sample of women aged 42–50 years who were followed for a 3-year period, that an increased prevalence of a complaint of sleep disturbance was not observed in those who were menopausal compared to those who were not, in a cross-sectional manner[30]. However, in another study of 12 603 women aged 40–55 years, menopause made an independent contribution to the prevalence of sleep disturbance[31]. Because women, during the initial years of menopause, sleep more than men, this increased complaint of sleep disturbance may be at least partially explained by the strong association between sleep complaints and mood changes.

Hormone replacement therapy

Clinically, it is commonly observed that HRT will decrease the symptoms associated with menopause, including the complaint of sleep disturbance. Recent data in terms of subjective reports appear to support this observation. No differences in terms of sleep disturbance at baseline were observed between pre- compared to postmenopausal women in a sample of 521 women aged 42–50 years[30]. However, those women who became postmenopausal during the follow-up and who were not taking HRT reported an increased prevalence of sleep disturbance. The recent Women's Health Initiative (WHI) study assessed the effects of estrogen and progesterone in a sample of 16 608 postmenopausal women[32]. In those randomly assigned to HRT, compared to those assigned to placebo, a decreased rate of sleep disturbance complaint was observed.

SLEEP DISORDERED BREATHING

Gender

Sleep disordered breathing, until recently, was assumed to be primarily a disorder associated with men. The typical patient with sleep apnea has been considered to be a male, aged 55 years old, obese, with excessive daytime sleepiness and hypertension. Several studies have recently demonstrated that the gender difference in favor of men in terms of prevalence is less than previously considered[5,33,34]. Most current epidemiological samples report that the difference in gender ratio is more in the range of 2 : 1 to 4 : 1. Recently, an incidence rate of approximately 2% per year was reported from the Cleveland Family Study[35]. This study further suggested that the significance of the incident sleep apnea (AHI ≥ 10) for men versus women declined with age, suggesting that older women had a higher incidence of sleep apnea than men.

Age

It was originally assumed that the prevalence of sleep apnea increased linearly with age (i.e. the elderly were most at risk). In the Penn State Cohort, we defined sleep apnea using criteria similar to those used clinically (AHI ≥ 10 plus daytime symptoms including daytime sleepiness, hypertension or some other cardiovascular problem)[4,5]. We observed that there was an age distribution that peaked in the sixth decade for men and in the seventh for women. We have also assessed the severity of sleep apnea in relation to age[4]. We employed minimum oxygen saturation ($Sa\mathrm{O}_2$) as a marker of severity. In men, we observed that, when we excluded those with sleep apnea (AHI ≥ 5), the minimum $Sa\mathrm{O}_2$ observed within our 8-h polysomnographic recording decreased with age. This was expected, as the efficiency of the respiratory system tends to decline with age. However, when we evaluated the minimum $Sa\mathrm{O}_2$ in those with sleep apnea (AHI ≥ 5), we observed that the minimum $Sa\mathrm{O}_2$ increased with age. Further, as we increased the threshold for sleep-disordered breathing (e.g. AHI ≥ 10), the slope of the best fitting line increased, suggesting that the most severe sleep-disordered breathing is observed in the young. This finding supports the hypothesis that sleep-disordered breathing has a genetic predisposition[36].

Menopause

It has been commonly assumed that premenopausal women are protected from sleep apnea and that postmenopausal women have a prevalence rate of sleep apnea that is similar to that of men. In our sample (Figure 2), we confirmed that premenopausal women were protected from sleep apnea and that menopause was a risk factor for sleep apnea[5]. This finding has been recently confirmed in the Wisconson Sleep Cohort[37]. Assuming that one of the major differences physiologically between pre- and postmenopausal women was associated with hormone levels, we further evaluated our data to assess the prevalence of sleep-disordered breathing in those postmenopausal women who were on HRT compared to those postmenopausal women who were not[5]. We observed that those postmenopausal women on HRT had a prevalence of sleep-disordered breathing which was similar to the prevalence in premenopausal women (Figure 2). Those not using HRT had a prevalence similar to men, although it remained significantly less when controlled for age and obesity. This finding has been recently confirmed in the Sleep Heart Health Study[38]. Further, in this study, the authors observed that the protective effect of HRT was strongest in those women aged 50–59 years and had lost its protective effect in those aged 70 years or older, suggesting the protective effect of HRT for sleep-disordered breathing may be limited in duration.

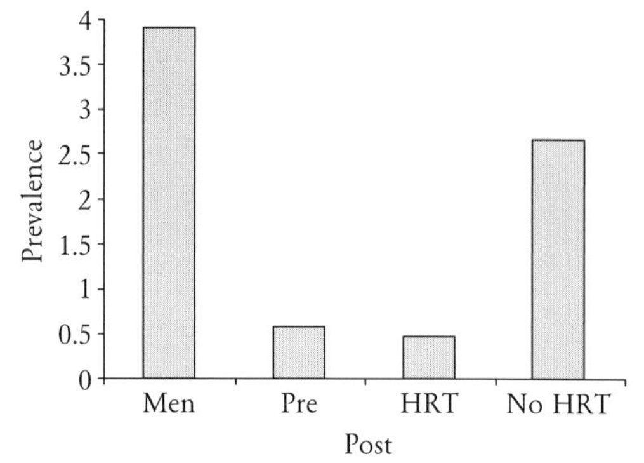

Figure 2 Prevalence of sleep apnea for women who are premenopausal, postmenopausal with hormone replacement therapy (HRT), and postmenopausal without HRT compared to men in the Penn State Cohort

Metabolic syndrome

It has been observed that metabolic factors play an important role in the clinical significance of sleep-disordered breathing[39]. The association of clinically significant sleep-disordered breathing is especially strong with visceral obesity, type 2 diabetes, and insulin resistance, all factors of the metabolic syndrome. Polycystic ovary syndrome (PCOS) is a common endocrine disorder in premenopausal women. This disorder includes hyperandrogenism, oligoanovulation, and insulin resistance. In a sample of women who were diagnosed with PCOS, Vgontzas and colleagues observed that the prevalence of sleep apnea was 30-fold higher than in the premenopausal women of the Penn State Cohort[40]. This finding has recently been confirmed[41,42]. In the sample reported by Vgontzas and colleagues, a multivariate analysis indicated that, in the PCOS patients, insulin and insulin-to-glucose ratio were independent predictors of sleep-disordered breathing. Age, body mass index and testosterone did not have such a strong association. Because PCOS is a common disorder observed in premenopausal women, it is reasonable to speculate that the presence of PCOS could at least partially account for those premenopausal women who have sleep-disordered breathing. We have recently confirmed this speculation within the Penn State Cohort. These findings add further support to the important role of metabolic factors in the clinical significance of sleep-disordered breathing.

Hypertension

There have now been four studies that have demonstrated that sleep-disordered breathing makes an independent contribution to the presence of hypertension when controlling for relevant confounding factors (e.g. age, body mass index, gender, menopause and HRT status, smoking and alcohol use, and race)[43-46]. One of these studies established that sleep-disordered breathing was an independent risk factor for the incidence of hypertension after only a 4-year follow-up[44]. Only in the Sleep Heart Health Study was a gender effect observed in terms of the association between sleep-disordered breathing and hypertension. In this sample, a significant association was observed between sleep-disordered breathing and hypertension in men but not in women. It must be remembered that the Sleep Heart Health Study is on an older cohort (46.7% $\geq$ 65 years) and also a much larger cohort (n = 6132). The effects of age on the strength of the association between sleep-disordered breathing and hypertension have been observed in both the Sleep Heart Health Study[45] and the Penn State Cohort[46]. In the Sleep Health Heart Study, a significant relationship was observed only in those individuals younger than 65 years. In the Penn State Cohort, we observed a significant negative relationship with age (i.e. the stronger association between sleep-disordered breathing and hypertension was in the young).

SUMMARY

Sleep disturbance as a subjective complaint is frequently associated with menopause, especially perimenopause. However, when sleep patterns are evaluated objectively in the sleep laboratory, the association between sleep deterioration and menopause is less clear. One reason is the lack of polysomnographic studies specifically designed to assess this transition. It is, however, well documented that objective sleep disturbance is observed in women who are currently experiencing hot flushes and that HRT will reduce this sleep disturbance. Another reason that objective polysomnographic evaluation of the association between menopause and sleep disturbance is unclear may be due to the confounding effects that aging and gender have on sleep. In general, sleep quantity and quality decrease with age, and women tend to sleep better than men (both in terms of quantity and quality). In contrast, women are more likely than men to complain of sleep disturbances, including chronic insomnia. Depression, especially dysthymic depression, is strongly associated with chronic insomnia, and women are also more likely to report depression than men. Thus, reports of sleep disruption associated with menopause could be a direct result of dramatic changes in the hormonal milieu associated with menopause, or these reports could be associated with other hormonally influenced processes, such as mood changes. Further studies specifically designed to address this question are needed. In any event, currently available data, although limited, do suggest that estrogens exert sleep-enhancing effects, while progesterone, in the doses employed in HRT, may not.

In contrast to sleep disturbance, women have a reduced risk for sleep apnea compared to men. For women, menopause is a strong risk factor for sleep apnea. Age is a confounding factor as the prevalence of sleep apnea increases with age, at least through the sixth decade in men and the seventh decade in women. In postmenopausal women who use HRT, the risk for sleep apnea appears to remain at the low premenopausal levels, in spite of the increased age of the postmenopausal women. The major risk associated with sleep apnea is hypertension and other cardiovascular events. Thus, postmenopausal women who use HRT appear to be at reduced risk for sleep apnea and thus at reduced risk for hypertension and associated cardiovascular events due to sleep apnea.

ACKNOWLEDGEMENTS

These studies were supported in part by the National Institutes of Health grants HL40916 and HL51931.

References

1. Ballinger CB. Subjective sleep disturbance at the menopause. *J Psychosom Res* 1976;20:509–13
2. Williams RL, Karacan I, Hursch CJ. *Electroencephalography (EEG) of Human Sleep: Clinical Applications*. New York: John Wiley & Sons, 1974
3. Kales A, Kales D. *Evaluation and Treatment of Insomnia*. New York: Oxford University Press, 1984
4. Bixler EO, Vgontzas AN, Ten Have T, *et al.* Effects of age on sleep apnea in men. I. Prevalence and severity. *Am J Respir Crit Care Med* 1998;157:144–8
5. Bixler EO, Vgontzas AN, Lin H-M, *et al.* Prevalence of sleep-disordered breathing in women: effects of gender. *Am J Respir Crit Care Med* 2001;163:608–13
6. Bixler EO, Vgontzas AN, Lin HM, *et al.* Normal sleep and sleep stage patterns: effects of age, BMI and gender. *Sleep* 2003;26:A61
7. Vgontzas AN, Bixler EO, Wittman AM, *et al.* Middle-aged men show higher sensitivity of sleep to the arousing effects of corticotropin-releasing hormone than young men: clinical implications. *J Clin Endocrinol Metab* 2001;86:1489–95
8. Peterson AG, Young T Finn LA, *et al.* Objective and subjective sleep quality in a population-based cohort of pre-, peri, and postmenopausal women. *Sleep* 2002;25:A61
9. Erlik Y, Tataryn IV, Meldrum DR, *et al.* Association of waking episodes with menopausal hot flushes. *J Am Med Assoc* 1981;245:1741–4
10. Thomson J, Oswald I. Effect of oestrogen on the sleep, mood, and anxiety of menopausal women. *Br Med J* 1977;2:1317–39
11. Woodward S, Freedman RR. The thermoregulatory effects of menopausal hot flashes on sleep. *Sleep* 1994;17:497–501
12. Bixler EO, Vgontzas AN, Lin H-M, *et al.* Women and sleep related disorders. *Eur Respir Mon* 2003;25:204–18
13. Moe KE, Larsen LH, Vitiello MV, *et al.* Estrogen replacement therapy moderates the sleep disruption associated with nocturnal blood sampling. *Sleep* 2001;24:886–94
14. Manber R, Armitage R. Sex, steroids, and sleep: a review. *Sleep* 1999;22:540–55
15. Bixler EO, Vgontzas AN, Lin H-M, *et al.* Insomnia in Central Pennsylvania. *J Psychosom Res* 2002; 53:589–92
16. Benca RM. Sleep in psychiatric disorders. *Neurol Clin* 1996;14:739–64
17. Nowell PD, Buysse DJ, Reynolds CF, *et al.* Clinical factors contributing to the differential diagnosis of primary insomnia and insomnia related to a mental disorder. *Am J Psychiatry* 1997;154: 1412–16
18. Reynolds CF, Hoch CC, Buysse DJ, *et al.* Sleep in late-life recurrent depression: changes during early continuation therapy with nortriptyline. *Neuropsychopharmacology* 1991;5:85–96
19. Lee JH, Reynolds CF, Hoch CC, *et al.* Electroencephalographic sleep in recently remitted, elderly depressed patients in double-blind placebo-maintenance therapy. *Neuropsychopharmacology* 1993;8:143–50
20. Gillin JC, Wyatt RJ, Fram D, *et al.* The relationship between changes in REM sleep and clinical improvement in depressed patients treated with amitriptyline. *Psychopharmacology* 1978;59:267–72
21. Thase ME, Buysse DJ, Frank E, *et al.* Which depressed patients will respond to interpersonal

psychotherapy? The role of abnormal EEG sleep profiles. *Am J Psychiatry* 1997;154:502–9
22. Wehr TA, Turner EH, Shimada JM, *et al.* Treatment of rapidly cycling bipolar patient by using extended bed rest and darkness to stabilize the timing and duration of sleep. *Biol Psychiatry* 1998;43:822–8
23. Nagtegaal JE, Laurant MW, Kerkhof GA, *et al.* Effects of melatonin on the quality of life in patients with delayed sleep phase syndrome. *J Psychosom Res* 2000;48:45–50
24. Ford DE, Kamerow DB. Epidemiologic study of sleep disturbances and psychiatric disorders: an opportunity for prevention?. *J Am Med Assoc* 1989; 262:1479–84
25. Breslau N, Roth T, Rosenthal L, *et al.* Sleep disturbance and psychiatric disorders: a longitudinal epidemiological study of young adults. *Biol Psychiatry* 1996;39:411–18
26. Bixler EO, Kales A, Soldatos CR, *et al.* Prevalence of sleep disorders in the Los Angeles metropolitan area. *Am J Psychiatry* 1979;136:1257–62
27. Robins LN, Reiger DA, eds. *Psychiatric Disorders in America: The Epidemiologic Catchment Area Study.* New York: The Free Press, 1991
28. Lugaresi E, Cirignotta F, Zucconi M, *et al.* Good and poor sleepers: an epidemiological survey of the San Marino population. In Guilleminault C, Lugaresi E, eds. *Sleep/Wake Disorders: Natural History, Epidemiology, and Long-Term Evolution.* New York: Raven Press, 1983
29. Brugge KL, Kripke DF, Ancoli-Israel S, *et al.* The association of menopausal status and age with sleep disorders. *Sleep Res* 1989;18:208
30. Owens JF, Matthews KA. Sleep disturbance in healthy middle-aged women. *Maturitas* 1998;30: 41–50
31. Kravitz, HM, Ganz PA, Bromberger J, *et al.* Sleep difficulty in women at midlife: a community survey of sleep and menopausal transition. *Menopause* 2003;10:19–28
32. Hays J, Ockene JK, Brunner RL, *et al.* Effects of estrogen plus progestin on health-related quality of life. *N Engl J Med* 2003;348:1839–54
33. Young T, Palta M, Dempsey J, *et al.* The occurrence of sleep-disordered breathing among middle-aged adults. *N Engl J Med* 1993;328:1230–5
34. Redline S, Kump K, Tishler PV, *et al.* Gender differences in sleep disordered breathing in a community-based sample. *Am J Respir Crit Care Med* 1994;149:722–6
35. Tishler PV, Larkin EK, Schluchter MD, *et al.* Incidence of sleep-disordered breathing in an urban adult population: the relative importance of risk factors in the development of sleep-disordered breathing. *J Am Med Assoc* 2003;289:2230–7
36. Palmer LJ, Buxbaum SG, Larkin E, *et al.* A whole genome scan for obstructive sleep apnea and obesity. *Am J Hum Genet* 2003;72:340–50
37. Young T, Finn L, Austin D, *et al.* Menopausal status and sleep-disordered breathing in the Wisconsin Sleep Cohort Study. *Am J Respir Crit Care Med* 2003;167:1181–5
38. Shahar E, Redline S, Young T, *et al.* Hormone replacement therapy and sleep-disordered breathing. *Am J Respir Crit Care Med* 2003;167:1186–92
39. Vgontzas AN, Bixler EO, Chrousos GP. Metabolic disturbances in obesity versus sleep apnea: the importance of visceral obesity and insulin resistance. *J Intern Med* 2003;254:1–13
40. Vgontzas AN, Legro RS, Bixler EO, *et al.* Polycystic ovary syndrome is associated with obstructive sleep apnea and daytime sleepiness: role of insulin resistance. *J Clin Endocrinol Metab* 2001;86:517–20
41. Fogel RB, Pillar G, Pittman SD, *et al.* Increased prevalence of obstructive sleep apnea syndrome in patients with polycystic ovarian syndrome. *J Clin Endocrinol Metab* 2001;86:1175–8
42. Gopal M, Duntley S, Uhles H, *et al.* The role of obesity in the increased prevalence of obstructive sleep apnea syndrome in patients with polycystic ovarian syndrome. *Sleep Med* 2003;in press
43. Young T, Peppard P, Palta M, *et al.* Population-based study of sleep-disordered breathing as a risk factor for hypertension. *Arch Intern Med* 1997; 157:1746–52
44. Peppard PE, Young T, Palta M, *et al.* Prospective study on the association between sleep-disordered breathing and hypertension. *N Engl J Med* 2000; 342:1378–84
45. Nieto FJ, Young TB, Lind BK, *et al.* Association of sleep-disordered breathing, sleep apnea, and hypertension in a large community-based study. *J Am Med Assoc* 2000;283:1829–36
46. Bixler EO, Vgontzas AN, Lin H-M, *et al.* Association of hypertension and sleep disordered breathing. *Arch Intern Med* 2000;160:2289–95

Sex hormones and headache

11

R. E. Nappi, G. Sances, F. Facchinetti, C. Tassorelli, S. Detaddei, M. Loi, F. Polatti and G. Nappi

INTRODUCTION

The goddess Athena was born from the skull of Zeus, who was suffering from severe recurrent headaches. Greek legend clearly exemplifies the evidence that headache has been considered a 'female disease' since ancient times. Women consistently have a greater incidence of headache than men in the cases of both migraine and tension-type headaches, with a life-time prevalence of 91% and 69%, respectively. The medical literature has linked gender to migraine, not only because of its predominance in women from puberty to menopause, but also because neuroendocrine events associated with reproductive stages and hormonal interventions, such as oral contraception and hormone replacement therapy, can cause a deep change in the clinical pattern of migraine itself. Studies of migraine prevalence have suggested that 17% of women are affected, compared with 6% of men, and a striking increase in migraine incidence in women occurs between ages 10 and 12 years, when hormonal events typical of female puberty take place[1-3].

In this chapter, we attempt to discuss critically some of the issues supporting the close linkage between sex homones and migraine within the female brain, with particular reference to reproductive milestones and hormonal interventions. The impact of hormone replacement therapy (HRT) on the course of primary headaches during the postmenopausal years is discussed in detail.

SEX HORMONES AND MIGRAINE

Several authors have investigated the link between sex hormones and migraine from both pathophysiological and clinicoepidemiological standpoints, but there is still a lack of clear evidence relating to the role of hormonal fluctuations in precipitating migraine attacks. The picture seems less complicated when considering menstrual migraine (MM), even though the complexity of neuroendocrine events occurring at the time of menstruation leads to the conclusion that hormones alone are unlikely to be directly responsible for triggering attacks, and an interrelationship of various steroid-dependent mechanisms, involving several neuronal and vascular pathways, should be taken into account to explain the vulnerability of menstruating women to migraine[4]. In addition, the concept of migraine as a bio-behavioral disorder in which predisposing and stressful factors may contribute to its occurrence emphasizes the importance of peculiar female adaptive abilities, and further complicates the network of hormonal influences on biochemical, neuroendocrine, autonomic, emotional and behavioral responses leading to the onset of migraine attacks[5]. Sex-steroid changes may contribute to insult the steady state of the brain, which could be in turn more susceptible to maladaptation in vulnerable women. Indeed, biochemical and neuroendocrine variations observed during the menstrual cycle in asymptomatic healthy women appear to be more pronounced, or to show a different chrono-organization, in patients with menstrually related migraine, reflecting a condition which predisposes to migraine attacks[6]. In addition, a higher sensitivity to pain stimuli has been observed during the luteal phase of the menstrual cycle, which probably results from a reduction in inhibitory descending control of the spinal nociceptive flexion reflex[7].

A large amount of data concerning the role of gonadal steroid cyclicity in modulating several systems probably involved in the over representation of migraine in women are available, and may be summarized as follows[8,9].

Opioid system

When injected during the luteal phase, naloxone, a μ-receptor antagonist, induces a maximal rise of circulating luteinizing hormone (LH) levels, while the lowest response is observed in the early follicular phase. This is because hypothalamic opioidergic tone, apart from being involved in analgesia and in affective/behavioral disorders related to adaptive responses to environmental and internal stimuli, controls gonadotropin secretion and is under the influence of gonadal steroids, in particular estrogens during the menstrual cycle. Patients with menstrually related migraine display a failure of the naloxone-induced LH release in close proximity to the attack, similar to that found in patients with premenstrual syndrome, free of any headache.

Hypothalamus-pituitary-adrenal system

The influence of the reproductive system upon stress response guarantees the female body a better adaptation during emergency situations. Indeed, hypothalamus-pituitary-adrenal (HPA) function is variable over the ovarian cycle, and estrogens modulate the HPA axis sensitivity to stress. In MM patients, the cortisol response to high doses of naloxone is inhibited in the luteal phase, while it is normal during the follicular phase of the menstrual cycle. On the other hand, women with premenstrual syndrome exhibit an exaggerated plasma cortisol response to a corticotropin-releasing hormone bolus, compared with asymptomatic controls, which is independent of the comorbidity with MM.

Adrenergic system

Several lines of evidence support the concept that the basal tone of sympathetic activity and its receptor sensitivity are modulated by menstrual cyclicity. An excessive fluctuation of dopamine β-hydroxylase plasma levels, with lower values in the late luteal period, has been reported in patients suffering from MM. As mentioned above, MM patients are characterized by a transient, cyclic failure of endogenous opioid activity. The evidence that the inhibitory effect of the opioid system at the central level is prevented by α2-adrenergic receptor blockers suggests a possible interaction between opioids and catecholamines in the naloxone-induced endocrine effect. In women suffering from MM, clonidine stimulates β-endorphin and growth hormone release during the follicular phase, and reduces 3-methoxy-4-hydroxyphenylglycol (MHPG) and norepinephrine plasma levels. Clonidine reduces MHPG and norepinephrine concentrations also in the late luteal phase, but the release of β-endorphin and growth hormone in the same patients is lost, suggesting a postsynaptic α2-adrenoreceptor hyposensitivity during the premenstrual period. The possible defective integration between gonadal steroids and catecholamines at the central level is also supported by the evidence that controls and non-menstrual migraine sufferers show a marked luteal increase in platelet norepinephrine, which is absent in menstrual migraine sufferers who also show a platelet epinephrine decrease in the luteal phase.

Serotoninergic system

Platelet function and 5-hydroxytryptamine (5-HT) have been extensively studied in migraine sufferers. In normal women, intraplatelet 5-HT does not change during other phases of the menstrual cycle, but shows an increase at menstruation. On the other hand, platelet 5-HT increases significantly during the premenstrual and menstrual phases of the cycle in menstrual migraine sufferers. Moreover, in patients with MM the mean values of platelet 5-HT drop significantly during the attack, in comparison with those found in basal conditions. Serotonin and monoamine oxidase B (MAO-B) appear to be compartmentalized together in neurons and platelets, and several studies suggest that MAO-B platelet activity is a good indicator of central serotoninergic activity. In addition, the endocrine milieu may play some role in the non-genomic regulation of MAO-B activity. Recent data suggest that in MM patients there could be a hypersensitivity of the serotoninergic system to hormonal modulation, since MAO-B activity is significantly increased in the luteal phase more than in asymptomatic control women.

Prostaglandins

There is a three-fold increase in prostaglandin levels in the uterine endometrium from the follicular to the luteal phase, with a further increase during menstruation, which stimulates uterine contractions. Endometrial prostaglandins are known to be increased in women with either dysmenorrhea or MM, and it is also known that plasma levels of some prostaglandins vary according to the phase of the menstrual cycle and during the migraine attack. In addition, prostaglandins modulate descending norepinephrine pain-control systems as well as the release of 5-HT by platelets or serotoninergic neurons in response to ischemic stimuli in the brain, a phenomenon under estrogenic control which probably contributes to the pathogenesis of MM. As well as platelet prostaglandins and serotoninergic metabolism, which are altered during the luteal phase of the cycle in MM, a direct involvement of other aspects of platelet function, such as aggregation, may be postulated, because also a change in platelet homeostasis, evident mainly in the luteal phase, has been found in MM.

Prolactin

Dopamine antagonists produce enhanced prolactin release throughout the luteal phase in all women, and during the entire menstrual cycle in women suffering from MM, even though basal plasma prolactin levels remain in the normal range in MM during the menstrual cycle. In addition, thyroid-releasing hormone (TRH) infusion enhances prolactin release, but not thyroid-stimulating hormone (TSH), during a migraine attack, and a supersensitivity of the dopaminergic system coupled to a serotoninergic hyperfunction has been postulated to explain this endocrine feature.

Melatonin

Nocturnal urinary melatonin excretion decreases in patients suffering from migraine in all phases of the menstrual cycle, and the normal rise in urinary melatonin excretion during the luteal phase is less evident in migraine sufferers. The significance of such subtle changes is not fully established, but it can be hypothesized that an impairment of melatonin function is related to nociceptive function, controlling circadian fluctuation of the pain threshold.

Nitric oxide

The pivotal role of nitric oxide in migraine pain and the outstanding observation that there is an estrogen-mediated enhancement of the activity and/or expression of endothelial nitric oxide synthase open a new field of investigation in the pathogenesis of MM. Indeed, it has recently been demonstrated that there is overactivation in the platelet arginine–nitric oxide pathway during the luteal phase of the cycle in women affected by MM. On the other hand, nitroglycerine, an organic nitrate that has been used in the treatment of cardiac diseases for over a century, consistently induces a specific headache attack in patients suffering from migraine. Preliminary data from our laboratory show that there is sexually dimorphic neuronal activation induced by systemic nitroglycerine injection, supporting the idea that estrogens significantly affect the (rat) brain structures implicated in the pathophysiology of migraine.

REPRODUCTIVE MILESTONES AND MIGRAINE

Hormonal milestones in reproductive life such as menarche, pregnancy and menopause often modulate the history of migraine in women[10]. Migraine with onset at menarche frequently develops a menstrual periodicity over the years, and pregnancy and menopause affect migraine positively. The reason may be related to the estrogen hypothesis, since the onset of menses brings cyclic changes in hormonal levels, pregnancy causes rising non-cyclic levels, while menopause results in declining non-cyclic levels. Indeed, over the centuries, 'natural' hormonal remedies against migraine, not considered standard practice, have been 'to be always pregnant' and 'to wait for the menopause'. This poor destiny for millions of women is supported by some studies from the literature, which are, however, limited, aged and usually retrospective[11].

The meaning of menstrual migraine (MM) is controversial, as elegantly revised by MacGregor in a recent report[12]. Indeed, she suggested that the definition of 'true' MM should be restricted to attacks starting exclusively on or within ± 2 days of cycle day 1, and related to estrogen withdrawal, as proposed by Sommerville several years ago[13]. The lack of unique criteria explains the high discrepancy in the prevalence of MM, which ranges from 4 to 73%. This is because the link between the menstrual cycle and migraine is not limited to menstruation, but potential mechanisms triggering hormone-related headaches are probably variable according to the complexity of the neuroendocrine control of reproductive function. In addition, the presence of menstrually related disorders, such as late luteal phase dysphoric disorder and dysmenorrhea, further complicates the picture. Indeed, the finding that a period of several days of exposure to high estrogen levels is necessary before estrogen withdrawal can result in migraine explains very well the so-called 'true' MM, but does not shed light on why women are prone to develop migraine throughout the entire menstrual cycle, pre- and post-menstrually and at the time of ovulation[14]. On the other hand, many clinicians are under the impression that migraine attacks related to menses are more severe, long-lasting and refractory to both acute and prophylactic treatment[15]. We have recently confirmed that in menstrually related migraine, peri-menstrual attacks are longer and less responsive to acute attack treatment than non-menstrual attacks (unpublished data).

As far as the pattern of migraine during pregnancy is concerned, 60–70% of women typically improve, in particular those affected by MM, probably because of the lack of hormonal fluctuations and/or the analgesic effects of β-endorphin which often increases in pregnancy. Conversely, migraine may occur for the first time in pregnancy or, if pre-existing, may worsen, particularly during the first trimester. However, most women become migraine-free later in pregnancy. Some women have no change in their headache pattern in pregnancy, in spite of the steady elevation in plasma estrogen levels. Following delivery, which is associated with a dramatic estrogen decline, a return of migraine to pre-pregnancy patterns is common, while sometimes migraine may start during the postpartum period or may worsen in parallel with successive pregnancies[2,16–20]. A recent prospective study that waits to be confirmed by data collected in a larger population of women reported that migraine sufferers showed an increase in attacks during the third trimester of gestation[21]. We have recently conducted a prospective study demonstrating that migraine improved in 46.8% of sufferers during the first trimester, in 83.0% during the second and in 87.2% during the third, with complete remission in 10.6%, 53.2% and 78.7% of the women, respectively. Migraine recurred during the first week after childbirth in 34.0% of the women and during the first month in 55.3%. In addition, we identified certain risk factors for lack of improvement of migraine during the first and third trimesters of pregnancy, such as the presence of menstrually related migraine before pregnancy. In addition, second-trimester hyperemesis, and a pathological pregnancy course, were associated with a lack of headache improvement in the second trimester. Bottle-feeding was found to be associated with migraine recurrence during the puerperium[22].

Nowadays, a bidirectional flow of information between neurologists and gynecologists is mandatory when facing the problem of migraine, because of the larger amount of hormonal tools available to manipulate fertility and reproductive aging in women. Indeed, common drugs from gynecological practice can influence the natural history of the disease, and in some cases can be proposed even in the treatment of migraine. Conflicting results on the use of hormonal preparations and migraine are not related only to the clinical setting, but mainly to the multitude of pharmacological combinations, and to their biochemical properties, dosages and routes of administration[23,24]. In a gynecological setting, headache is the most common side-effect of oral contraceptives, but only studies from neurological and migraine clinics have clearly documented an increased incidence and severity of migraine in women who use oral contraceptives and are established migraine sufferers. In particular, a trend towards an increased incidence of attacks during the drug-free interval of the cycle may be present, and hormones may contribute to the occurrence of neurological symptoms. Oral contraceptives may trigger the first migraine attack, more often in women with a family history of migraine, and such new onset may occur in the early cycles of use or even after prolonged use. Sometimes no improvement may be observed following discontinuation of treatment, while in some women with a history of intractable migraine the pill may be proposed as an attempt to reduce the frequency of attacks. The mechanisms whereby manipulation of gonadal steroids influence migraine are still unknown, but the abrupt fall in plasma estrogen levels just before menstruation is a well-known critical factor explaining why women suffer especially in the drug-free week. Such estrogen-withdrawal headache may be concomitant with other headache attacks during the taking of the pill, supporting the hypothesis that treatment strategies should be aimed at preventing not only a fall in plasma estrogen levels at the time of menstruation but also substantial fluctuations in endogenous plasma estrogen levels throughout the entire menstrual cycle. On the other hand, the notion that oral contraceptive use and migraine might interact in predisposing young women to ischemic stroke has to be kept in mind when prescribing the pill or any hormonal supplementations, in order to choose the lowest effective dose of synthetic estrogens and to stop the treatment if migraine changes from common (without aura) to classical (with aura)[25-27]. Some hormonal tricks, such as tricycling the pill, altering the ratio of estrogens to progestins, blocking the menstrual cycle at the hypothalamus-pituitary level by the use of gonadotropin-releasing hormone (GnRH) analogs associated with so-called 'add-back therapy', interfering with the menstrual cycle by using danazol, an androgen derivative, tamoxifen, an anti-estrogen, or bromocriptine, a dopamine receptor agonist which inhibits prolactin release, or using estrogen supplementation during the pill-free week, have been proposed to relieve migraine[8]. In our experience, transdermal estradiol supplementation during the pill-free interval of the cycle can be effective in ameliorating not only the intensity of the migraine attack but also its response to unsuccessful treatments, confirming previous data obtained using percutaneous estradiol gel applied just before and throughout menses (unpublished data).

COURSE OF PRIMARY HEADACHES AT MENOPAUSE AND DURING HORMONE REPLACEMENT THERAPY

Migraine incidence generally decreases with advancing age, and at the time of the menopause may either regress or worsen. Indeed, the menopause has a variable effect on migraine depending on the neuroendocrine adjustment to the new hormonal environment, involving mainly the adrenergic and opioidergic pathways. Erratic estrogen secretion and unbalanced estrogen exposure due to anovulatory cycles and/or progesterone deficiency may worsen or even initiate migraine during the perimenopausal period, and such endocrine aberrations often precede by several years the stable and low plasma levels of gonadal steroids typical of the postmenopausal period. In addition, the intensity of climacteric symptomatology such as hot flushes, palpitations, night sweats, disturbed sleep, negative emotions, etc. may contribute more or less to the triggering or aggravation of migraine attacks[28].

MacGregor has recently reported that the perimenopausal years are extremely critical for first consultations, meaning that migraine becomes a problem for women later in fertile life[29]. On the other hand, an indirect clue of the low prevalence of migraine at the menopause emerged from a retrospective study indicating that only about 12%, of 1300 women suffering from migraine, referred to a headache center during the postmenopausal years[10].

The controversy about the actual role played by menopause in the natural history of migraine may also be ascribed to the observation that neurologists and gynecologists have often carried out studies from different points of view. Indeed, migraine sufferers referred to headache centers are not representative of the general population, and are probably those who worsen with menopause, while patients recruited in menopause clinics may lack accurate diagnostic criteria, since the 'headache' symptom is commonly included in the majority of scales assessing menopausal well-being[30]. We reported that the postmenopausal course of headache with a premenopausal onset differed according to the type of headache and type of menopause. While migraine improved in almost two-thirds of cases, tension-type headache worsened or was unchanged in 70% of cases. On the other hand, women who underwent a physiological menopause experienced a more favorable course of migraine than women who underwent a surgical menopause with bilateral oophorectomy, suggesting the abrupt estrogen withdrawal to be a well-defined aggravating factor of migraine, probably coupled to the emotional impact of hysterectomy[31].

As far as HRT at the time of the menopause is concerned, very few controlled studies have been conducted in recent times. In clinical practice, it is very common to observe a benefit from HRT when women are in the perimenopausal period because the treatment prevents erratic hormonal secretion, particularly when stable plasma estrogen levels are provided by the use of a continuous regimen. On the other hand, the cyclic administration of progestins, which is mandatory in non-hysterectomized women, may induce migraine attacks[32]. In these cases, on the basis of their clinical experience, Silberstein and Merriam suggested the use of a progestin with low androgenic properties, natural progesterone or even a combined estrogen-progestin continuous therapy[24]. MacGregor, in a preliminary uncontrolled retrospective study, suggested that transdermal estradiol was associated with more improvement in migraine than oral conjugated estrogens[33]. In addition, high doses of exogenous estrogens may induce migraine with aura, as happens during pregnancy and hormonal contraception[34]. Hodson and colleagues found that headache is a substantial problem at the menopause and in HRT users, since 259 women out of 1000 reported a worsening of the number of attacks. In addition, by using logistic regression models, the same authors showed reported history of migraine and more difficulty coping with stress to be strong predictors for worse headache at menopause and with HRT[35].

In a prospective study recently conducted by our group, we found that HRT significantly affects the course of migraine, but not of episodic tension-type headache, in postmenopausal women[36]. This observation fits with the common knowledge that migraine is more sensitive to hormones in comparison with tension-type headache, which is probably more affected by psychological distress and coping strategies[37]. Moreover, it was of paramount interest to observe different effects exerted by the different routes of administration of HRT on the course of migraine. In particular, the oral route of administration significantly worsened head pain already at the 3rd month of treatment. Both frequency of attacks ($F = 8.5; p < 0.001$) and days with headache ($F = 6.9; p < 0.001$) increased significantly during HRT in the subgroup taking an oral formulation. In contrast, no changes in the same parameters were found in the group receiving transdermal treatment. Furthermore, while severity of migraine was unaffected by HRT, analgesic consumption was significantly increased in the subgroup on oral treatment ($F = 6.3; p = 0.001$)[36]. Our results allowed the suggestion that the best method of hormonal replacement for a postmenopausal woman suffering from migraine, even preserving the physiological pattern of ovarian hormones, is the transdermal route of estrogen administration. Indeed, in a recent prospective study, we confirmed that the oral route of HRT administration progressively increased attack frequency (from 2.2 ± 1.0 to 3.8 ± 1.3, $p < 0.001$), days with headache (from 3.4 ± 1.3 to 4.9 ± 1.9, $p < 0.001$) and analgesic consumption (from 3.4 ± 1.3 to 5.6 ± 2.2, $p < 0.001$) after 6 months. However, the increase in number of days with headache and number of analgesics used was smaller in the group receiving the continuous combined regimen than in the other two groups[38].

CONCLUSION

The close linkage between headaches and sex steroids implies a multidisciplinary approach to improving the clinical management of such a common women's disease. Rigorous diagnosis and the early identification of hormone-sensitive headaches form the basis of appropriate treatment during the reproductive life span. Further studies are need to clarify the impact of hormonal manipulations on the clinical expression of headaches.

References

1. Lipton RB, Stewart WF. Migraine in the United States: a review of epidemiology and health care use. *Neurology* 1993;43:S6–10
2. Rasmussen BK. Migraine and tension-type headache in a general population: precipitating factors, female hormones, sleep pattern and relation to lifestyle. *Pain* 1993;53:65–72
3. Mortimer MJ, Kay J, Jaron A. Childhood migraine in general practice: clinical features and characteristics. *Cephalalgia* 1992;12:238–43
4. MacGregor EA. Menstruation, sex hormones, and migraine. *Neurol Clin* 1997;15:125–41
5. Nappi G, Costa A, Tassorelli C, *et al.* Migraine as a complex disease: heterogeneity, comorbidity and genotype–phenotype interactions. *Funct Neurol* 2000;15:87–93
6. Silberstein SD. The role of sex hormones in headache. *Neurology* 1992;42:37–42
7. Tassorelli C, Sandrini G, Proietti Cecchini A, *et al.* Changes in nociceptive flexion reflex threshold across the menstrual cycle in healthy women. *Psychosom Med* 2002;64:621–6
8. Nappi RE, Veneroni F, Chiapparini I, *et al.* Gonadal hormones and migraine: a tight bondage within the female brain. *Semin Headache Manage* 1999;4:11–15
9. Fioroni L, Martignoni E, Facchinetti F. Changes of neuroendocrine axes in patients with menstrual migraine. *Cephalalgia* 1995;15:297–300
10. Granella F, Sances G, Zanferrari C, *et al.* Migraine without aura and reproductive like events: a clinical epidemiological study in 1300 women. *Headache* 1993;33:385–9
11. Massiou H, Bousser M-G. Influence of female hormones on migraine. In Olesen J, Tfelt-Hansen P, Welch KMA, eds. *The Headache*, 2nd edn. Philadelphia: Lippincott Williams & Wilkins, 2000:261–7
12. MacGregor A. Migraine associated with menstruation. *Funct Neurol* 2000;15:143–53
13. Sommerville BW. Estrogen-withdrawal migraine. *Neurology* 1975;25:239–44
14. Nappi G, Facchinetti F, Rossi F, eds. Headache and menstrually related disorders: in search of a consensus. *Cephalalgia* 1997;17(Suppl 20)
15. Silberstein SD, Lipton RB, Goadsby PJ. *Headache in Clinical Practice.* Oxford: Isis Medical Media, 1998:61–90
16. Callaghan N. The migraine syndrome in pregnancy. *Neurology* 1968;18:197–201
17. Somerville BW. A study of migraine in pregnancy. *Neurology* 1972;22:824–8
18. Cupini LM, Matteis M, Troisi E, *et al.* Sex-hormone-related events in migrainous females. A clinical comparative study between migraine with aura and migraine without aura. *Cephalalgia* 1995;15:140–4
19. Maggioni F, Alessi C, Maggino T, *et al.* Headache during pregnancy. *Cephalalgia* 1997;17:765–9
20. Granella F, Sances G, Pucci E, *et al.* Migraine with aura and reproductive life events: a case control study. *Cephalalgia* 2000;20:701–7
21. Scharff L, Marcus DA, Turk DC. Headache during pregnancy and in the postpartum: a prospective study. *Headache* 1997;37:203–10
22. Sances G, Granella F, Nappi RE, *et al.* Course of migraine during pregnancy and postpartum. A prospective study. *Cephalalgia* 2003;23:197–205
23. Kudrow L. The relationship of headache frequency to hormone use in migraine. *Headache* 1975;15:36–40
24. Silberstein SD, Merriam GR. Estrogens, progestins and headache. *Neurology* 1991;41:786–93
25. MacGregor EA, de Lignieres B. The place of combined oral contraceptives in contraception. *Cephalalgia* 2000;20:157–63
26. Bousser MG, Conard J, Kittner S, *et al.* Recommendations on the risk of ischaemic stroke associated with use of combined oral contraceptives and hormone replacement therapy in women with migraine. The International Headache Society Task Force on Combined Oral Contraceptives and Hormone Replacement Therapy. *Cephalalgia* 2000;20:155–6

27. Massiou H, MacGregor EA. Evolution and treatment of migraine with oral contraceptives. *Cephalalgia* 2000;20:170–4
28. Fettes I. Migraine in the menopause. *Neurology* 1999;53:S29–33
29. MacGregor A. Gynecological aspects of migraine. *Rev Contemp Pharmacother* 2000;11:75–90
30. MacGregor EA, Barnes D. Migraine in a specialist menopause clinic. *Climacteric* 1999;2:218–23
31. Neri I, Granella F, Nappi RE, *et al.* Characteristics of headache at menopause: a clinico-epidemiological study. *Maturitas* 1993;17:31–7
32. de Lignieres B, MacGregor EA. Risks and benefits of hormone replacement therapy. *Cephalalgia* 2000; 20:164–9
33. MacGregor EA. Effect of oral and transdermal estrogen replacement on migraine. *Cephalalgia* 1999;19:124–5
34. MacGregor EA. Estrogen replacement and migraine aura. *Headache* 1999;39:674–8
35. Hodson J, Thompson J, Al-Azzawi F. Headache at menopause and in hormone replacement therapy users. *Climacteric* 2000;3:119–24
36. Nappi RE, Cagnacci A, Granella F, *et al.* Course of primary headaches during hormone replacement therapy. *Maturitas* 2001;38:157–63
37. Bono G, Neri, I, Granella F, *et al.* Factors associated with pain complaints in a clinical sample of postmenopausal women. *J Psychosom Obstet Gynecol* 1995;16:117–21
38. Facchinetti F, Nappi RE, Tirelli A, *et al.* Hormone supplementation differently affects migraine in postmenopausal women. *Headache* 2002;42: 924–9

Gender differences in affective disorders: a brief review

12

J. Angst and A. Gamma

GENDER AND DEPRESSION

There is no controversy about a preponderance of depressive women over men in the community: the cross-national epidemiological analysis of Weissman and colleagues[1] demonstrated clearly that women showed higher rates of depression than men across nine countries, comprising approximately 38 000 community subjects. Also, the World Health Organization (WHO) monograph of Picinelli and associates[2], reviewing the epidemiological literature on gender differences, stated clearly: 'Although prevalence rates of major depression and dysthymia vary by country, a consistent finding is that rates are higher in females compared to males, with about a twofold gender difference on average.' The review also concluded that the gender difference is not due to case definition, measurements, recall bias or differential mortality.

The preponderance of women, also confirmed by the reviews of Bebbington[3] and Kessler[4,5], was found not only in major depression and dysthymia but also in minor depression[6] and recurrent brief depression[7]. Finally, this is also true for the number of reported depressive symptoms[6].

Data from the Netherlands Mental Health Survey and Incidence Study (NEMESIS) in the community ($n = 7076$) are in line with the general knowledge; it found a 1-month prevalence of Depression Scale-III-Revised (DSM-III-R) major depression in 1.9% of men and 5.0% of women (lifetime prevalence rates 10.9% and 20.1%, respectively); dysthymia was found over lifetime in 3.8% of men and 8.9% of women[8].

Conclusion

Depression is twice as common among women than among men. O'Keane[9] recently stated: 'This is a universal finding and thus cannot be explained by socio-political factors alone . . .'. Nonetheless, not much is known about the gender difference in relation to age, an issue dealt with below.

GENDER AND BIPOLAR DISORDERS

In sharp contrast with the above observations about depression, there is evidence for a more or less equal distribution of bipolar disorders between the sexes[5]. Historically, this is not new: the dichotomy between depression and bipolar disorder, which was reintroduced in 1966, was partially founded on an equal morbidity risk for mood disorders among male and female relatives of bipolar patients, in contrast with relatives of depressive patients, where affected females prevailed strongly[10].

In the Epidemiologic Catchment Area (ECA) Study, the 1-year prevalence rate of manic episodes was 0.5% for men and 0.7% for women (lifetime prevalence rates 0.7% in men and 0.9% in women). This study also provided data on bipolar I disorder (lifetime prevalence: men 0.7%, women 0.9%) and bipolar II disorder (men 0.4%, women 0.5%) suggesting a small gender difference[11]. More important, a cross-national comparison of seven countries, including the ECA data, found no gender difference in prevalence rates of bipolar disorders[1]. The large National Comorbidity Survey (NCS) in the USA identified a lifetime prevalence of 1.6% for manic episodes among males and 1.7% among females[12]. A longitudinal study of a young population sample in Munich ($n = 4263$) found higher rates of bipolar I and bipolar II disorders among females (BP-I 1.7%,

BP-II 0.7%) than among males (BP-I 1.1%, BP-II 0.2%)[13]. The NEMESIS study in The Netherlands found a lifetime prevalence for bipolar disorders in 1.6% of men and 2.2% of women; most of them (41 of 50) were bipolar I cases[14]. The following 1-month prevalence rates were determined: males 0.4%, females 0.8%[8]. A Hungarian study ($n = 2953$) found equal lifetime rates by gender for hypomania and bipolar II disorders and a mild gender difference in bipolar I disorders (males 1.3%, females 1.6%)[15].

Conclusion

There is no clear evidence for a gender difference in bipolar I and bipolar II disorders.

WHY IS FURTHER EPIDEMIOLOGICAL RESEARCH ON GENDER DIFFERENCES NECESSARY?

The findings mentioned above are well established, but may be too global and insufficient for further research into the causes of gender differences. Prior to any speculations and hypotheses about causes of the female preponderance, it is necessary to analyze carefully the gender distribution among subtypes of mood disorders, including subgroups of bipolar disorders, on the basis of large community and clinical studies.

Depression is not a homogeneous syndrome, which raises serious methodological problems. Mood disorders comprise a wide range of manifestations varying in severity (major, minor), symptomatology (melancholic versus atypical depression), chronicity (minor depression versus dysthymia) and bipolarity (bipolar I, bipolar II, minor bipolar disorders versus cyclothymia). We must examine carefully whether the gender ratios vary between these subgroups to any considerable extent. Depression may be heterogeneous from another point of view: atypical depression, which is characterized by mood reactivity, rejection sensitivity, overeating, oversleeping and leaden paralysis, seems to prevail very strongly among women[16]. Most epidemiological studies have provided little data on just a few of these subgroups, and breaking down the samples by gender, age and typology of mood disorders usually results in rather small inconclusive cell frequencies.

Most important is that the data on bipolar disorders may be seriously flawed, because definitions of hypomania given by the currently used diagnostic manuals may be inadequate, and the instruments for its assessment invalid[17]. There is actually much controversy about the definition of hypomania, which is considered by experts to be too strict as given by DSM-IV and ICD-10 criteria[18]. Modern definitions shift up to 50% of all depressives into the bipolar spectrum[19]. Therefore, depression may be overdiagnosed to a major extent. Hypomania may be grossly underdiagnosed by the currently used diagnostic instruments, focusing in their stem questions too strongly on mood symptoms and omitting hypomanic overactivity; in addition, hypomanics usually feel well, not ill, and may not answer questions focusing on psychopathology[20].

NEW RESEARCH TRENDS AND FINDINGS ON GENDER DIFFERENCES IN DEPRESSION

Is the gender difference of depression dependent on women's reproductive age?

Little is known about gender differences of depression across the life cycle. Jorm[21] and Bebbington and colleagues[22] hypothesized that the high gender ratio female/male of depression would be restricted to the period of female fertility and, later, even reverse. The hypothesis of Bebbington was built on solid data from the National Survey of Psychiatric Morbidity in Great Britain ($n = 9792$). The study showed a preponderance of depression among women only up to age 44; the gender ratio became almost equal in the age group 45–54 years and reversed into a preponderance of male depression in the group of 55–64 years (Figure 1). Unfortunately, this exciting finding could not be reproduced. In contrast with the British National Survey there was no reversal of gender ratio in the large and representative epidemiological depression in Europe (EURODEP) study ($n = 78\,458$), which included six European countries[23,24]. Major depressive episodes occurred twice as often among

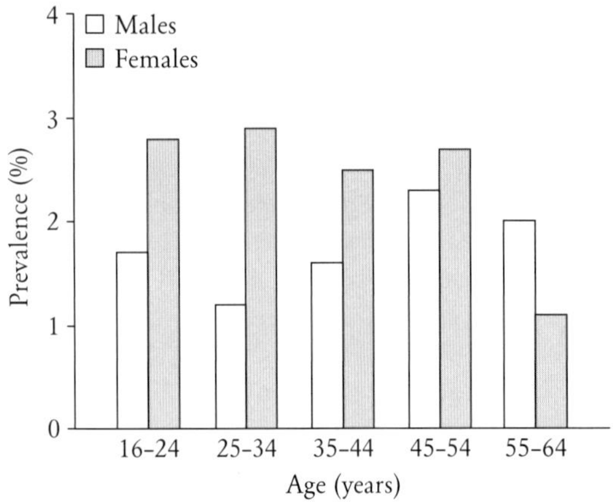

Figure 1 Reversal of sex differences in depression in older age: prevalence of depressive episodes according to age group. Reproduced from Bebbington PE, Dunn G, Jenkins R, Lewis G, Brugha T, Farnell M, Meltzer H. The influence of age and sex on the prevalence of depressive conditions: report from the National Survey of Psychiatric Morbidity. *Psychol Med* 1988;28:9–19[22], with permission from Cambridge University Press

women than among men across all age groups, also in the elderly. In contrast with this, the 6-month prevalence rate of minor depression was only slightly higher among women than among men, but again there was no change with increasing age[25]. Both findings were consistently present across all six countries.

Is there a peak of depression around the menopause?

In the EURODEP study the highest 6-month prevalence rate of major depression was present in the age group 45–54 years, and this period of course coincides with the menopause. But the finding was present to the same extent in women and men. More detailed ongoing analyses show that the peak of prevalence around the age of 50 is present for all diagnostic depressive symptoms and also for depression-induced impairment; but again there is no clear gender difference[26]. The existence of a special subtype of menopausal psychosis (severe depression or schizophrenia) was also rejected by Bleuler in his large monograph on endocrinological psychiatry, although he clearly described emotional symptoms[27].

Is severity of depression associated with gender difference?

The answer to this question is 'Yes'. From the NCS study[6] and from the EURODEP study there is convincing evidence for a correlation between severity of depression, measured by sum of the nine criterial symptoms, and gender.

Figure 2 demonstrates the small gender difference in minor compared with major depression. Furthermore, in community studies, compared with cases with major depression alone, women prevailed strongly among patients with more than one diagnosis of depression (double depression = major depression (MD) + dysthymia (DYST); combined depression = MD + recurrent brief depression (RBD); triple depression = (MD + DYST + RBD)[28].

Is atypical depression mainly a form of female depression?

There are no sound epidemiological data yet available on atypical depression. In the epidemiological Zurich cohort study, a slightly modified definition of atypical depression was developed (not including the hierarchical position of the symptom 'mood reactivity'), and it could be demonstrated that atypical major depressive episodes (MDE) showed about a four-fold higher prevalence rate than non-atypical syndromes. This was true whether we applied DSM-IV criteria or Zurich criteria for atypical depression[16]. The lifetime prevalence rates for MDE at the age of 35 were as follows: atypical MDE: men 1.6%, women 6.3%, ratio female/male 3.94; non-atypical MDE: men 11.3%, women 13.1%, ratio female/male 1.16. Figure 3 demonstrates that one-third of women with MDE suffered from atypical MDE with a high gender ratio, and that the gender ratio of non-atypical MDE was very low. These data require replication by another study, but raise interesting questions about the causes of gender differences of depression. In this context one should consider that other authors have described symptoms of atypical depression among twins[29] and relatives[30], suggesting that genetic factors may be involved.

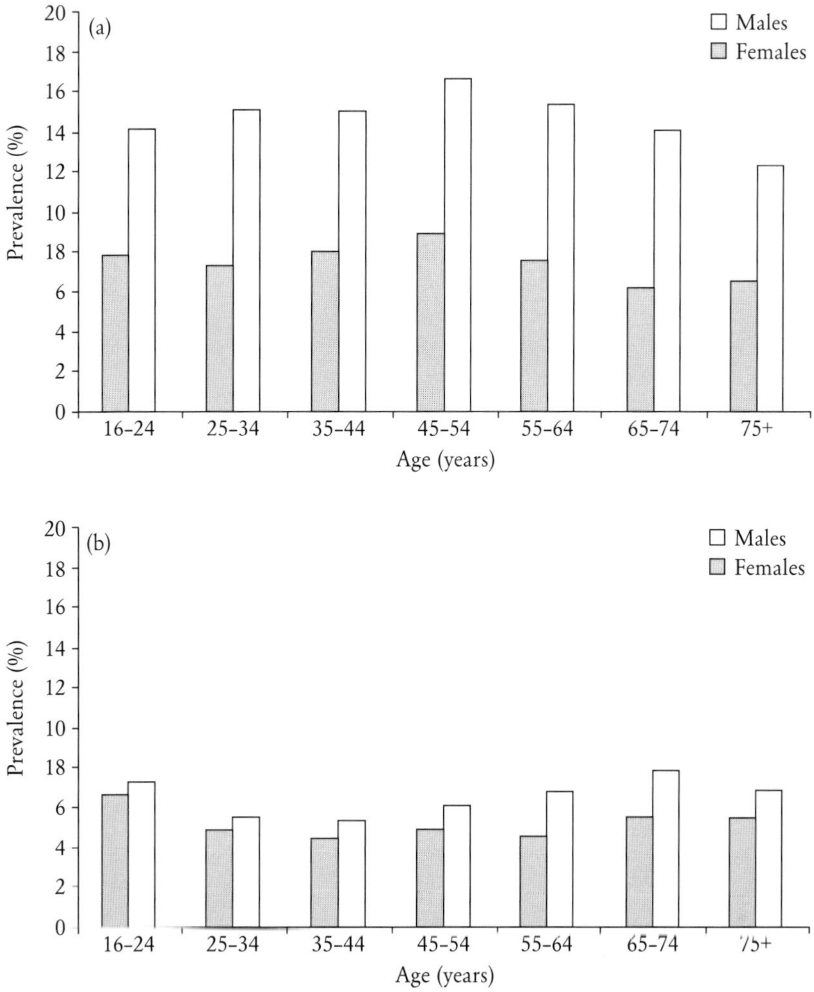

Figure 2 Gender-specifc prevalence rates of (a) major and (b) minor depression for different age groups. Reproduced from Angst J, Gamma A, Gastpar M, Lépine J P, Mendlewicz J, Tylee A. Gender differences in depression. Epidemiological findings from European DEPRES I and II studies. *Eur Arch Psychiatr Clin Neurosci* 2002;252:201–9[25], with permission from Steuinkopf Verlag

NEW RESEARCH TRENDS AND FINDINGS ON GENDER DIFFERENCES IN BIPOLAR SPECTRUM DISORDERS

As mentioned above, published epidemiological findings on bipolar II disorders may be problematic owing to invalid case definition.

In this context, we present new findings of the Zurich cohort study defining hypomania in a 'soft' way by the presence of hypomanic symptoms[20]. Diagnosis of bipolar II disorders required the presence of a major depressive episode and hypomanic symptoms. Figure 4 shows that the odds ratio (OR) of the gender difference was 1.7 for MDE; the dichotomy of MDE into unipolar major depression (UP) and bipolar II disorder gave an OR of 2.0 for UP and 1.5 for BP-II disorders. The finding on BP-II disorders is interesting. It suggests that the gender ratio in BP-II disorders may take an intermediate position (OR = 1.5) between depression (OR = 2.0) and BP-I disorder (OR according to the literature of 1.0). More important is the high prevalence rate of bipolar II disorders, which comes close to the

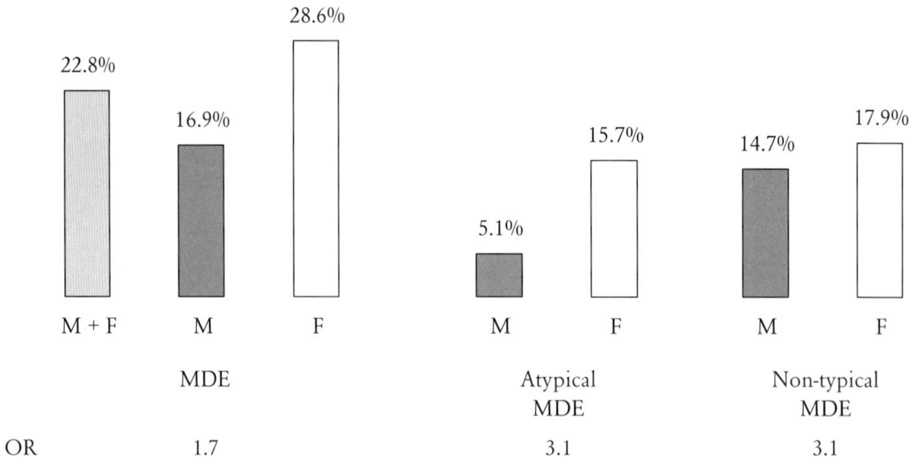

Figure 3 Gender differences in atypical versus non-atypical major depressive episodes (MDE): prevalence rates and odds ratios (OR). M, males; F, females

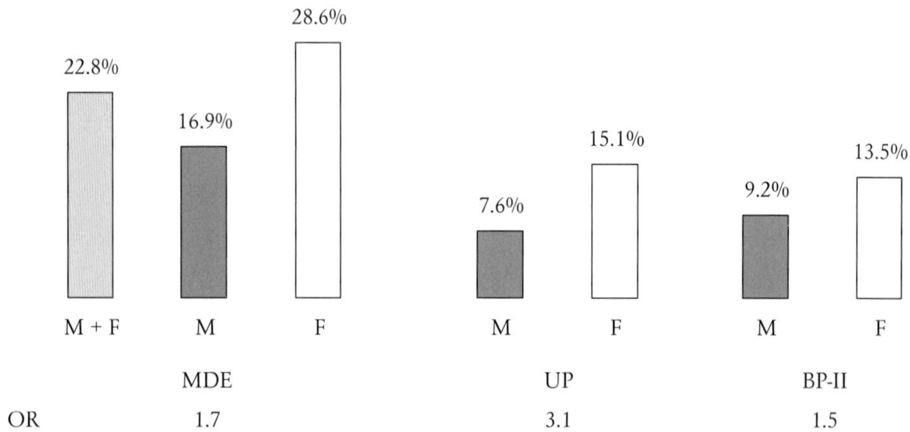

Figure 4 Gender differences in unipolar (UP) versus bipolar II (BP-II) major depressive episodes (MDE): prevalence rates and odds ratios (OR). M, males; F, females

prevalence of unipolar major depression. Women represented 58.4% of BP-II ($n = 89$) disorders, 59.0% ($n = 59$) of minor bipolar disorders and 67.0% of UP ($n = 101$). Men suffered significantly more than women from a hypomanic syndrome with social consequences (66.3% men, gender ratio female/male 0.5). This finding suggests the hypothesis that men may be more prevalent among cases with M/Md (pure mania (M) or mania + minor depression (Md)), and that bipolar I disorder would take an intermediate position in gender ratio between Md and bipolar II disorder.

CONCLUSIONS

Gender differences in affective disorders are universally present across cultures, and raise major questions about their origins. The overall statement that major depression is about two-fold more prevalent in women is correct, but probably not very helpful for research into its causation. Depression is a heterogeneous syndrome: atypical depression is about four-fold more common among women than among men, and seems to explain a large proportion of the gender difference in depression. Genetic research in this area seems promising. New research into subgroups of depression suggests the hypothesis of a continuous distribution of the gender ratio of affective disorders, with a maximum in atypical depression and a decrease by severity from major depressive disorder to minor depression.

Research into gender differences in bipolar disorders is less advanced, and hampered by major unsolved methodological problems in its assessment and definition. A gender difference has not been found to date, although is perhaps present in subgroups. Within the bipolar spectrum an elevated gender ratio may be present in bipolar II disorder, followed by bipolar I disorder with major mania and major depression and bipolar I disorder with a preponderance of mania. Mania and hypomania without a diagnosis of depression seem to be more common among males than among females.

References

1. Weissman MM, Bland RC, Canino GJ, *et al.* Cross-national epidemiology of major depression and bipolar disorder. *J Am Med Assoc* 1996;276:293–9
2. Piccinelli M, Gomez Homen F, Tansella M. *Gender Differences in the Epidemiology of Affective Disorders and Schizophrenia*. Geneva: World Health Organization, 1997
3. Bebbington PE. Sex and depression [Editorial]. *Psychol Med* 1998;28:1–8
4. Kessler RC. Gender differences in major depression. Epidemiological findings. In Frank E, ed. *Gender and its Effects on Psychopathology*. Washington, DC: American Psychiatric Press, 1999:61–84
5. Kessler RC. Gender differences in the prevalence and correlates of mood disorders in the general population. In Steiner M, Yonkers KA, Eriksson E, eds. *Mood Disorders in Women*. London: Martin Dunitz, 2000:15–33
6. Kessler RC, Zhao S, Blazer DG, Swartz M. Prevalence, correlates, and course of minor depression and major depression in the National Comorbidity Survey. *J Affect Disord* 1997;45:19–30
7. Ernst C, Angst J. The Zurich Study: XII. Sex differences in depression. Evidence from longitudinal epidemiological data. *Eur Arch Psychiatry Clin Neurosci* 1992;241:222–30
8. Bijl RV, van Zessen G, Ravelli A. Psychiatrische morbiditeit onder volwassenen in Nederland: het NEMESIS-onderzoek. II. Prevalentie van psychiatrische stoornissen. *Ned Tijdschr Geneeskd* 1997; 141:2453–60
9. O'Keane V. Unipolar depression in women. In Steiner M, Yonkers KA, Eriksson E, eds. *Mood Disorders in Women*. London: Martin Dunitz, 2000:119–35
10. Angst J. *Zur Aetiologie und Nosologie endogener depressiver Psychosen. Eine genetische, soziologische und klinische Studie.* Berlin: Springer, 1966
11. Weissman MM, Leaf PJ, Tischler GL, *et al.* Affective disorders in five United States communities. *Psychol Med* 1988;18:141–53
12. Kessler RC, McGonagle KA, Zhao S, *et al.* Lifetime and 12-month prevalence of DSM-III-R psychiatric disorders in the United States. Results from the National Comorbidity Survey. *Arch Gen Psychiatry* 1994;51:8–19
13. Wittchen H-U, Nelson CB, Lachner G. Prevalence of mental disorders and psychosocial impairments in adolescents and young adults. *Psychol Med* 1998, 28:109–26
14. ten Have M, Vollebergh W, Bijl R, Nolen WA. Bipolar disorder in the general population in The Netherlands (prevalence, consequences and care utilisation): results from The Netherlands Mental Health Survey and Incidence Study (NEMESIS). *J Affect Disord* 2002;68:203–13
15. Szadoczky E, Papp Z, Vitrai J, Rihmer Z, Füredi J. The prevalence of major depressive and bipolar disorders in Hungary. Results from a National Epidemiologic Survey. *J Affect Disord* 1998;50: 153–62
16. Angst J, Gamma A, Sellaro R, Zhang H, Merikangas K. Toward validation of atypical depression in the community: results of the Zurich cohort study. *J Affect Disord* 2002;72:125–38
17. Kessler RC, Wittchen H-U, Abelson JM, *et al.* Methodological studies of the Composite International Diagnostic Interview (CIDI) in the US National Comorbidity Survey (NCS). *Int J Meth Psychiatr Res* 1998;7:33–55

18. Akiskal H, Bourgeois ML, Angst J, Post R, Möller H-J, Hirschfeld R. Re-evaluating the prevalence of and diagnostic composition within the broad clinical spectrum of bipolar disorders. *J Affect Disord* 2000;59(Suppl 1):5–30
19. Benazzi F, Akiskal H. Refining the evaluation of bipolar II: beyond the strict SCID-CV guidelines for hypomania. *J Affect Disord* 2003;73:33–8
20. Angst J, Gamma A, Benazzi F, Ajdacic V, Eich D, Rössler W. Toward a re-definition of subthreshold bipolarity: epidemiology and proposed criteria for bipolar-II, minor bipolar disorders and hypomania. *J Affect Disord* 2003;73:133–46
21. Jorm AF. Sex and age differences in depression: a quantitative synthesis of published research. *Aust NZ J Psychiatry* 1987;21:46–53
22. Bebbington PE, Dunn G, Jenkins R, *et al.* The influence of age and sex on the prevalence of depressive conditions: report from the National Survey of Psychiatric Morbidity. *Psychol Med* 1998;28:9–19
23. Tylee A, Gastpar M, Lépine J-P, Mendlewicz J. DEPRES II (Depression Research in European Society II): a patient survey of the symptoms, disability and current management of depression in the community. *Int Clin Psychopharmacol* 1999;14:139–51
24. Lépine J-P, Gastpar M, Mendlewicz J, Tylee A. Depression in the community: the first pan-European study DEPRES (Depression Research in European Society). *Int Clin Psychopharmacol* 1997;12:19–29
25. Angst J, Gamma A, Gastpar M, Lépine J-P, Mendlewicz J, Tylee A. Gender diffferences in depression. Epidemiological findings from European DEPRES I and II studies. *Eur Arch Psychiatry Clin Neurosci* 2002;252:201–9
26. Angst J, Gamma A, Gastpar M, Lépine J-P, Mendlewicz J, Tylee A. Age and gender differences in depression. Epidemiological findings from the European DEPRES I study. *Eur Arch Psychiatr Neurol Sci* 2003;in preparation
27. Bleuler M. *Endokrinologische Psychiatrie.* Stuttgart: Georg Thieme Verlag, 1954
28. Angst J. Comorbidity of mood disorders: a longitudinal prospective study. *Br J Psychiatry* 1996; 168(Suppl 30):31–7
29. Kendler KS, Eaves LJ, Walters EE, Neale MC, Heath AC, Kessler RC. The identification and validation of distinct depressive syndromes in a population-based sample of female twins. *Arch Gen Psychiatry* 1996;53:391–9
30. Stewart JW, McGrath PJ, Rabkin JG, Quitkin FM. Atypical depression. A valid clinical entity? *Psychiatr Clin North Am* 1993;16:479–95

Androgen-insufficiency syndrome and women's sexuality 13

R. E. Nappi, I. Abbiati, F. Ferdeghini, P. Sampaolo, F. Albani, A. Salonia, F. Montorsi and F. Polatti

INTRODUCTION

Sexual health is considered a crucial issue in determining the well-being of a woman and her partner during the entire life span. Women's sexuality is multidimensional; indeed, the net expression of sexuality before and after the menopause is the result of a complex interplay among physical, psychological and sociocultural dynamics, and hormonal deficiency cannot be the sole factor to explain the multitude and the rate of climacteric complaints, including sexual symptoms, in different cultures and countries[1-3]. On the other hand, some women adjust very well to the crucial step of the menopause, and a pre-existing healthy relationship with their partner, and good general health of both partners and relatives together with the absence of negative life circumstances, contribute positively to sexual function[4,5]. However, sex hormones play a crucial role in maintaining the anatomical and functional integrity of all the structures involved in women's sexual response. While the role of estrogen in the activity of neuroendocrine circuitries and in the trophism of genital organs has been well established, the contribution of androgens to female physical and mental well-being is still a matter of debate[6-8].

Female sexual dysfunction has recently been defined as a persistent or recurring reduction of sex drive or aversion to sexual activity, difficulty becoming aroused, inability to reach orgasm and pain during sexual intercourse[9]. Because of the complex nature of female sexual dysfunction, it is often difficult to determine the major symptom, the leading factor primarily responsible for the symptom and the most adequate therapeutic strategy to resolve the symptom[10].

This chapter attempts to discuss critically some of the issues supporting the relevance of androgens to women's sexuality, with particular regard to androgen-insufficiency syndrome. The effects of tibolone and the combination of estrogen–androgen therapy on sexual function during the postmenopausal years are discussed in detail.

ANDROGENS IN WOMEN

The major androgens in women include dehydroepiandrosterone sulfate (DHEAS), dehydroepiandrosterone (DHEA), androstenedione, testosterone and dihydrotestosterone (DHT). However, DHEAS, DHEA and androstenedione are considered to be proandrogens, because they must be converted to testosterone to express their effects. Androgen biosynthesis occurs in both the ovary and the adrenal gland under stimulation by luteinizing hormone (LH) and adrenocorticotropic hormone (ACTH), respectively, together with intraglandular paracrine and autocrine regulatory mechanisms. Two key enzymes are involved in androgen biosynthesis: P450 SCC and P450 c17, required for DHEA and androstenedione production from pregnenolone and progesterone, respectively. Substantial androgen production originates from circulating DHEAS, which is a unique secretory steroid of the adrenal zona reticularis, in target tissues[11]. The most potent androgen, testosterone, is secreted by the adrenal zona fasciculata (25%) and the ovarian stroma (25%), while the remaining amount (50%) derives from peripheral conversion of circulating androstenedione[12]. Plasma testosterone levels are in the range 0.2–0.7 ng/ml (0.6–2.5 nmol/l), with significant fluctuations related to the phase of the menstrual cycle, being highest at ovulation, lowest during the early follicular phase and higher during the luteal phase in relation to the early follicular phase. In addition, testosterone shows circadian variations, with a peak in the early morning hours. Testosterone is converted to DHT in target tissues; DHT is the principal ligand to androgen receptors, but it can also be aromatizable to estradiol[13].

Plasma testosterone levels fall slowly with age[14], and both free testosterone and androstenedione are produced in lesser quantities at mid-cycle in older women[15], without significant changes of testosterone during the menopausal transition[16]. At physiological menopause, the cessation of follicular activity is characterized by a significant decline of ovarian production of androstenedione, more than testosterone, and the progressive fall of plasma testosterone concentration is the consequence of reduced peripheral conversion from its major precursor[17] and from DHEA and DHEAS, which decline with age[18]. Indeed, plasma testosterone and androstenedione levels at age 60 are about half those in women aged 40 years. As far as surgical menopause is concerned, bilateral oophorectomy both premenopausally and postmenopausally leads to a sudden 50% fall in circulating testosterone levels[19]. Recent data suggest that, during postmenopause, approximately 100% of active sex steroids derive from the peripheral conversion of precursors, mainly DHEA and DHEAS, to estrogens and androgens[20]. These data support the concept that target tissues may represent a local source of testosterone and estradiol, starting from circulating ovarian and adrenal precursors. The key tissue-specific enzyme responsible for peripheral conversion is represented by the various forms of 17β-hydroxysteroid dehydrogenase (HSD). Therefore, circulating levels may not even reflect the action of sex steroids in different target tissues[21]. Finally, it is important to note that sex steroid hormone-binding globulin (SHBG), the protein binding circulating testosterone, seems to be significantly reduced throughout the menopause, with a consequent increase in free androgen index (FAI)[16]. Such an observation was not confirmed in surgical menopause in a cross-sectional study conducted in older women[22]. On the other hand, oral administration of estrogens substantially increases circulating SHBG, with a consequent fall in free testosterone concentrations[23], while transdermal estradiol exerts minimal effects on circulating androgens[24].

ANDROGENS AND WOMEN'S SEXUALITY

During the entire reproductive life span, sex hormones exert both organizational and activational effects, which are relevant to sexual behavior, and their actions are mediated by non-genomic as well as direct and indirect genomic pathways[25,26]. Androgens are essential for the development of reproductive function, and the growth and maintenance of secondary sex characteristics directly or throughout their conversion to estrogens. However, they modulate the physiological function of many tissues and organs, including the central nervous system, the cardiovascular system, the musculoskeletal apparatus, the immune system, etc., in both sexes[27].

The androgen influence over female sexual response has long been hypothesized, but only in recent years has basic research in laboratory animals and clinical trials with androgenic compounds contributed towards an understanding of the role of androgens in libido and sexual arousal in women.

Circulating testosterone is aromatized to estradiol within the central nervous system, and binds to the androgen receptor (AR) following conversion to DHT[28]. A further non-genomic action by testosterone metabolites on sexual receptivity has been described at the hypothalamic level[26]. Estradiol influences sexual receptivity by acting on its own receptor α (ERα)[29], and by increasing progesterone receptor (PR) expression, which takes part in sexual response[30]. In addition, estradiol stimulates oxytocin release and the expression of its receptor[31], and facilitates the lordosis reflex by stimulating noradrenaline α_1 receptor (NAα1R)[32]. Some neurosteroids are involved in the lordosis reflex at hypothalamic levels by interfering with γ-aminobutyric acid (GABA)ergic funcion[33].

Apart from modulating cortical co-ordinating and controlling centers, interpreting what sensations are to be perceived as sexual, and issuing appropriate commands to the rest of the nervous system, sex hormones affect the sensitivity of both genital organs and hypothalamic–limbic structures, where they elicit conscious perception and pleasurable reactions by influencing the release of specific neurotransmitters and neuromodulators[34]. Androgens modulate vaginal and clitoral physiology by influencing the muscular tone of erectile tissue and of the vaginal walls. Androgen receptors are located in both the proximal and the distal vagina and in the clitoris, and their expression is specifically regulated by androgens and estrogens. In addition, androgens interact with the synthesis and release of nitric oxide synthase (NOS) in the proximal vagina by facilitating vaginal and clitoral smooth muscle relaxation response to electric field stimulation[35]. On the other hand, androgens down-regulate arginase activity by reducing L-arginine concentrations, a substrate for NOS. Basic research in laboratory animals demonstrates a modulatory role for vasoactive intestinal peptide (VIP) and nitric oxide (NO) in vaginal lubrication and genital sensation. VIP causes dose-dependent relaxation of rabbit clitoral cavernous bodies and vaginal smooth muscle *in vitro*, similar to NO donors such as nitroprussiate and L-arginine[36]. NO has been identified in clitoral smooth muscle, and the enzyme responsible for cyclic guanosine monophosphate (cGMP) degradation, phosphodiesterase type V, has been isolated in culture from smooth muscle cells of clitoral origin, and is inhibited by sildenafil, which causes a dose-dependent relaxation of smooth muscle strips from rabbit clitoris and vagina. The aging process and surgical castration induce a reduction of vaginal NO in female rats, and cause an increase of vaginal fibrosis, both of which are dependent on estrogens and androgens[37,38]. The recent evidence of phosphodiesterase type V activity in the anterior wall of the human vagina allows the hypothesis that the NO system is highly operative in women at the anatomical site corresponding to the so-called G spot[39]. Even neuropeptide Y (NPY) has been identified in human vagina and clitoris with vasoconstrictive activity, as well as calcitonin gene-related peptide (CGRP), substance P, pituitary adenilate-cyclase activating peptides (PACAP), methionine histidine peptide (PHM), etc., with unclear effects[40]. Collectively, these data suggest that vaginal wall vasocongestion occurs throughout estrogen-dependent VIP activity (arterial vasodilatation) and probably throughout NPY activity (venous constriction), both inducing a neurogenic transudate which lubricates the vagina. Similarly, the labia minora are able to release a transudate by the same means, while NO plays a dominant androgen- and estrogen-dependent role in clitoral cavernous body vasocongestion by regulating, together with prostaglandins, clitoral and vaginal smooth muscle tone[41].

In clinical practice, an inadequate hormonal-dependent vaginal receptivity is the precipitating factor of dyspareunia, which in turn may cause other sexual symptoms that contribute to amplify pain during coital activity. Indeed, it is extremely common to observe a decline of libido following a history of dyspareunia; the consequent reduction of orgasmic capacity, then, may reduce sexual satisfaction, which negatively influences sexual motivation in a kind of self-sustaining 'loop'. This model clearly explains the high degree of co-morbidity displayed by sexual symptoms in women[42].

Studies conducted in women of fertile age found an increase in establishing interpersonal relationship and exchanging sexual pleasure during the periovulatory period, corresponding to the plasma androgenic peak, even though no clear correlation has been reported between plasma androgen levels and the entity of sexual response[43–45]. However, we should keep in mind that the strong motivation for sexual activity at the time of ovulation may be due to the estradiol peak.

Estrogen–progestin use, particularly as a monophasic regimen, seems to interfere with the spontaneous expression of sexual desire, but even the effects of the contraceptive pill on mental well-being may play a role in sexual motivation[46,47]. There is no doubt that hormonal contraception increases plasma SHBG levels and reduces free and total testosterone, as well as resulting in the absence of marked endogenous estradiol fluctuations, but how these features relate to sexual function remains to be established[48]. Some authors have reported that serum testosterone levels are related to genital response and to subjective physical sensation (lubrication and breast sensitivity), in response to visual erotic stimulation, in both premenopause and postmenopause[49]. Moreover, antiandrogen administration has been associated with low libido in females[50]. Further evidence suggests that circulating free testosterone is related to sexual desire and masturbation in young women[51]. Finally, 5α-reductase activity is significantly impaired in target tissues in those women reporting low libido following the menopause[52], while a significant correlation has been found between high levels of circulating testosterone and androstenedione and a lower index of vaginal atrophy[53].

ANDROGEN-INSUFFICIENCY SYNDROME

Surgical menopause is associated with the so-called androgen-deficiency syndrome, an increasingly accepted clinical entity comprising specific symptoms[54]. Women report low libido, persistent and inexplicable fatigue, blunted motivation and a general reduced sense of well-being. The first-line treatment is always represented by estrogen replacement therapy to restore adequate plasma estradiol levels, to secure the vaginal environment. As a second therapeutic step, after excluding other organic and psychorelational issues, androgen supplementation may be proposed. The major problem with such a syndrome is that, in spite of growing interest in the treatment of sexual dysfunction with androgens in clinical practice, no cut-off level for a normal range of testosterone has been agreed. The lack of consensus on the definition of low testosterone levels is related to difficulties with sensitive assays for total and free testosterone in women, and fluctuations during the menstrual cycle and in different stages of life[55]. For these reasons, a better term to define this clinical condition is androgen-insufficiency syndrome, and bearing in mind the present state of knowledge it is reasonable to use values at or below the lowest quartile of the normal range for women in their reproductive years to support the diagnosis. Other signs of androgen insufficiency include reduced pubic hair, bone mass and muscle mass, poor quality of life and more frequent vasomotor symptoms, insomnia, depression and headache[56]. Apart from surgical menopause, other causes of androgen insufficiency include normal aging (physiological menopause with not enough benefits from conventional hormone replacement therapy and premenopausal women reporting low libido and with circulating free testosterone levels at lower limits of detection), ovarian insufficiency (unilateral oophorectomy, hysterectomy, spontaneous premature ovarian failure or after chemotherapy or radiotherapy, hypothalamic amenorrhea), adrenal insufficiency (adrenal failure or surgery), combined (hypopituitarism, autoimmune adrenal and ovarian failure) and iatrogenic (treatment with exogenous oral estrogens, antiandrogen therapy, oral contraceptives, gonadotropin-releasing hormone agonist therapy, chronic exogenous corticosteroid administration)[57].

THERAPEUTIC STRATEGIES FOR SEXUAL DYSFUNCTION IN POSTMENOPAUSAL WOMEN

A recent systematic review including all randomized and placebo-controlled trials of treatment for sexual dysfunction in postmenopausal women concluded that many treatments used in practice are not supported by adequate evidence[10]. Only one trial of hormone replacement therapy (HRT) was randomized and placebo-controlled and investigated the effects of estrogen and progestin on sexual desire, arousal and mood in healthy postmenopausal women, without assessing frequency of sexual activity and orgasm. Sherwin concluded that there was a significant improvement of sexual desire and arousal on a short-term basis[58]. The most interesting findings on positive sexual effects of sex hormones at the menopause come from studies of oral and transdermal combinations of estrogens and exogenous testosterone[59-61], even though only two trials were randomized and placebo-controlled. The first trial conducted in a small sample of subjects ($n = 20$) reported that sexual desire, satisfaction and frequency in postmenopausal women taking hormonal therapy were improved significantly by combined estrogen-androgen therapy, but not by estrogen or estrogen-progestin therapy. Sexual function improved with estrogen-androgen therapy, even though circulating estrogen levels were lower than those measured during previous estrogen therapy, leading to the conclusion that androgens play a pivotal role in sexual function, with estrogens not having a significant impact on levels of sexual drive and enjoyment[62]. The second trial was conducted following surgical menopause with two doses of transdermal testosterone (150 and 300 μg/day) versus placebo, and reported a significant improvement in sexual function with a further increase in scores for frequency of sexual activity and orgasm when women were taking the higher dose. However, there was an extremely strong response of sexual function in women taking placebo, and 24% of study participants withdrew from the trial because of androgen-related adverse side-effects[63]. Therefore, the use of androgens in clinical management of the menopause needs a certain degree of caution, because the long-term effects of such preparations on women's general health are still unknown. In addition, estro-androgenic treatments are still unavailable in several countries. In Europe, long-term experience in the treatment of climacteric symptoms and low mood and libido is available for tibolone, a synthetic steroid with tissue-specific estrogenic, progestogenic and androgenic properties[64,65]. Apart from direct effects of its metabolites in the vagina and in brain areas relevant to well-being[66,67], tibolone lowers SHBG, thus increasing free estradiol, testosterone and DHEAS levels[68]. In randomized studies versus placebo or estradiol-norethisterone acetate, tibolone treatment (2.5 mg/day) alleviated vaginal dryness and dyspareunia, ameliorating libido, arousal and sexual satisfaction in postmenopausal women to a greater extent[69,70]. Moreover, tibolone shows a positive effect on sexuality which is superimposable on that observed with estro-androgenic preparations[71]. These data, together with the recent observation that tibolone significantly increases vaginal pulse amplitude at baseline and following erotic stimulation, compared with placebo[72], further support the notion that such a tissue-specific compound is a good therapeutic option for the relief of low libido and improvement of arousability and lubrication at the menopause because of both its estrogenic and its androgenic properties.

CONCLUSION

Further studies are needed to clarify the relevance of androgens to women's sexuality and the impact of hormonal treatments on the clinical expression of sexual symptoms. An adequate diagnostic and therapeutic approach will necessarily involve a multidisciplinary team to avoid dangerous body mind separations. However, the role of the clinician in identifying all possible biological factors leading to low androgen levels is mandatory in the design of therapeutic strategies tailored to women's needs.

References

1. Sarrel PM, Whitehead MI. Sex and menopause: defining the issue. *Maturitas* 1985;7:217–24
2. Dennerstein L. Well-being, symptoms and menopausal transition. *Maturitas* 1996;23:147–57
3. Nappi RE, Baldaro Verde J, Polatti F, *et al.* Self-reported sexual symptoms in women attending menopause clinics. *J Obstet Gynecol Invest* 2002; 53:181–7
4. Bachmann GA, Leiblum SR. Sexuality in sexagenarian women. *Maturitas* 1991;13:43–50
5. Avis NE, Stellato R, Crawford S, *et al.* Is there an association between menopause status and sexual functioning? *Menopause* 2000;7:297–309
6. Semmers J, Wagner G. Estrogen deprivation and vaginal function in postmenopausal women. *J Am Med Assoc* 1982;248:445–8

7. Dennerstein L, Dudley EC, Hopper JL, *et al.* A prospective population-based study of menopausal symptoms. *Obstet Gynecol* 2000;93:351–8
8. Rosen R, Bachmann G, Leiblum S, *et al.*, eds. Androgen insufficiency in women: the Princeton Conference. *Fertil Steril* 2002;77(Suppl 4)
9. Basson R, Berman J, Burnett A, *et al.* Report of the international consensus development conference on female sexual dysfunction: definitions and classifications. *J Urol* 2000;163:888–93
10. Modelska K, Cummings S. Female sexual dysfunction in postmenopausal women: systematic review of placebo-controlled trials. *Am J Obstet Gynecol* 2003;188:286–93
11. Burger HG. Androgen production in women. *Fertil Steril* 2002;77(Suppl 4):S3–5
12. Longcope C. Adrenal and gonadal androgen secretion in normal females. *J Clin Endocrinol Metab* 1986;15:213–27
13. Abraham GE. Ovarian and adrenal contribution to peripheral androgens during the menstrual cycle. *J Clin Endocrinol Metab* 1974:39:340–6
14. Zumoff B, Strain GW, Miller LK, *et al.* Twenty-four-hour mean plasma testosterone concentration declines with age in normal premenopausal women. *J Clin Endocrinol Metab* 1995;80:1429–30
15. Mushayandebvu T, Castracane VD, Gimpel T, *et al.* Evidence for diminished midcycle ovarian androgen production in older reproductive aged women. *Fertil Steril* 1996;65:721–3
16. Burger HG, Dudley EC, Cui J, *et al.* A prospective longitudinal study of serum testosterone, dehydroepiandrosterone sulphate and sex hormone binding globulin levels through the menopause transition. *J Clin Endocrinol Metab* 2000;85: 2832–938
17. Adashi EY. The climacteric ovary as a functional gonadotropin driven androgen producing gland. *Fertil Steril* 1994;62:20–7
18. Zumoff B, Rosenfield RS, Strain GW, *et al.* Sex differences in the twenty-four hour mean plasma concentrations of DHA and DHAS and DHA to DHAS ratio in normal adults. *J Clin Endocrinol Metab* 1995;51:330–3
19. Davis S. Androgen replacement therapy: a commentary. *J Clin Endocrinol Metab* 1999;84: 1886–91
20. Labrie F, Luu-The V, Labrie C, *et al.* DHEA and its transformation into androgens and estrogens in peripheral target tissues: intracrinology. *Front Neuroendocrinol* 2001;22:185–212
21. Labrie F, Belanger A, Simard J, *et al.* DHEA and peripheral androgen and estrogen formation: intracrinology. *Ann NY Acad Sci* 1995;774:16–28
22. Laughlin GA, Barrett-Connor E, Kritz-Silverstein D, *et al.* Hysterectomy, oophorectomy, and endogenous sex hormone levels in older women: the Rancho Bernardo Study. *J Clin Endocrinol Metab* 2000;85:645–51
23. Casson PR, Elkind-Hirsch KE, Buster JE, *et al.* Effect of postmenopausal estrogen replacement on circulating androgens. *Obstet Gynecol* 1997;90: 995–8
24. Kraemer GR, Kraemer RR, Ogden BW, *et al.* Variability of serum estrogens among postmenopausal women treated with the same transdermal estrogen therapy and the effect on androgens and sex hormone binding globulin. *Fertil Steril* 2003;79:534–42
25. McEwen BS. Clinical review 108: The molecular and neuroanatomical basis for estrogen effects in the central nervous system. *J Clin Endocrinol Metab* 1999;84:1790–7
26. Frye CA. The role of neurosteroids and non-genomic effects of progestins and androgens in mediating sexual receptivity of rodents. *Brain Res Rev* 2001;37:201–22
27. Davis SR, Burger H. Androgen and postmenopausal women. *J Clin Endocrinol Metab* 1996; 81:2759–63
28. Roselli CE, Resko JA. Aromatase activity in the rat brain: hormone regulation and sex differences. *J Steroid Biochem Mol Biol* 1993;44:499–508
29. Ogawa S, Chan J, Chester AE, *et al.* Survival of reproductive behaviours in estrogen receptor β gene-deficient male and female mice. *Proc Natl Acad Sci USA* 1999;96:12887–92
30. Etgen AM. Estrogen induction of progestin receptors in the hypothalamus of male and female rats which differ in their ability to exhibit cyclic gonadotropin secretion and female sexual behavior. *Biol Reprod* 1981;25:307–13
31. Bale TL, Pedersen CA, Dorsa DM. CNS oxytocin receptor mRNA expression and regulation by gonadal steroids. *Adv Exp Med Biol* 1995;395: 269–80
32. Kow LM, Weesner GD, Pfaff DW. α_1-Adrenergic agonists act on the ventromedial hypothalamus to cause neuronal excitation and lordosis facilitation: electrophysiological and behavioral evidence. *Brain Res* 1992;588:237–45
33. Frye CA, Bayon LE, Pursnani NK, *et al.* The neurosteroids, progesterone and 3α,5α-THP, enhance sexual motivation, receptivity, and proceptivity in female rats. *Brain Res* 1998;808:72–83
34. Bancroff J. *Human Sexuality and its Problems*, 2nd edn. London: Churchill Livingstone, 1989
35. Traish AM, Kim N, Min K, *et al.* Role of androgens in female genital sexual arousal: receptor expression, structure and function. *Fertil Steril* 2002;77(Suppl 4):S11–18
36. Levine RJ. Sex and the human female reproductive tract, what really happens during and after coitus. *Int J Impotence Res* 1998;10:S14–21

37. Berman JR, Berman L, Goldstein I. Female sexual dysfunction: incidence, pathophysiology, evaluation, and treatment options. *Urology* 1999;54: 385-91
38. Goldstein I, Berman J. Vasculogenic female sexual dysfunction: vaginal engorgement and clitoral erectile insufficiency syndrome. *Int J Impotence Res* 1998;10:S84-90
39. D'Amati G, di Gioia CR, Bologna M, *et al.* Type 5 phosphodiesterase expression in the human vagina. *Urology* 2002;60:191-5
40. Goldstein I. Female sexual arousal disorder: new insights. *Int J Impotence Res* 2000;12:S152-7
41. Munarriz R, Kim NN, Goldstein I, *et al.* Biology of female sexual function. *Urol Clin North Am* 2002;29:685-93
42. Laumann EO, Paik A, Rosen RC. Sexual dysfunction in the United States: prevalence and predictors. *J Am Med Assoc* 1999;281:537-44
43. Morrel M, Dixen J, Carter S, *et al.* The influence of age and cyclic status on sexual arousability in women. *Am J Obstet Gynecol* 1984;148:66-71
44. Persky H, Dreisbach L, Miller WR, *et al.* The relation of plasma androgen levels to sexual behavior and attitudes in women. *Psychosom Med* 1982;44:305-10
45. Nappi RE, Ferdeghini F, Verticale M, *et al.* Hormones and sexuality. Presented at the *XIII International Society of Psychosomatic Obstetrics and Gynecology World Congress*, Buenos Aires, Argentina, April 2001
46. Warner P, Bancroft J. Mood, sexuality, oral contraceptives and the menstrual cycle. *J Psychosom Res* 1988;32:417-27
47. McCoy NL, Matyas JR. Oral contraceptives and sexuality in university women. *Arch Sex Behav* 1996;25:73-90
48. Bancroft J, Sherwin BB, Alexander GM, *et al.* Oral contraceptives, androgens, and the sexuality of young women: II. The role of androgens. *Arch Sex Behav* 1991;20:121-35
49. Myers LS, Morokoff PJ. Physiological and subjective sexual arousal of pre- and postmenopausal women taking hormone replacement therapy. *Psychophysiology* 1986;23:283-92
50. Appelt H, Strauss B. The psychoendocrinology of female sexuality: a research project. *Geriatr J Psychol* 1986;6:19-29
51. Vermeulen A. Plasma androgens in women. *J Reprod Med* 1998;43:725-33
52. Kennedy RG, Davies T, Al-Azzawi F. Sexual interest in postmenopausal women is related to 5α-reductase activity. *Hum Reprod* 1997;12:209-13
53. Leiblum S, Bachmann G, Kemmann E, *et al.* Vaginal atrophy in the postmenopausal woman. The importance of sexual activity and hormones. *J Am Med Assoc* 1983;249:2195-8
54. Davis S, Tran J. Testosterone influences libido and well-being in women. *Trends Endocrinol Metab* 2001;12:33-7
55. Braunstein GD. Androgen insufficiency in women: summary of critical issues. *Fertil Steril* 2002;77 (Suppl 4):S94-9
56. Bachmann GA. The hyperandrogenic woman: pathophysiologic overview. *Fertil Steril* 2002;77 (Suppl 4):S72-6
57. Davis SR. When to suspect androgen deficiency other than at menopause. *Fertil Steril* 2002;77 (Suppl 4):S68-71
58. Sherwin BB. The impact of different doses of estrogen and progestin on mood and sexual behavior in postmenopausal women. *J Clin Endocrinol Metab* 1991;72:336-43
59. Studd J, Collins WP, Chakravarti S. Oestradiol and testosterone implants in the treatment of psychosexual problems in postmenopausal women. *Br J Obstet Gynaecol* 1977;84:314-15
60. Sherwin B, Gelfand M. The role of androgen in the maintenance of sexual functioning in oophorectomized women. *Psychosom Med* 1987;49:397-409
61. Davis SR, McCloud P, Strauss BJ, *et al.* Testosterone enhances estradiol's effects on postemnopausal bone density and sexuality. *Maturitas* 1995;21: 227-36
62. Sarrel P, Dobay B, Wiita B. Estrogen and estrogen-androgen replacement in postmenopausal women dissatisfied with estrogen-only therapy. Sexual behavior and neuroendocrine responses. *J Reprod Med* 1998;43:847-56
63. Shifren J, Braunstein G, Siman J, *et al.* Transdermal testosterone treatment in women with impaired sexual function after oophorectomy. *N Engl J Med* 2000;343:682-8
64. Kloosterboer HJ. Tibolone: a steroid with a tissue-specific mode of action. *Steroid Biochem Mol Biol* 2001;76:231-8
65. Davis SR. The effects of tibolone on mood and libido. *Menopause* 2002;9:162-70
66. Rymer J, Chapman MG, Fogelman I, *et al.* A study of the effect of tibolone on the vagina in postmenopausal women. *Maturitas* 1994;18:127-33
67. Genazzani AR, Petraglia F, Facchinetti F, *et al.* Effects of Org OD14 on pituitary and peripheral β-endorphin in castrated rats and postmenopausal women. *Maturitas* 1987;1:S35-48
68. Doren M, Rubig A, Coelingh Bennink HK, *et al.* Differential effects on the androgen status of postmenopausal women treated with tibolone and continuous combined estradiol and norethindrone acetate replacement therapy. *Fertil Steril* 2001;75: 554-9
69. Palacios S, Menendez C, Jurado AR, *et al.* Changes in sex behaviour after menopause: effects of tibolone. *Maturitas* 1995;22:155-61

70. Nathorst-Boos J, Hammar M. Effect on sexual life – a comparison between tibolone and a continuous estradiol-norethisterone acetate regimen. *Maturitas* 1997;26:15–20
71. Castelo-Branco C, Vicente JJ, Figueras F, *et al.* Comparative effects of estrogens plus androgens and tibolone on bone, lipid pattern and sexuality in postmenopausal women. *Maturitas* 2000;34:161–8
72. Laan E, van Lunsen RH, Everaerd W. The effects of tibolone on vaginal blood flow, sexual desire and arousability in postmenopausal women. *Climacteric* 2001;4:28–41

Estrogen replacement therapy and mood: the brain as a target tissue of sex steroids

14

S. L. Berga

Abundant evidence supports the notion that the brain is a primary target tissue for sex steroids (for reviews, see references 1 and 2). The role of sex steroids in regulating traditional reproductive processes such as implantation, lactation and reproductive behavior has been extensively chronicled and is widely appreciated. The commonplace symptoms that accompany the climacteric, namely hot flushes, sleep disturbances and irritability, suggest that parts of the brain subserving functions other than solely reproductive ones are critically impacted upon by the presence or absence of sex steroids[3]. Sex steroids have both organizational and activational influences upon the brain. These and other observations underlie the concept that postmenopausal hormone use will preserve cognitive functions and protect from dementia. At a minimum, the following central nervous system outputs are modulated by sex steroid exposure.

(1) Affective state and mood, including sleep[4], libido[5–12] and social behavior[13,14];

(2) Cognitive functioning, especially verbal memory, speed of processing and spatial ability[1,15–20];

(3) Motor co-ordination, including balance and psychomotor speed[1,15,18];

(4) Neuronal excitability and vulnerability to epilepsy[1];

(5) Pain sensitivity[1];

(6) Auditory threshold (which is lower in women than in men).

Multiple mechanisms mediate the impact of sex steroids upon neuronal plasticity, function and integrity. Sex steroids modulate the following neurotransmitter systems (for reviews, see references 1, 2 and 21):

(1) Basal forebrain dopaminergic system, which regulates attention;

(2) Forebrain cholinergic system, which regulates memory and learning[22];

(3) Midbrain noradrenergic system, which is implicated in the modulation of arousal;

(4) Midbrain serotonergic system[23], which subserves mood, affect, cognition, attention and the integration of cognition and emotionality into complex social behaviors;

(5) Midbrain dopaminergic system, which mediates reward.

Sex steroids regulate synaptic density and neuronal and glial viability by a variety of mechanisms (for reviews, see references 1 and 2). In short, sex steroids have important organizational (anatomical) and activational (functional) effects upon neural substrates.

In addition to the abundant cellular and molecular evidence demonstrating a critical role for sex steroids in modulating and preserving brain function, epidemiological data also support the notion that hormone replacement therapy (HRT) use will reduce the likelihood of two common and debilitating conditions linked with the menopause and aging, namely depression and dementia. Although it is not commonly appreciated, dementia is typically accompanied by mood dysregulation. Likewise, mood dysregulation and stress can mimic and enhance the likelihood of dementia. This clinically recognized interaction between mood and cognition is yet another example of the brain as a target tissue of sex steroids. Dementia affects, to some extent, approximately 50% of those above 80 years of age. Alzheimer's disease is the most common type. In addition to loss of cognitive abilities and working memory, dementia impairs mood and social integration[24]. Even when accounting for the increased longevity of women, Alzheimer's dementia is more common in women than in men[25]. It is also worth noting that the incidence of Parkinson's disease was increased in women who underwent a surgical menopause relative to women experiencing a natural menopause[26]. Depression is also a common late-life disorder, and can increase the risk of and masquerade as dementia[27]. The epidemiological data on the neuroprotective effects of estrogen were reviewed recently[18]. The authors included 29 studies and addressed two domains. One was the cognitive effects of HRT use and the other was the association between HRT use and risk of dementia. Women who were symptomatic from the menopause had improvements in verbal memory, vigilance, reasoning and motor speed when given HRT.

In that symptomatic postmenopausal women were found to benefit most in the short term from HRT, the conclusion of LeBlanc and colleagues[18] is similar to the recently reported results from the Heart and Estrogen/progestin Replacement Study (HERS)[28]. Women in the HERS trial had active cardiovascular disease and were randomized to placebo versus continuous 0.625 mg conjugated equine estrogens combined with 2.5 mg medroxyprogesterone acetate. Participants were followed for 3 years, and quality of life was monitored with three inventories, the Duke Activity Status, the RAND scale and the Burnham screening scale. Women with hot flushes who were given HRT had improved mental health and fewer depressive symptoms, compared with women given placebo. Asymptomatic women given HRT had greater declines in physical functioning and energy, with no change in depressive symptoms when compared with those given placebo. Of note, the asymptomatic women also had very low depression scores at the time of randomization. Thus, it was unlikely that their mood would further improve (a ceiling effect), and it is noteworthy that postmenopausal estrogen therapy did not worsen mood. With regard to mood, a cross-sectional analysis of 6602 white women over age 71 years, which employed the short form of the Geriatric Depression Scale, found the odds ratio of depression in estrogen replacement therapy (ERT) users to be 0.7, with a confidence interval of 0.5–0.9[29]. For postmenopausal ERT users, the odds ratio was 0.8 (0.5–1.4). These and other studies have led to the view that estrogen therapy may improve mood in those in whom it is compromised, and may reduce the risk or aid in the treatment of late-life depression.

Much of the confusion regarding the neuroprotective effects of estrogen comes from the trial in which conjugated equine estrogens (which may not readily transgress the blood–brain barrier) were given to women with established mild dementia[30]. No benefit was observed. However, by the time dementia is clinically evident, there has been a significant loss of neurons and glia, and it is unrealistic to expect HRT to revive dead tissues. Thus, the more relevant question is whether ERT or postmenopausal ERT has a role in primary prevention of dementia. As noted above, this question was addressed by a meta-analysis of 29 observational studies[18]. The conclusion was that HRT decreased the risk of dementia. The summary odds ratio was 0.66, with a 95% confidence interval of 0.53–0.82. More recently, Zandi and colleagues[25] reported the results of a prospective, observational study of 1357 elderly men and 1889 elderly women residing in Cache County, Utah with an average age at enrolment of about 74 years. The incidence of dementia increased after age 80, and the relative risk for women compared with men was 2.11 (1.22–3.86). This is shown in Figure 1a. More instructive, however, is Figure 1b, which shows rates of dementia in women according to duration of HRT use. Those women who had used HRT for > 10 years had rates of dementia approximating those of men, while those who had used HRT for < 10 years had higher rates. However, for HRT to confer protection, it had to be started at least 10 years before the onset of dementia. In summary, extant epidemiological data fulfil the criteria of being generally consistent across studies and mechanistically plausible. Needless to say, a long-term, prospective, randomized clinical trial

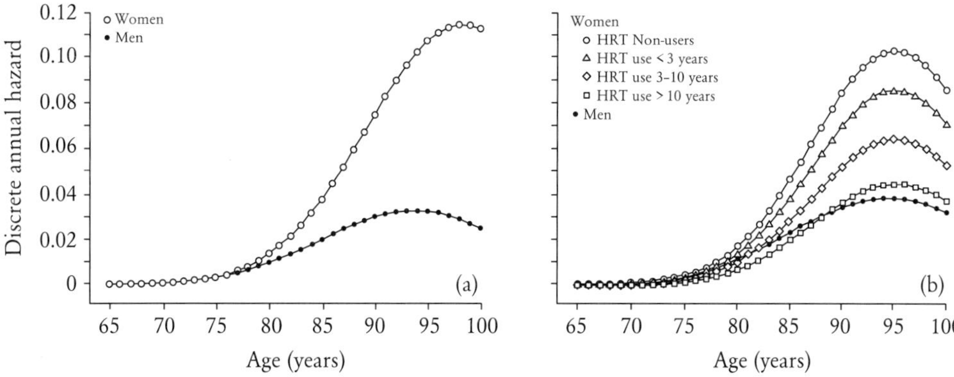

Figure 1 Estimated discrete annual hazard of Alzheimer's disease for men and women (a) by age, and (b) by duration of hormone replacement therapy (HRT) use for women. Reproduced from reference 25 with permission

has not been done and would be difficult, if not impossible, to do. It has been suggested that randomized clinical trials cannot be performed to assess risks and benefits remote from the time of exposure[31]. While dementia is common, it does not present typically until after age 80. Thus, its presentation is remote from the time of menopause. If preventing or delaying the onset of dementia is a goal, the Cache County data suggest that maximal protection is afforded by > 10 years of use. However, to maintain the full complement of central nervous system outputs, available molecular, physiological and neuroimaging evidence suggests the need for persistent use[19,20,32]. For instance, short-term transdermal estradiol therapy has been demonstrated to enhance memory after many years of hypoestrogenism[20,33]. In a study of elderly postmenopausal women who had not used hormones for at least 7 years, Wolf and associates found that a 2-week exposure to transdermal estradiol increased memory, but only when circulating estradiol levels exceeded 29 pg/ml (Figure 2). In short, the epidemiological data support the concept that HRT can be used for primary neuroprotection against dementia, but not for secondary prevention once dementia is clinically apparent.

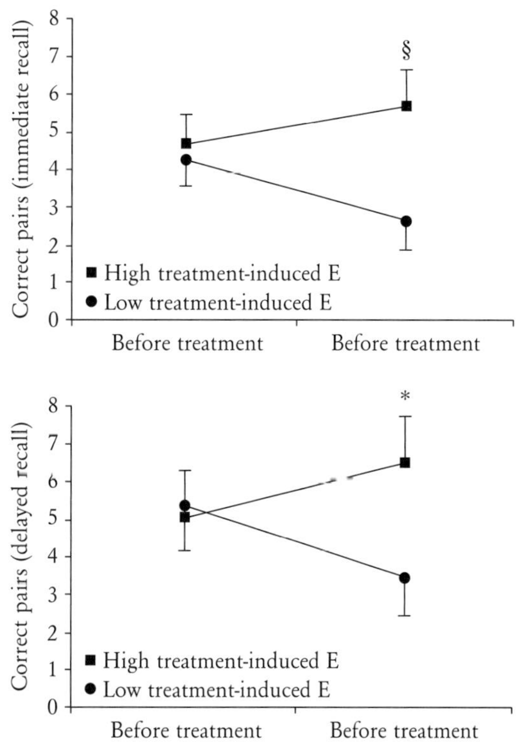

Figure 2 Indices of verbal memory in postmenopausal women treated with transdermal estradiol (E). $^{*}p < 0.05$, $^{\S}p < 0.10$, significant difference. Reproduced from reference 20 with permission from Elsevier © 1999

An area of uncertainty is whether hormone types or formulations differ in their effects. Investigative attention has primarily focused on estrogen types. The brain centers subserving cognition express both types of estrogen receptors, namely ERα and ERβ[2]. Using the powerful technique of selectively deleting each estrogen receptor subtype to create a 'knock-out' mouse model, Dubal and colleagues[33] showed that ERα occupation was required to limit neuronal death in the face of ischemic insult. Cholinergic neurons, which are critically involved in memory and learning, are heavily invested with ERα[34]. In rats, cholinergic neurons mediate estrogen's preservation of memory after ovariectomy[22]. These and other molecular data have led to the notion that full neuroprotection requires estrogen occupation and activation of ERα. This would also mean that the hormone preparation in question must lead to levels in the circulation of an estrogen that can transgress the blood-brain barrier and gain access to the central nervous system. In this regard, cognitive preservation was more strongly associated with bioavailable estradiol than with total estradiol[35]. These and similar data suggest that complete neuroprotection might not be garnered by the use of agents that are ERα antagonists (such as currently available selective estrogen receptor modulators (SERMs) or aromatase inhibitors) or mainly ERβ agonists, such as phytoestrogens[19]. The molecular underpinnings of neuroprotection are being carefully studied, and it is anticipated that future data may provide further insights into whether a particular estrogen preparation, dose or route of administration provides better neuroprotection. Other than the study by Wolf and colleagues[20] showing benefit if circulating levels of estradiol exceed 29 pg/ml, current data do not suggest dose recommendations for prevention of dementia. Patients should be advised that other strategies, such as cognitive enrichment, tobacco cessation, good nutrition, exercise, stress management, aspirin, antioxidants and remediation of depression also might reduce the likelihood of dementia or delay its onset. In summary, current data suggest, but do not prove, that postmenopausal estrogen use will reduce the risk of dementia and will safeguard important brain functions needed for negotiating the tasks of daily living. The estrogen type and dose, and impact of progestins have not been established.

References

1. McEwen BS. The molecular and neuroanatomical basis for estrogen effects in the central nervous system. *J Clin Endocrinol Metab* 1999;84:1790–7
2. Wang L, Andersson S, Warner M, Gustafsson JA. Estrogen actions in the brain. *Science's* STKE 2002, http://www.stke.org/cgl/content/full/sigtrans; 2002/138/pe29
3. Stadberg E, Mattson LA, Milsom I. The prevalence and severity of climacteric symptoms and the use of different treatment regimens in a Swedish population. *Acta Obstet Gynecol Scand* 1997;76:442–8
4. Hollander LE, Freeman EW, Sammel MD, Berlin JA, Grisso JA, Battistini M. Sleep quality, estradiol levels, and behavioral factors in late reproductive age women. *Obstet Gynecol* 2001;98:391–7
5. Barrett-Connor E, Young R, Notelovitz M, *et al.* A two-year, double blind comparison of estrogen-androgen and conjugated estrogens in surgically menopausal women. Effects on bone mineral density, symptoms and lipid profiles. *J Reprod Med* 1999;44:1012–20
6. Castelo-Branco C, Vicente JJ, Figueras F, *et al.* Comparative effects of estrogens plus androgens and tibolone on bone, lipid pattern, and sexuality in postmenopausal women. *Maturitas* 2000;34: 161–8
7. Graham CA, Janssen E, Sanders SA. Effects of fragrance on female sexual arousal and mood across the menstrual cycle. *Psychophysiology* 2000; 37:76–84
8. Insel TR, Young L, Wang Z. Central oxytocin and reproductive behaviors. *Rev Reprod* 1997;2:28–37
9. Matteo S, Rissman EF. Increased sexual activity during the midcycle portion of the human menstrual cycle. *Horm Behav* 1984;18:249–55
10. Pfaff DW. Hormones, genes, and behavior. *Proc Natl Acad Sci USA* 1997;94:14213–16
11. Savic I, Berglund H, Gulyas B, Roland P. Smelling of odorous sex hormone-like compounds causes sex-differentiated hypothalamic activations in humans. *Neuron* 2001;31:661–8
12. Warner P, Bancroft J. Mood, sexuality, oral contraceptives, and the menstrual cycle. *J Psychosom Res* 1988;32:417–27
13. Finkelstein JW, Susman EJ, Chinchilli VM, *et al.* Estrogen or testosterone increases self-reported aggressive behaviors in hypogonadal adolescents. *J Clin Endocrinol Metab* 1997;82:2433–8

14. Finkelstein JW, Susman EJ, Chinchilli VM, *et al.* Effects of estrogen or testosterone on self-reported sexual responses and behaviors in hypogonadal adolescents. *J Clin Endocrinol Metab* 1998;83:2281-5
15. Birge SJ. HRT and cognitive function: what are we to believe? *Menopause* 2002;9:221-3
16. Duka T, Tasker R, McGowan JF. The effects of 3-week estrogen hormone replacement on cognition in elderly healthy females. *Psychopharmacology* 2000;149:129-39
17. Hogervost E, Williams J, Budge M, Riedel W, Jolles J. The nature of the effect of female gonadal hormone replacement therapy on cognitive function in post-menopausal women: a meta-analysis. *Neuroscience* 2000;101:485-512
18. LeBlanc ES, Janowsky J, Chan BKS, Nelson HD. Hormone replacement therapy and cognition. *J Am Med Assoc* 2001;285:1489-99
19. Resnick SM, Maki PM. Effects of hormone replacement therapy on cognitive and brain aging. *Ann NY Acad Sci* 2001;949:203-14
20. Wolf OT, Kudielka BM, Hellhammer DH, Torber S, McEwen BS, Kirschbaum C. Two weeks of transdermal estradiol treatment in postmenopausal elderly women and its effect on memory and mood: verbal memory changes are associated with the treatment induced estradiol levels. *Psychoneuroendocrinology* 1999;24:727-41
21. Smith YR, Zubieta JK. Neuroimaging of aging and estrogen effects on central nervous system physiology. *Fertil Steril* 2001;76:651-9
22. Gibbs RB. Basal forebrain cholinergic neurons are necessary for estrogen to enhance acquisition of a delayed matching-to-position T-maze task. *Horm Behav* 2002;42:245-57
23. Moses EL, Drevets WC, Smith G, *et al.* Effects of estradiol and progesterone administration on human serotonin 2A receptor binding: a PET study. *Biol Psychiatry* 2000;48:854-60
24. Shepherd JE. Effects of estrogen on cognition, mood, and degenerative brain diseases. *J Am Pharmacol Assoc* 2001;41:221-8
25. Zandi PP, Carlson MC, Plassman BL, *et al.* Hormone replacement therapy and incidence of Alzheimer disease in older women. *J Am Med Assoc* 2002;288:2123-9
26. Benedetti MD, Maraganore DM, Bower JH, *et al.* Hysterectomy, menopause, and estrogen use preceding Parkinson's disease: an exploratory case-control study. *Mov Disord* 2001;16:830-7
27. Seeman TE, McEwen BS, Singer BH, Albert MS, Rowe JW. Increase in urinary cortisol excretion and memory declines: MacArthur studies of successful aging. *J Clin Endocrinol Metab* 1997;82:2458-65
28. Hlatky MA, Boothroyd D, Vittinghoff E, Sharp P, Whooley MA. Quality-of-life and depressive symptoms in postmenopausal women after receiving hormone therapy. *J Am Med Assoc* 2002;287:591-7
29. Whooley MA, Grady D, Cauley JA. Postmenopausal estrogen therapy and depressive symptoms in older women. *J Gen Intern Med* 2000;15:535-41
30. Mulnard RA, Cotman CW, Kawas C, *et al.* Estrogen replacement therapy for treatment of mild to moderate Alzheimer disease: a randomized, clinical trial. Alzheimer's Disease Cooperative Study. *J Am Med Assoc* 2000;283:1007-15
31. Marchbanks PA, McDonald JA, Wilson HG, *et al.* Oral contraceptives and the risk of breast cancer. *N Engl J Med* 2002;346:2025-32
32. Tang MX, Jacobs D, Stern Y, *et al.* Effect of oestrogen during menopause on risk and age at onset of Alzheimer's disease. *Lancet* 1996;348:429-32
33. Dubal DB, Zhu H, Yu J, *et al.* Estrogen receptor α, not β, is a critical link in estradiol-mediated protection against brain injury. *Proc Natl Acad Sci USA* 2001;98:1952-7
34. Shughrue PJ, Scrimo PJ, Merchenthaler I. Estrogen binding and estrogen receptor characterization (ERα and ERβ) in the cholinergic neurons of the rat basal forebrain. *Neuroscience* 2000;96:41-9
35. Yaffe K, Liu LY, Grady D, Cauley J, Kramer J, Cummings SR. Cognitive decline in relation to non-protein-bound oestradiol concentrations. *Lancet* 2000;356:708-12

Progestogens and menopause: effect on mood and quality of life 15

I. Björn, T. Bäckström, M. Wang, L. Andreé, M. Bixo, I. Sundström-Poromaa, V. Birzniece, I.-M. Johansson, P. Lundgren, S. Nyberg, I.-S. Ödmark and A.-C. Wihlbäck

HORMONE REPLACEMENT THERAPY AND COMPLIANCE

The reasons for poor compliance with hormone replacement therapy (HRT), in particular drug-related reasons, have not yet been fully elucidated. In spite of beliefs that estrogen therapy increases well-being, several reports describe low compliance[1,2]. One out of three women discontinue HRT within a year[3]. In studies of osteoporosis and treatment with hormones, 40–50% were not taking the prescribed drug 8–12 months after initiation of treatment[4,5]. When women are treated with 0.625 mg conjugated estrogen (CE) plus 2.5 mg medroxyprogesterone (MPA), adherence declines to 81% after a year, and after 6 years only 45% continue therapy[6]. It seems a contradiction that on the one hand HRT improves well-being and is believed to have beneficial effects on health, but on the other hand discontinuation rates are high. There is reason to assume that women are not fully satisfied with the treatment, and that explanations might be found in unwanted side-effects owing to modes of treatment. Discontinuation is partly explained by irregular bleeding and fear of cancer[7,8], but other factors should be considered. Studies of effects on mood induced by the addition of a progestogen to an estrogen have been inconclusive, and many questions remain unanswered. In a cohort study of peri- and postmenopausal women, Björn and Bäckström[9] have investigated why women discontinue HRT, even when great effort has been made to inform and fulfil the demands of the patient. In total, 356 women who were prescribed HRT received a questionnaire and 92% replied; 2% of them never started HRT and 75% continued the therapy for more than 3 years. Reasons for discontinuing HRT were negative side-effects (35%), desire to find out if climacteric symptoms had ended (26%), fear of cancer and thrombosis (25%), weariness of bleeding (19%) and a wish to deal with the problems 'naturally' (15%). The authors thus concluded that compliance with HRT can be high if adequate information is given and follow-ups are made, but one main reason for poor compliance was negative side-effects, most likely progestogen-related. Among the symptoms reported as negative side-effects, depression, irritability and tension were significantly more often reported by patients who discontinued, compared with those who continued.

ESTROGEN–PROGESTOGEN REPLACEMENT THERAPY AND MOOD

Approximately 30% of women treated with hormones will experience negative mood changes (depression and irritability) related to the progestogen component in sequential HRT[9]. The onset of symptoms occurs shortly after the progestogen addition, and symptoms continue to increase in severity until the end of treatment. The symptoms usually remain 1–3 days after termination of the progestogen addition[10–12]. A meta-analysis of depression and mood changes in women receiving HRT revealed that estrogen alone was associated with symptom improvement, whereas progesterone given in combination with an estrogen counteracted the beneficial effect of the estrogen[13]. Review papers describe negative side-effects and therapeutic problems with the progestogen addition during HRT[14–16], and there are a number of clinical trials sustaining these statements[10–12,17–19].

In a 6-month placebo-controlled study, 54 asymptomatic postmenopausal women without a psychiatric history were randomly assigned to estrogen treatment either alone or in combination with cyclic medroxyprogesterone. Mood ratings were obtained every day for 30 days prior to treatment and during the last 30 days of treatment. The women randomized to estrogen plus MPA exhibited significant increases in daily depression, anxiety, cramping and breast tenderness. Although the increases were significant, they were mild and did not interfere with normal functioning[20]. In our studies where symptom ratings were recorded daily for 5 months and a cross-over design was used, mood and physical symptoms changed significantly when a progestogen was added. The mood changes affected the daily life of the women, but not daily functioning with their partner, family or work. Among women who dropped out from three of our studies, several reported severe premenstrual syndrome like side-effects, with an extensive influence on daily functioning[12,19,21].

At odds with these findings are studies reporting no adverse mood effects with a progestogen addition. In a 3-year prospective, double-blind placebo-controlled study, participants were assigned to placebo, daily CE, CE plus cyclical MPA, CE plus daily MPA or CE plus cyclical micronized progesterone. Fifty-two symptoms were self-reported on a checklist at 1 and 3 years. Progestogen-containing regimens were significantly associated with higher levels of breast discomfort, but anxiety, cognitive and affective symptoms did not differ according to treatment assignment[22]. Symptoms were, however, not reported daily, but intermittently. In addition, the study was designed as a parallel study, not a cross-over study. In a second trial, 23 non-depressed early-postmenopausal women participated in a single-blind pilot study with the following sequence of treatments: 1 week of no substance; 2 weeks of placebo; 2 weeks of progestogen only; 1 week of placebo; and 2 months of sequential standard HRT consisting of continuous 0.625 mg CE and an addition of progestogen 2 weeks per month. Half of the group received 5 mg MPA as a progestogen addition and the other half 200 mg of micronized progesterone. Daily assessments of mood and somatic symptoms were made. None of the hormone treatments had a detectable effect on mood. MPA users reported more breast tenderness and vaginal bleeding than the progesterone users. The authors conclude: 'In contrast with the widely held belief among psychiatrists that progesterone depresses mood, neither of the progestogens we used in normal, non-depressed and non-anxious women showed this effect'[23]. Again, mood symptoms were assessed between treatment groups rather than within individuals. In surgically postmenopausal women, no adverse side-effect was noted of sequential oral MPA given in conjunction with transdermal estrogen[24]. This study was, however, conducted only during one treatment cycle, and as the positive effects of estrogen treatment for postmenopausal vasomotor symptoms increase continuously during the first treatment cycle[18,21,25], this might blunt negative effects of MPA at the end of the first treatment cycle. The cyclical pattern would hereby be concealed.

The discrepancies between our studies and the above-cited studies with contradictory results are most likely a result of the design of the studies. It is clear that intraindividual studies, where comparisons within individuals are made, are a superior way of evaluating mood scores rather than parallel studies. Furthermore, we have shown that women with a prior history of premenstrual syndrome (PMS) are more affected by HRT than women with no prior PMS, and this might have enhanced the mood-provoking effects by the progestogen addition in our studies in which women with a PMS history as well as women without were included.

MPA given alone has been studied in one placebo-controlled, double-blind cross-over study. Prior and co-workers[26] found no adverse effects of MPA treatment in postmenopausal women. In this study, no estrogen was added, and the results suggest that MPA together with estrogen has a different, negative mood-provoking effect compared with MPA alone.

IMPORTANCE OF PROGESTOGEN DOSE

Magos and colleagues found a significant increase in behavioral changes with 7 days' addition of

5 mg of norethisterone acetate (NETA) to subcutaneous estradiol and testosterone treatment. However, the addition of 2.5 mg NETA or placebo did not induce negative side-effects[11]. The authors concluded that there seemed to be an increase in negative mood with increasing dosage of the progestogen[11]. The dose of progestogen added to an estrogen appears to have an impact on mood response. Surprisingly, women with a PMS history showed more positive mood with the addition of 20 mg MPA compared with 10 mg MPA. Negative mood was less provoked during 20 mg of MPA compared with 10 mg, in women with or without a history of PMS. Physical symptoms did not differ between the two MPA doses[19]. Postmenopausal women taking 2 mg estradiol continuously and sequential vaginal progesterone responded with more negative mood when treated with 400 mg/day compared with 800 mg/day[27]. A similar influence on negative mood has been reported in women using oral contraceptives[28,29]. Also, using oral contraceptives, women feel worse on lower compared with higher doses of progestogen[28].

ESTROGEN, PROGESTOGENS AND MOOD

Quality of life, well-being and depressed mood related to the menopause improve when women with climacteric symptoms are treated with estrogen[21,30-32]. Hot flushes, sleeping disturbances and vaginal dryness are all improved by estrogen[33]. Asymptomatic women without vasomotor symptoms, however, do not report increased well-being with unopposed estrogen treatment[20,34]. When women are treated with cyclical estrogen alone, no mood deterioration is noticed at the end of treatment, while with a sequential regimen, significant mood deterioration occurs when the progestogen is added[10]. In our studies, well-being is at its best during the estrogen-only phase of sequential HRT[12,27]. Similar results have been found in women treated with CE plus cyclic MPA, compared with women treated with CE and placebo, in a 1-year randomized study[35].

The combination of estradiol and a progestogen appears to be essential for negative mood provocation. We have also investigated whether different doses of estrogen during sequential HRT affect mood and physical symptoms[21]. Postmenopausal women who completed a randomized double-blind cross-over study started with either 2 or 3 mg of estradiol continuously during three 28-day cycles, with an addition of 10 mg MPA on days 17–28. Thereafter, a cross-over to the other estrogen dose was made for two more 28-day cycles. The women recorded daily prospective symptom scores of physical, negative and positive mood symptoms. Menstrual bleeding, hot flushes, libido and influence on daily life were also monitored using the scales. When treated with the higher estradiol dose (3 mg), tension, irritability and depressed mood were all significantly augmented compared with when 2 mg estradiol was used, but only during the progestogen phase. Likewise, during treatment with the higher estrogen dose, physical symptoms increased during the progestogen phase. Positive mood symptoms were less affected, but friendliness decreased significantly during treatment with 3 mg estradiol. Our conclusion is that an increase of the estrogen dose accentuates negative mood and physical symptoms during the progestogen phase with sequential hormonal therapy[21]. There is some support in the literature for this interpretation. In a study of serum estradiol levels and mood during HRT, Klaiber and co-workers found that women with higher treatment serum estradiol levels had significantly more dysphoria when receiving a combination of estrogen plus progestogen than did the women with lower serum estradiol levels[36].

DIFFERENCES BETWEEN NORETHISTERONE ACETATE, MEDROXYPROGESTERONE ACETATE AND PROGESTERONE IN MOOD-PROVOKING EFFECTS

From the studies we have performed so far, some conclusions regarding women with prior PMS and progestogen type and dose can be drawn. The type of progestogen seems to be of minor importance to women with a history of PMS. While controls responded with increased negative mood and decreased positive mood scores when treated with NETA compared with MPA[12], the mood response in women with prior PMS was more inconsistent. In a study aimed towards investigating change in well-being during the first month of continuous combined HRT, CE-MPA was compared with estradiol (E_2)-NETA in a double-blind randomized study. Women who had not used HRT before the start of the study ('starters') improved significantly in scores of hot flushes and well-being during the first week of treatment, but deteriorated in scores of abdominal bloating and breast tenderness. Surprisingly, the positive effects on well-being vanished after the first week of treatment. In fact, at the end of the first month of treatment, women reported mood scores similar to those before treatment[25]. The women who switched from previous sequential HRT improved significantly regarding hot flushes, but deteriorated in terms of physical symptoms, energy, cheerfulness, depression and effect on daily life. Women treated with CE-MPA reported better well-being than women treated with E_2-NETA. 'Switchers', in particular, reported more deterioration of well-being when treated with E_2-NETA compared with CE-MPA, suggesting that 'starters' and 'switchers' respond differently to the onset of HRT[25]. Furthermore, we found that a history of PMS had a significant predictive value for deterioration of symptoms of well-being during the first month of treatment[25]. However, at odds with these results, Smith and co-workers found that cyclical NETA during continuous estrogen treatment was more likely to cause pain than either MPA or dydrogesterone, but less likely to cause negative affect symptoms[37].

It has been suggested that PMS might be treated with MPA, but the beneficial effect of MPA therapy is the consequence of total inhibition of hormone production rather than the result of ovulation suppression only[38]. When the menstrual cycle is totally disrupted, ovarian estradiol and progesterone production are inhibited, but when only ovulation is inhibited, the production of estradiol continues, and with addition of exogenous MPA a similar situation develops to that observed during combined estrogen-progestogen treatment. NETA was reported to have no beneficial effects compared with placebo; in fact, some women withdrew from the study owing to adverse effects[38].

SIGNS OF VULNERABILITY IN DIFFERENT PATIENT GROUPS

Women with a history of PMS seem to be more vulnerable to adverse mood effects induced by HRT than women without prior PMS. The PMS diagnosis of women participating in postmenopausal studies is of course a difficulty, since they are already postmenopausal when consulting for climacteric symptoms. Therefore, women with a retrospective diagnosis should be regarded as having had cyclical negative mood symptoms, which decreased or disappeared at the onset of bleeding, rather than premenstrual dysphoric disorder (PMDD) according to the *Diagnostic and Statistical Manual of Mental Disorders* (DSM IV)[39]. Fifty-two per cent of the women in our clinical trials reported experiences of premenstrual symptoms, whereas only 2-6% of the female fertile population suffers from severe PMDD[12,40]. The number of women with self-reported, retrospective PMS symptoms in our studies is similar to that found in population-based studies with retrospective self-reported data[40]. However, when counselling women with climacteric problems, the only PMS diagnosis that can be obtained at that point is retrospective and based on self-report.

There seems to be a relationship between experiencing negative mood symptoms during progestogen treatment and a history of PMS. Women with PMS during their fertile life respond with lower mood scores during the progestogen addition to estrogen than women without a history of PMS, as shown in one of our double-blind randomized clinical trials[12].

SEX HORMONES AND PREMENSTRUAL SYNDROME

The following discusses some of what is known about the relationship between sex steroid hormones and PMS. The pattern of mood changes during sequential HRT has resemblances to the pattern of premenstrual cyclic mood swings. If menopause was induced in women with or without PMS by treatment with a gonadotropin-releasing hormone (GnRH) agonist, add-back therapy with estradiol and/or progesterone provoked a significant recurrence of symptoms in women with PMS. However, for women without PMS, no mood changes occurred[41]. In fertile women, the presence of premenstrual symptoms requires ovulation, formation of a corpus luteum and both estrogen and progesterone production. PMS symptoms disappear during anovulatory cycles where progesterone and allopregnanolone, a γ-aminobutyric acid type A ($GABA_A$) receptor-active progesterone metabolite (see below), levels are low[42–44]. Symptoms develop in close connection with the increased secretion of progesterone and allopregnanolone during the early luteal phase[42,45]. During the preovulatory estrogen peak when progesterone and allopregnanolone levels are low, women are at their phase of highest well-being[45]. During the luteal phase when progesterone and allopregnanolone levels are high, estrogen seems to deteriorate well-being and is related to the severity of negative mood symptoms in women with PMS[46,47] . If women with moderate to severe PMS are treated with estrogen during the luteal phase, mental and physical symptoms of PMS are aggravated[48]. Finally, women with PMS are more susceptible to mood provocation during treatment with oral contraceptives than healthy controls[49]. Another sign indicating that women suffering from PMS have different neurosteroid sensitivity is that the sedative response to intravenous pregnanolone (a progesterone metabolite acting as a $GABA_A$ receptor agonist) was reduced during the luteal phase of PMS patients compared with controls[50]. In addition, patients with severe premenstrual symptoms were less sensitive to the administered pregnanolone compared with patients with more moderate symptoms[50]. Similar results were obtained when benzodiazepines were given, suggesting that patients with PMS have a tolerance for $GABA_A$ receptor allosteric agonists[51–53].

MECHANISMS OF PROGESTOGEN AND ESTROGEN EFFECTS ON MOOD

The exact mechanism behind the induction of negative mood symptoms is still not completely understood. It is clear, however, that the deterioration of mood is related to the progestogen addition to estrogen in postmenopausal replacement therapy. Estrogen given alone seems also to have a different effect, compared with when given in combination with progestogens, as discussed below. The most pronounced effect of progesterone and progestogens in the central nervous system (CNS) is that of their 5α-3α-hydroxy metabolites. Pregnanolone and allopregnanolone (3α-OH-5α/β-pregnan-20-one) are major metabolites of progesterone, and very potent positive allosteric modulators of the $GABA_A$ receptor in the brain[54,55]. The GABA system is the largest inhibitory system in the brain and the target system for benzodiazepines, barbiturates and many of alcohol's effects. The GABA system is also most likely to be involved in mood responses to HRT. Progestogens such as MPA are metabolized into GABA-active metabolites as well, although their potency is lower than that of the progesterone metabolites[56]. It has been shown that the anesthetic effect of progesterone is mediated via its metabolite allopregnanolone, through modulation of the $GABA_A$ receptor[57].

It is of interest that several $GABA_A$ receptor agonists such as benzodiazepines, barbiturates, alcohol and the progesterone metabolite allopregnanolone seem to have biphasic effects on CNS-related symptoms in both humans and animals. In high doses, one type of effect (inhibition) is seen, while low doses result in the opposite effect (disinhibition). Allopregnanolone has anxiolytic, sedative and antiepileptic effects, some seen in both humans and animals, others only in animals[50,57–61].

In addition, the $GABA_A$ receptor agonists including allopregnanolone have been shown to inhibit learning and memory[62,63], increase appetite[64–66], disturb motor function[67–69] and worsen petit mal epilepsy[70,71], and in very high dosages a drug abuse potential has been seen[72,73].

In contrast, a low dose of allopregnanolone given to rats produces a conditioned place aversion while a higher dose has no effect or gives a place preference effect[73,74]. Allopregnanolone, which has similarities to alcohol, increases aggression in rats up to a certain level, after which a further increased dose of allopregnanolone and/or alcohol decreases aggressive behavior[75]. Moreover, a low dose of diazepam given to humans and animals elicits more negative mood and aggression than placebo, even under experimental conditions[76-79]. Induction of severe negative mood reactions by barbiturates has been found in 2.5–6% of patients undergoing amobarbital injections as a work-up for epilepsy surgery, and milder emotional reactions seem even more common[80-82]. The prevalence of severe reactions (2.5–6%) to barbiturates is interesting, as it is similar to the prevalence of PMDD (2–6%)[39].

The $GABA_A$ receptor modulators, allopregnanolone, alcohol, barbiturates and benzodiazepines, also have effects via indirect changes in the function of the $GABA_A$ system, by induction of tolerance. An animal model resembling HRT has been developed. In this model, progesterone and its metabolite allopregnanolone induce changes in the α_4 subunit of the $GABA_A$ receptor in the hippocampus, parallel to the induction of anxiety[83]. Several papers report changes in $GABA_A$ receptor subunit composition and decreased GABA function after long-term exposure of $GABA_A$ receptor agonists[84-88]. A reduced sensitivity to benzodiazepine, alcohol and pregnanolone is also seen in women with PMDD who have a reduced benzodiazepine, alcohol and pregnanolone sensitivity during the luteal phase[50,53,89].

If continuous exposure to a $GABA_A$ receptor agonist is interrupted, a withdrawal effect will occur. An example of conditions that may be influenced by this withdrawal/abstinence phenomenon is epilepsy, in which the patient has an epileptic focus in the cerebral cortex where a worsening takes place by the time of the hormone withdrawal period during menstruation. Another example is menstrually related migraine[90-98]. It is plausible that this phenomenon also occurs at the end of the progestogen phase in sequential hormone therapy.

The serotonin system is also likely to be responsive to mood effects of sex steroids. Recently, Alves and colleagues found that estrogen treatment significantly increased progesterone receptor expression in the midbrain raphe where serotonin neurons originate[99]. Birzniece and colleagues[100] gave adult ovariectomized female rats estradiol alone or in combination with progesterone for 2 weeks. Serotonin type 1A (5-HT(1A)) receptor mRNA levels were analyzed by *in situ* hybridization in the dorsal hippocampus, dorsal and median raphe nuclei and entorhinal cortex. Chronic estradiol treatment alone reduced 5-HT(1A) gene expression, while the combined treatment increased 5-HT(1A) gene expression in the hippocampus. Concomitantly, 5-HT(1A) mRNA expression was decreased in the ventrolateral part of the dorsal raphe[100]. Also, 5-HT(2A) and 5-HT(2C) receptor mRNA changed with estradiol plus progesterone treatment in the hippocampus but not in the frontal cortex. The direction of changes varied in different subregions and with estradiol alone or estradiol plus progesterone treatment[101].

The urinary metabolite of serotonin, 5-hydroxyindole acetic acid (5-HIAA), increased significantly during estrogen-only treatment, whereas estradiol in combination with NETA abolished this effect[102]. Blood platelet serotonin content and imipramine binding are peripheral markers of serotonin activity. Continuous treatment with CE and MPA is suggested to increase platelet [^{3}H] imipramine binding and improve mood in postmenopausal women[103]. However, other studies have not been able to show any effects of unopposed estradiol or HRT in terms of peripheral markers of serotonin activity on healthy postmenopausal women[104].

Treatment with a GnRH agonist in PMDD patients relieved their premenstrual symptoms, compared with placebo. In the above study, the binding of paroxetine to platelet serotonin uptake sites was analyzed. The number of paroxetine binding sites was higher in the follicular phase in untreated PMDD patients compared with controls, and when women were successfully treated with GnRH agonist, the difference disappeared. The results are consistent with the hypothesis that changes in serotoninergic transmission could be a trait in PMDD[105].

It is obvious that ovarian steroids influence the serotonin system; however, general conclusions can sometimes be difficult to draw as the interactions differ from brain region to brain region and effects also depend on the time course of treatment (short-term versus long-term effects).

We know that estrogen also exerts its CNS effects via enhancing the excitatory effect of glutamate[106-108]. The glutamate system is the largest excitatory system in the brain, and is the excitatory counterpart to the inhibitory GABA system. The glutamate system is known to be involved in the induction of depression, and glutamate antagonists are used as antidepressants[109]. A situation in which the recall of unpleasant depressant/anxiogenic memories is enhanced by estrogen-induced stimulation of the glutamate system, combined with disinhibition of the GABA system, may allow negative emotional memories to surface. In such a concept, the effects of progestogens and estrogen, as shown by the results of studies to date, are understandable. Estradiol treatment alone would consequently not induce negative mood symptoms, but instead enhance pleasant mood feelings.

ACKNOWLEDGEMENTS

Work presented here has been supported by the Swedish Medical Research Council (project 4X-11198), Wallenberg Foundation, Umeå sjukvård, spjutspetsanslag, Visare Norr, Samverkansnämnden, Norra Regionen, EU-regional fund Objective 1, Umeå University foundations, Västerbottens läns landsting and Umeå Kommun.

References

1. Cano A. Compliance to hormone replacement therapy in menopausal women controlled in a third level academic centre. *Maturitas* 1994;20: 91-9
2. Kotzan JA, Martin BC, Wade WE. Persistence with estrogen therapy in a postmenopausal Medicaid population. *Pharmacotherapy* 1999; 19:363-9
3. Wren BG, Brown L. Compliance with hormonal replacement therapy. *Maturitas* 1991;13:17-21
4. Ryan PJ, Harrison R, Blake GM, Fogelman I. Compliance with hormone replacement therapy (HRT) after screening for postmenopausal osteoporosis. *Br J Obstet Gynaecol* 1992;99:325-8
5. Torgerson DJ, Donaldson C, Russell IT, Reid DM. Hormone replacement therapy: compliance and cost after screening for osteoporosis. *Eur J Obstet Gynecol Reprod Biol* 1995;59:57-60
6. Hulley S, Furberg C, Barrett-Connor E, *et al.*, HERS Research Group. Noncardiovascular disease outcomes during 6.8 years of hormone therapy: Heart and Estrogen/progestin Replacement Study follow up (HERS II). *J Am Med Assoc* 2002;288:99-101
7. Dören M, Reuther G, Minne HW, Schneider HP. Superior compliance and efficacy of continuous combined oral estrogen-progestogen replacement therapy in postmenopausal women. *Am J Obstet Gynecol* 1995;173:1446-51
8. Stadberg E, Mattsson L-Å, Milsom I. Women's attitudes and knowledge about the climacteric period and its treatment. A Swedish population-based study. *Maturitas* 1997;27;109-16
9. Björn I, Bäckström T. Compliance to estrogen and progestins in treatment of peri- and postmenopausal women. The significance of negative side effects. *Maturitas* 1999;32:77-86
10. Hammarbäck S, Bäckström T, Holst J, von Schoultz B, Lyrenäs S. Cyclical mood changes as in the premenstrual tension syndrome during sequential estrogen-progestagen postmenopausal replacement treatment. *Acta Obstet Gynecol Scand* 1985;64:393-7
11. Magos AL, Brewster E, Sing R, O'Dowd TM, Studd JW. The effect of norethisterone in postmenopausal women on oestrogen therapy: a model for the premenstrual syndrome. *Br J Obstet Gynaecol* 1986;93:1290-6
12. Björn I, Bixo M, Nöjd KS, Nyberg S, Bäckström T. Negative mood changes during hormone replacement therapy: a comparison between two progestogens. *Am J Obstet Gynecol* 2000;183: 1419-26
13. Zweifel JE, O'Brien WH. A meta-analysis of the effect of hormone replacement therapy upon depressed mood. *Psychoneuroendocrinology* 1997; 22:189-212
14. von Schoultz B. Climacteric complaints as influenced by progestogens. *Maturitas* 1986;8: 107-12
15. Panay N, Studd J. Progestogen intolerance and compliance with hormone replacement therapy

in menopausal women. *Hum Reprod Update* 1997; 3:159–71
16. Sherwin BB. Progestogens used in menopause. Side effects, mood and quality of life. *J Reprod Med* 1999;44:227–32
17. Klaiber EL, Broverman DM, Vogel W, Peterson LG, Snyder MB. Individual differences in changes in mood and platelet monoamine oxidase (MAO) activity during hormonal replacement therapy in menopausal women. *Psychoneuroendocrinology* 1996;21:575–92
18. Holst J, Bäckström T, Hammarbäck S, von Schoultz B. Progestogen addition during oestrogen replacement therapy – effects on vasomotor symptoms and mood. *Maturitas* 1989;11:13–20
19. Björn I, Bixo M, Nöjd KS, *et al.* The impact of different doses of medroxyprogesterone acetate on mood symptoms in sequential hormonal therapy. *Gynecol Endocrinol* 2002;16:1–8
20. Girdler SS, O'Briant C, Steege J, Grewen K, Light KC. A comparison of the effect of estrogen with or without progesterone on mood and physical symptoms in postmenopausal women. *J Women Health Gend Based Med* 1999;8:637–46
21. Björn I, Bixo M, Nyberg S, Bäckström G, Sundström-Poromaa I, Bäckström T. Increase of estrogen dose deteriorates mood during progestin phase in sequential hormonal therapy. *J Clin Endocrinol Metab* 2003;in press
22. Greendale GA, Reboussin BA, Hogan P, *et al.* Symptoms relief and side effects of postmenopausal hormones: results from the Postmenopausal Estrogen/Progestin Interventions Trial. *Obstet Gynecol* 1998;92:982–8
23. Cummings JA, Brizendine L. Comparison of physical and emotional side effects of progesterone or medroxyprogesterone in early postmenopausal women. *Menopause* 2002;9:253–63
24. Kirkham C, Hahn PM, Van Vugt DA, Carmichael JA, Reid RL. A randomized, double-blind, placebo-controlled, cross-over trial to assess the side effects of medroxyprogesterone acetate in hormone replacement therapy. *Obstet Gynecol* 1991;78:93–7
25. Ödmark I-S, Bixo M, Jonsson B, Bäckström T. Well-being in postmenopausal women at the onset of two different continuous combined therapies. Presented at the *Nordic Federation of Societies of Obstetricians and Gynecologists (NFOG) XXXIII Congress*, Umeå, Sweden, June 2002 abstr 169 (http://www.nfog.org)
26. Prior JC, Alojado N, McKay DW, Vigna YM. No adverse effects of medroxyprogesterone treatment without estrogen in postmenopausal women: double blind, placebo-controlled, crossover trial. *Obstet Gynecol* 1994;83:24–8
27. Andréen L, Bixo M, Nyberg S, Sundström-Poromaa I, Bäckström T. Progesterone effects during sequential hormone replacement therapy. *Eur J Endocrinol* 2003;in press
28. Cullberg J. Mood changes and menstrual symptoms with different gestagen/estrogen combinations. A double blind comparison with a placebo. *Acta Psychiatr Scand Suppl* 1972;236:1–86
29. Bancroft J, Sanders D, Warner P, Loudon N. The effects of oral contraceptives on mood and sexuality: comparison of triphasic and combined preparations. *J Psychosom Obstet Gynaecol* 1987; 7:1–8
30. Derman RJ, Danwood MY, Stone S. Quality of life during sequential hormone replacement therapy – a placebo-controlled study. *Int J Fertil Menopausal Stud* 1995;40:73–8
31. Rebar RW, Trabal J, Mortola J. Low-dose esterified estrogens (0.3 mg/day): long-term and short-term effects on menopausal symptoms and quality of life in postmenopausal women. *Climacteric* 2000;3:176–82
32. Schmidt PJ, Nieman L, Danaceau MA, *et al.* Estrogen replacement in perimenopause-related depression: a preliminary report. *Am J Obstet Gynecol* 2000;183:414–20
33. Wiklund I, Berg G, Hammar M, Karlberg J, Lindgren R, Sandin K. Long-term effect of transdermal therapy on aspects of quality of life in postmenopausal women. *Maturitas* 1992;14: 225–36
34. Skarsgard C, Berg G, Ekblad S, Wiklund I, Hammar M. Effects of estrogen therapy on well-being in postmenopausal women without vasomotor complaints. *Maturitas* 2000;36:123–30
35. Sherwin BB. The impact of different doses of estrogen and progestin on mood and sexual behaviour in postmenopausal women. *J Clin Endocrinol Metab* 1991;72:336–43
36. Klaiber EL, Broverman DM, Vogel W, Peterson LG, Snyder MB. Relationships of serum estradiol levels, menopausal duration, and mood during hormonal replacement therapy. *Psychoneuroendocrinology* 1997;22:549–58
37. Smith RN, Holland EF, Studd JW. The symptomatology of progestogen intolerance. *Maturitas* 1994;18:87–91
38. West CP. Inhibition of ovulation with oral progestins – effectiveness in premenstrual syndrome. *Eur J Obstet Gynecol Reprod Biol* 1990;34:119–28
39. American Psychiatric Association. *Diagnostic and Statistical Manual of Mental Disorders*, 4th edn. Washington, DC: Department of Health and Human Services, 1994:714–18
40. Sveinsdottir H, Bäckström T. Prevalence of menstrual cycle symptom cyclicity and premenstrual dysphoric disorder in a random sample of women using and not using oral contraceptives. *Acta Obstet Gynecol Scand* 2000;79:405–13

41. Schmidt PJ, Nieman LK, Danaceau MA, Adams LF, Rubinow DR. Differential behavioral effects of gonadal steroids in women with and in those without premenstrual syndrome. *N Engl J Med* 1998;338:209-16
42. Hammarbäck S, Bäckström T. Induced anovulation as treatment of premenstrual tension syndrome. A double-blind cross-over study with GnRH-agonist versus placebo. *Acta Obstet Gynecol Scand* 1988;67:159-66
43. Hammarbäck S, Ekholm UB, Backstrom T. Spontaneous anovulation causing disappearance of cyclical symptoms in women with the premenstrual syndrome. *Acta Endocrinol* 1991;125:132-7
44. Wang M, Seippel L, Purdy RH, Bäckström T. Relationship between symptom severity and steroid variation in women with premenstrual syndrome: study on serum pregnenolone, pregnenolone sulfate, 5α-pregnane-3,20-dione and 3α-hydroxy-5α-pregnan-20-one. *J Clin Endocrinol Metab* 1996;81:1076-82
45. Bäckström T, Sanders D, Leask R, Davidson D, Warner P, Bancroft J. Mood, sexuality, hormones, and the menstrual cycle. II. Hormone levels and their relationship to the premenstrual syndrome. *Psychosom Med* 1983;45:503-7
46. Hammarbäck S, Damber JE, Bäckström T. Relationship between symptom severity and hormone changes in women with premenstrual syndrome. *J Clin Endocrinol Metab* 1989;68:125-30
47. Seippel L, Bäckström T. Luteal-phase estradiol relates to symptom severity in patients with premenstrual syndrome. *J Clin Endocrinol Metab* 1998;83:1988-92
48. Dahr V, Murphy BE. Double-blind randomized crossover trial of luteal phase estrogens (Premarin) in the premenstrual syndrome (PMS). *Psychoneuroendocrinology* 1990;15:489-93
49. Cullberg J. Mood changes and menstrual symptoms with different gestagen/estrogen combinations. A double blind comparison with placebo. *Acta Psychiatr Scand* 1972;236(Suppl):1-84
50. Sundström I, Andersson A, Nyberg S, *et al.* Patients with premenstrual syndrome have a different sensitivity to a neuroactive steroid during the menstrual cycle compared to control subjects. *Neuroendocrinology* 1998;67:126-38
51. Sundström I, Ashbrook D, Bäckström T. Reduced benzodiazepine sensitivity in patients with premenstrual syndrome: a pilot study. *Psychoneuroendocrinology* 1997;22:25-38
52. Sundström I, Nyberg S, Bäckström T. Patients with premenstrual syndrome have reduced sensitivity to midazolam compared to control subjects. *Neuropsychopharmacology* 1997;17:370-81
53. Nyberg S, Sundström-Poromaa I, Bäckström T. Patients with premenstrual dysphoric disorder have a decreased sensitivity to alcohol in the luteal phase. Presented at the *Nordic Federation of Societies of Obstetricians and Gynecologists (NFOG) XXXIII Congress*, Umeå, Sweden, June 2002: abstr 187 (http://www.nfog.org)
54. Majewska MD, Harrison NL, Schwartz RD, Barker JL, Paul SM. Steroid hormone metabolites are barbiturate-like modulators of the GABA receptor. *Science* 1986;232:1004-7
55. Korkmaz S, Wahlström G. The EEG burst suppression threshold test for the determination of CNS sensitivity to intravenous anaesthetics in rats. *Brain Res Protocols* 1997;1:378-84
56. Meyerson BJ. Relationship between the anesthetic and gestagenic action and estrus behavior-inducing activity of different progestins. *Endocrinology* 1967;81:369-74
57. Mok WM, Krieger NR. Evidence that 5α-pregnan-3α-ol-20-one is the metabolite responsible for progesterone anesthesia. *Brain Res* 1990;533:42-5
58. Bäckström T, Zetterlund B, Blom S, Romano M. Effects of intravenous progesterone infusions on the epileptic discharge frequency in women with partial epilepsy. *Acta Neurol Scand* 1984;69:240-8
59. Landgren S, Aasly J, Backstrom T, Dubrovsky B, Danielsson E. The effect of progesterone and its metabolites on the interictal epileptiform discharge in the cat's cerebral cortex. *Acta Physiol Scand* 1987;131:33-42
60. Wieland S, Lan NC, Mirasedeghi S, Gee KW. Anxiolytic activity of the progesterone metabolite 5α-pregnan-3α-ol-20-one. *Brain Res* 1991;565:263-8
61. Carl P, Hogskilde S, Nielsen JW, *et al.* Pregnanolone emulsion. A preliminary pharmacokinetic and pharmacodynamic study of a new intravenous anaesthetic agent. *Anaesthesia* 1990;45:189-97
62. Mayo W, Dellu F, Robel P, *et al.* Infusion of neurosteroids into the nucleus basalis magnocellularis affects cognitive processes in the rat. *Brain Res* 1983;607:324-8
63. Johansson IM, Birzniece V, Lindblad C, Olsson T, Bäckström T. Allopregnanolone inhibits learning in the Morris water maze. *Brain Res* 2002;934:125-31
64. Chen SW, Rodriguez L, Davies MF, Loew GH. The hyperphagic effect of 3α-hydroxylated pregnane steroids in male rats. *Pharmacol Biochem Behav* 1996;53:777-82
65. Both-Orthman B, Rubinow DR, Hoban MC, Malley J, Grover GN. Menstrual cycle phase-related changes in appetite in patients with premenstrual syndrome and in control subjects. *Am J Psychiatry* 1988;145:628-31
66. Reddy DS, Kulkarni SK. The role of $GABA_A$ and mitochondrial diazepam-binding inhibitor receptors on the effects of neurosteroids on food intake in mice. *Psychopharmacology* 1998;137:391-400

67. Gasior M, Carter RB, Goldberg SR, Witkin JM. Anticonvulsant and behavioral effects of neuroactive steroids alone and in conjunction with diazepam. *J Pharmacol Exp Ther* 1997;282:543-53
68. Khisti RT, Mandhane SN, Chopde CT. The neurosteroid 3α-hydroxy-5α-pregnan-20-one induces catalepsy in mice. *Neurosci Lett* 1998; 251:85-8
69. Wieland S, Belluzzi JD, Stein L, Lan NC. Comparative behavioral characterization of the neuroactive steroids 3α-OH,5α-pregnan-20-one and 3α-OH,5β-pregnan-20-one in rodents. *Psychopharmacology* 1995;118:65-71
70. Banerjee PK, Snead OC III. Neuroactive steroids exacerbate γ-hydroxybutyric acid-induced absence seizures in rats. *Eur J Pharmacol* 1998;359:41-8
71. Grunewald RA, Aliberti V, Panayiotopoulos CP. Exacerbation of typical absence seizures by progesterone. *Seizure* 1992;1:137-8
72. Finn DA, Phillips TJ, Okorn DM, Chester JA, Cunningham CL. Rewarding effect of the neuroactive steroid 3α-hydroxy-5α-pregnan-20-one in mice. *Pharmacol Biochem Behav* 1997;56:261-4
73. Franklin KBJ, Biskin RS, Bossert JM. *Systemic administration of allopregnanolone, but not other neurosteroid metabolites, induces a place preference in rats.* Program no. 607.17.2002, Abstract Viewer/ Itinerary Planner. Washington, DC: Society for Neuroscience, 2002 (http://sfn.scholarone.com/ itin2002/index.html)
74. Beauchamp MH, Ormerod BK, Jhamandas K, Boegman RJ, Beninger RJ. Neurosteroids and reward: allopregnanolone produces a conditioned place aversion in rats. *Pharmacol Biochem Behav* 2000;67:29-35
75. Fish EW, Faccidomo S, DeBold JF, Miczek KA. Alcohol, allopregnanolone and aggression in mice. *Psychopharmacology* 2001;153:473-83
76. Wenzel RR, Bartel T, Eggebrecht H, Philipp T, Erbel R. Central-nervous side effects of midazolam during transesophageal echocardiography. *J Am Soc Echocardiogr* 2002;15:1297-300
77. Miczek KA, Weerts EM, DeBold JF. Alcohol, benzodiazepine-$GABA_A$ receptor complex and aggression: ethological analysis of individual differences in rodents and primates. *J Stud Alcohol* 1993;(Suppl 11):170-9
78. Ferrari PF, Parmigiani S, Rodgers RJ, Palanza P. Differential effects of chlordiazepoxide in mice. *Psychopharmacology* 1997;134:258-65
79. Ben-Porath DD, Taylor SP. The effects of diazepam (valium) and aggressive disposition on human aggression: an experimental investigation. *Addict Behav* 2002;27:167-77
80. Kurthen M, Linke DB, Reuter BM, Hufnagel A, Elger CE. Severe negative emotional reactions in intracarotid sodium amytal procedures: further evidence for hemisphere asymmetries? *Cortex* 1991;27:333-7
81. Lee GP, Loring DW, Meador KJ, Flanigin HF, Brooks BS. Severe behavioral complications following intracarotid sodium amobarbital injection: implications for hemisphere asymmetry of emotion. *Neurology* 1988;38:1233-6
82. Masia SL, Perrine K, Westbrook L, Alper K, Devinsky O. Emotional outbursts and post-traumatic stress disorder during intracarotid amobarbital procedure. *Neurology* 2000;54:1691-3
83. Gulinello M, Gong QH, Li X, Smith SS. Short-term exposure to a neuroactive steroid increases α_4 GABA(A) receptor subunit levels in association with increased anxiety in the female rat. *Brain Res* 2001;910:55-66
84. Friedman LK, Gibbs TT, Farb DH. γ-Aminobutyric acid A receptor regulation: heterologous uncoupling of modulatory site interactions induced by chronic steroid, barbiturate, benzodiazepine, or GABA treatment in culture. *Brain Res* 1996;707:100-9
85. Yu R, Ticku MK. Chronic neurosteroid treatment decreases the efficacy of benzodiazepine ligands and neurosteroids at the γ-aminobutyric acid A receptor complex in mammalian cortical neurons. *J Pharmacol Exp Ther* 1995;275:784-9
86. Yu R, Follesa P, Ticku MK. Down-regulation of the GABA receptor subunits mRNA levels in mammalian cultured cortical neurons following chronic neurosteroid treatment. *Brain Res Mol Brain Res* 1996;41:163-8
87. Marshall FH, Stratton SC, Mullings J, *et al.* Development of tolerance in mice to the sedative effects of the neuroactive steroid minaxolone following chronic exposure. *Pharmacol Biochem Behav* 1997;58:1-8
88. Concas A, Mostalino MC, Porcu P, *et al.* Role of brain allopregnanolone in the plasticity of γ-aminobutyric acid type A receptor in rat brain during pregnancy and after delivery. *Proc Natl Acad Sci USA* 1998;95:13284-9
89. Sundström I, Ashbrook D, Bäckström T. Reduced benzodiazepine sensitivity in patients with premenstrual syndrome: a pilot study. *Psychoneuroendocrinology* 1997;22:25-38
90. Laidlaw J. Catamenial epilepsy. *Lancet* 1956; 271:1235-7
91. Bäckström T. Epileptic seizures in women related to plasma estrogen and progesterone during the menstrual cycle. *Acta Neurol Scand* 1976;54: 321-47
92. Herzog AG, Klein P, Ransil BJ. Three patterns of catamenial epilepsy. *Epilepsia* 1997;38:1082-8
93. MacGregor EA. 'Menstrual' migraine: towards a definition. *Cephalalgia* 1996;16:11-21
94. Voiculescu V, Hategan D, Manole E, Ulmeanu A. Increased susceptibility to audiogenic seizures

following withdrawal of progesterone. *Rom J Neurol Psychiatry* 1994;32:131–3
95. Gallo MA, Smith SS. Progesterone withdrawal decreases latency to and increases duration of electrified prod burial: a possible rat model of PMS anxiety. *Pharmacol Biochem Behav* 1993; 46:897–904
96. Moran MH, Smith SS. Progesterone withdrawal I: pro-convulsant effects. *Brain Res* 1998;807: 84–90
97. Smith SS, Gong QH, Hsu FC, Markowitz RS, ffrench-Mullen JM, Li X. GABA(A) receptor α_4 subunit suppression prevents withdrawal properties of an endogenous steroid. *Nature (London)* 1998;392:926–30
98. Rosciszewska D. Analysis of seizure dispersion during menstrual cycle in women with epilepsy. *Monogr Neural Sci* 1980;5:280–4
99. Alves SE, McEwen BS, Hayashi S, Korach KS, Pfaff DW, Ogawa S. Estrogen-regulated progestin receptors are found in the midbrain raphe but not in hippocampus of estrogen receptor α (ERα) gene-disrupted mice. *J Comp Neurol* 2000;427: 185–95
100. Birzniece V, Johansson IM, Wang MD, Seckl JR, Backstrom T, Olsson T. Serotonin 5-HT(1A) receptor mRNA expression in dorsal hippocampus and raphe nuclei after gonadal hormone manipulation in female rats. *Neuroendocrinology* 2001;74:135–42
101. Birzniece V, Johansson IM, Wang MD, Bäckström T, Olsson T. Ovarian hormone effects on 5-hydroxytryptamine(2A) and 5-hydroxytryptamine(2C) receptor mRNA expression in the ventral hippocampus and frontal cortex of female rats. *Neurosci Lett* 2002;319:157–61
102. Mueck AO, Seeger H, Kasspohl-Buts S, Teichmann AT, Lippert TH. Influence of norethisterone acetate and estradiol on the serotonin metabolism of postmenopausal women. *Horm Metab Res* 1997;29:80–3
103. Bukulmez O, Al A, Gurdal H, Yarali H, Ulug B, Gurgan T. Short-term effects of the continuous hormone replacement therapy regimens on platelet tritiated imipramine binding and mood scores: a proscpective randomized trial. *Fertil Steril* 2001;75:737–43
104. Wihlbäck AC, Sundström-Poromaa I, Allard P, Mjörndal T, Spigset O, Bäckström T. Influence of postmenopausal hormone replacement therapy on platelet serotonin uptake site and serotonin 2A receptor binding. *Obstet Gynecol* 2001;98:450–7
105. Bixo M, Allard P, Bäckström T, *et al.* Binding of [3H]paroxetine to serotonin uptake sites and of [3H]lysergic acid diethylamide to 5-HT2A receptors in platelets from women with premenstrual dysphoric disorder during gonadotropin releasing hormone treatment. *Psychoneuroendocrinology* 2001;26:551–64
106. Smith SS, Waterhouse BD, Woodward DJ. Locally applied estrogens potentiate glutamate-evoked excitation of cerebellar Purkinje cells. *Brain Res* 1988;475:272–82
107. Smith SS. Estrogen administration increases neuronal responses to excitatory amino acids as a long-term effect. *Brain Res* 1989;503:354–7
108. McEwen B. Estrogen actions throughout the brain. *Recent Prog Horm Res* 2002;57:357–84
109. Krystal JH, Sanacora G, Blumberg H, *et al.* Glutamate and GABA systems as targets for novel antidepressant and mood-stabilizing treatments. *Mol Psychiatry* 2002;7(Suppl):71–80

Δ^5-Androgen replacement therapy: a new piece of the mosaic

16

A. R. Genazzani, F. Bernardi, M. Stomati, N. Pluchino, I. di Bono, L. Rovati, M. Palumbo, A. D. Genazzani and M. Luisi

INTRODUCTION

Although much attention has been given to study of the postmenopause and the options in hormone replacement treatment (i.e. estrogens and progestins), relatively less attention has been paid to the activity of endogenous or exogenous androgens in women. However, middle-age in women is characterized by a combination of menopause and adrenopause that can both participate in creating the so-called androgen-deficiency syndrome.

Androgens are produced in women by both the ovaries and the adrenals, which synthesize androstenedione, testosterone and dehydroepiandrosterone (DHEA). The adrenal glands also produce DHEA sulfate (DHEAS), while testosterone is also obtained from the conversion of active precursors (mainly androstenedione)[1]. In the ovaries, androgens are secreted by the thecal cells under the control of luteinizing hormone (LH). Serum androstenedione and testosterone levels have a relative cyclicity, with a first rise in circulating levels of both hormones close to ovulation and a second rise in only androstenedione level in the late luteal phase[2]. Only 1-2% of circulating testosterone and androstenedione are free and biologically active on target tissues. Both these androgens are mainly bound (98–99%) to a specific circulating protein, sex hormone-binding globulin (SHBG) or albumin. The affinity of steroid hormones for SHBG is higher in the cases of dihydrotestosterone, testosterone and androstenedione than in the case of DHEA[3]. In humans, modification of SHBG levels, induced by a specific or non-specific mechanism, produces several effects on free plasma androgen levels. For instance, increased levels of estradiol and thyroid hormones induce an increase of SHBG, while glucocorticoids, growth hormone and insulin decrease SHBG levels. As a consequence, states associated with (relative or absolute) high estrogen levels, such as pregnancy or estrogen replacement therapy, can induce androgen deficiency.

DHEA and its sulfate ester, DHEAS, are the major circulating adrenal cortex products[4,5]. DHEAS is synthesized from the conversion of free DHEA, which is mainly secreted by the adrenals (70–80%) and only in part (20%) by the ovaries. Both Δ^5-androgens (DHEA and DHEAS) are peripherally converted into androstenedione, testosterone, dihydrotestosterone (DHT) and estrogens. Adrenocorticotropic hormone (ACTH) acutely administered stimulates DHEA release, with a prompt increase in the venous adrenal blood and in the peripheral circulation[6,7]. On the other hand, DHEAS, which has a long plasma half-life, does not increase with ACTH stimulation. Several physiological or pathological conditions may modify the synthesis and release of $\Delta 5$-androgens. Adrenal androgen levels are suppressed in acute stress, severe systemic illness, anorexia nervosa and states associated with high cortisol levels[8-10].

The climacteric and the postmenopause are characterized by several endocrine, neuroendocrine and metabolic modifications that produce various short- and long-term symptoms. The short-term consequences are represented by vasomotor instability (hot flushes and sweats), mood or 'neurogenic' disturbances (depression, anxiety, migraine/headaches, insomnia) and dyslipidemia. Long-term consequences are represented by atrophic vaginitis, dyspareunia, decrease of libido, urinary disturbances (stress incontinence, nocturia), osteoporosis and increased risk of cardiovascular and cerebral diseases. Estrogen–progestin replacement therapy is considered to be the most effective approach to relieve symptoms, although several studies have focused on androgen replacement therapy, especially for those patients suffering from sexual disorders, loss of pubic and axillary hair, loss of well-being and energy, mood disorders and metabolic and bone mass effects; all of these symptoms are part of the androgen-deficiency syndrome.

ANDROGENS AND MENOPAUSE

Several studies have investigated the effect of the menopausal transition on androgen synthesis and circulating levels. A significant reduction in testosterone circulating levels occurs in premenopausal women, when compared with fertile women; circulating levels of testosterone in women in their 40s are 50% of those of women in their 20s[11]. Concerning the postmenopause, both unchanged, and a small but significant decrease in, testosterone, androstenedione and SHBG levels have been reported in the first 6 months after the menopause[12,13]. However, after a spontaneous menopause the ratio of testosterone/SHBG did not show any change[13,14], even though in surgical menopause both testosterone and androstenedione decreased (about 50%)[15], suggesting an important role of the ovaries in testosterone secretion also after the menopause. Nevertheless, in the postmenopause the principal source of circulating testosterone derives from the peripheral conversion of androstenedione and DHEA(S).

Starting from the third decade of life, independent of menopausal transition, circulating Δ^5-androgen levels fall linearly with age. After 70 years of age, DHEA(S) levels are 20% or less of the maximum plasma concentrations, cortisol levels being unchanged[16]. It has been hypothesized that, in postmenopausal women, a reduction of 17,20-desmolase activity, the enzyme that dictates the biosynthesis of the Δ^5-adrenal pathway, may induce modifications in DHEA(S) synthesis[17,18]. The decline in Δ^5-androgens and parallel increase in the cortisol/DHEA(S) ratio has been reported to be in part responsible for physiological and/or physiopathological age-related changes[19,20].

It can be suggested that the decline of circulating androgens results from a combination of two events: ovarian failure and aged-related decline in adrenal androgen synthesis. The relative androgen deficiency in postmenopausal women may provoke an impairment in sexual function, well-being and energy, and may contribute to bone mass reduction. However, the decline in circulating testosterone, androstenedione and in particular DHEA(S) levels begins in the decades that precede the menopause, and sometimes the above-mentioned symptoms are detected in the perimenopausal years, as a consequence of so-called adrenopause. Just as the menopause is characterized by a decline in gonadal function, the adrenopause is characterized by an age-related diminishing of the Δ^5-adrenal pathway.

To understand the androgen-deficiency syndrome it is important to emphasize that androgens play a key role in female sexuality and libido. A reduction of androgen levels contributes to the decline in sexual interest experienced by many women[21]. Very little improvement in libido is described in women treated with estrogen replacement therapy[22,23]. Although estrogen administration improves sexual satisfaction by acting on vaginal dryness and dyspareunia, it seems not to induce a modification of libido in women without coital discomfort[24,25]. In these cases, characterized by normal estrogenization, androgens may represent a relevant component in the management of replacement therapy. To date, the majority of studies related to androgen replacement have been performed using testosterone therapy in selected patients, but new perspectives are surely offered by Δ^5-androgen (namely DHEA) administration[24–31].

Δ^5-ANDROGENS AND POSTMENOPAUSE

Epidemiological studies have shown a relationship between the progressive decrease in circulating DHEA(S) levels and increases in cardiovascular morbidity in men[32] and breast cancer in women[33,34], and a decline of immune competence in both sexes[35]. An association between low DHEAS levels and an increase in mortality in men but not in women has also been demonstrated[36].

Experimental studies have shown an improvement in the insulin/glucose balance and a reduction of atherosclerotic plaque formation in aging animals treated with DHEA[37-40]. In rodents, a protective role of DHEA in the development of spontaneous carcinomas[41,42] and an up-regulation of the immune system[31,43,44] have also been reported.

Clinical studies have investigated the effects of DHEA(S) administration in men and women of various ages. Earlier trials reported different and non-comparable metabolic effects in young and old men and women treated with very high doses of DHEA (1600 mg/day)[19,45-47]. At this dose, DHEA induced a hyperandrogenic state, while lower doses of DHEA (50–100 mg/day) led to a restoration in circulating DHEA and DHEAS levels close to physiological values[19], but a two-fold increase in circulating levels of androgens (androstenedione, testosterone and DHT) and no changes in estradiol, estrone and SHBG in either sex[19]. In addition, it was demonstrated that DHEA administration was associated with a dose-dependent increase in plasma androgens and estrogens, particularly estradiol, in subjects affected by panhypopituitarism[48]. A positive correlation between DHEA(S) and bone mineral density (BMD) in aging women[49,50] has been reported, but it is unclear whether this effect is direct or indirect via DHEA(S) transformation to estrogen or other androgen molecules[51].

However, only a few studies have been conducted in humans to investigate the physiological function of DHEA(S) and the possible role of this molecule in the central nervous system (CNS). DHEA administration at 50 mg/day induced an improvement in psychological and physical well-being in postmenopausal women[19], thus suggesting a specific role for DHEA supplementation in CNS function. Recently, it has been shown that the oral administration of DHEA (50 mg/day) tends to determine an increase in well-being and mood only in women[52]. Moreover, further data relating to short-term treatment (30–90 mg/day for 4 weeks) imply that DHEA(S) has an antidepressant function in middle-aged and elderly patients with major depression and low basal DHEA(S) levels[53].

The mechanisms of action of DHEA are not clear, but it is important to emphasize that it serves as a precursor for peripheral conversion to estrogens and other androgens. However, it cannot be excluded that it has its own genomic and non-genomic effects. The latter effects have been investigated by our group using an endothelial cell model. Endothelial cells are primary targets of steroids that regulate endothelial function through transcriptional as well as via rapid, non-transcriptional mechanisms[54]. Estradiol stimulates nitric oxide (NO) synthesis via induction of endothelial nitric oxide synthase (eNOS) expression[55], as well as through non-genomic enhancement of its activity[56]. In part, the effects of DHEA probably depend on conversion to estrogens and androgens, and on the recruitment of their respective receptors. This might also be true for vessels, as shown by a report indicating that a reduction of atherosclerotic lesions by DHEA administration in rabbits may be related to its conversion to estrogens[57]. However, there is evidence to suggest that DHEA may have its own receptor(s). This has been implicated at the vascular level, where DHEA binds with high affinity to non-human endothelial cell membranes, without being displaced by structurally related steroids[57]. DHEA binding to endothelial cell membranes is associated with $G\alpha_{i2}$ and $G\alpha_{i3}$ proteins and eNOS activation[58].

Since endothelial-derived NO has anti-inflammatory and antiatherogenic actions[59], we tested the hypothesis that DHEA may exert direct regulatory actions on the vessel wall, through induction of endothelial NO synthesis[60] (Figure 1). We therefore characterized the genomic and non-genomic actions of DHEA *in vitro*, in human endothelial cells, as well as *in vivo*, in Wistar rats. Our data support the hypothesis that DHEA administration triggers NO synthesis in human endothelial cells, owing to enhanced expression and stabilization of eNOS. Additionally, DHEA rapidly activates eNOS, through a non-transcriptional mechanism which depends on ERK1/2 mitogen-activated protein kinases (MAPK) but not on phosphatidylinositol 3-OH kinase/Akt. DHEA is not converted to estrogens or androgens by endothelial cells, and its genomic

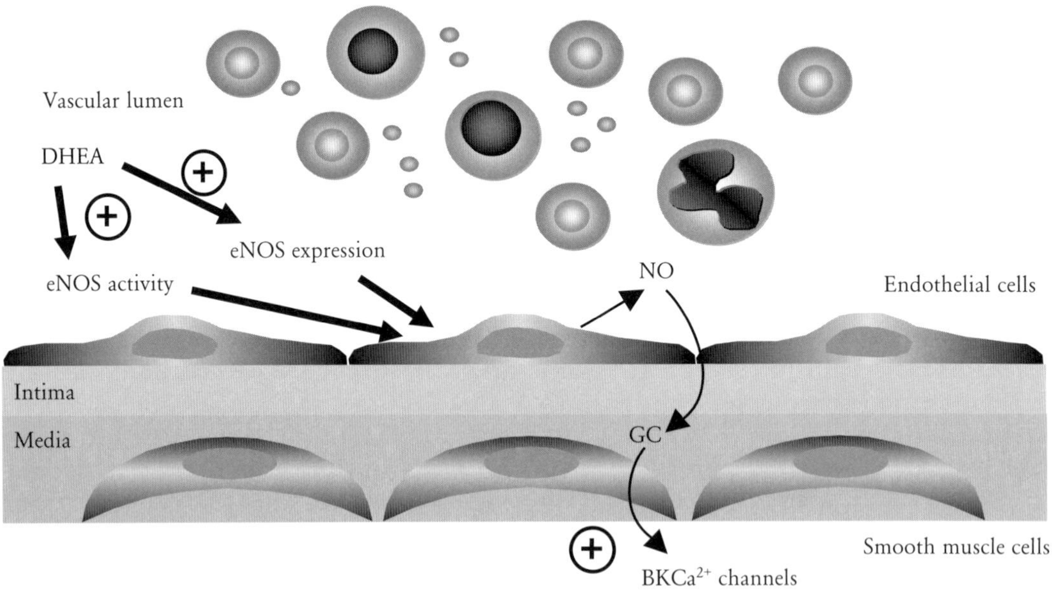

Figure 1 Dehydroepiandrosterone (DHEA) may have direct genomic and/or non-genomic protective effects on the vascular wall via endothelial nitric oxide synthase (eNOS) activation and induction

and/or non-genomic effects are not blocked by antagonists of the estrogen, progesterone, glucocorticoid or androgen receptors, suggesting that DHEA acts through a specific receptor. Oral DHEA administration restores aortic eNOS amounts and eNOS activity in ovariectomized Wistar rats in a dose-dependent fashion, confirming DHEA effects in an *in vivo* animal model. These data suggest that DHEA may have direct genomic and/or non-genomic protective effects on the vascular wall via eNOS activation and induction, which are not mediated by other steroid hormone receptors[60].

It is important to remember that DHEA and DHEAS are also considered as 'neurosteroids', because they are produced in the CNS and they may directly affect central function(s). The concentration of DHEA(S) in the CNS is 5-10 times greater than plasma levels, and experimental studies indicate that the mammalian brain contains steroid precursors, such as cholesterol and lipid derivatives[61,62], and is able to metabolize steroids coming from the peripheral circulation. The enzyme involved in the cleavage of cholesterol to pregnanolone and progesterone, cytochrome P450, is localized in the mitochondria of glial cells. This enzyme is encoded by the same P450 gene that is expressed in the adrenals and gonads, and has been identified in rodents, cows and human brain. The origin of DHEA in the brain is unknown, since the adult rat brain does not have 17α-hydroxylase activity and cannot convert pregnanolone or progesterone, or C21 or C19 steroids, to hydroxylated compounds[63]. However, the concentrations of DHEA(S) in rat brain remain unchanged for a long time after removal of the gonads and adrenals. The synthesis of classical neurosteroids, including DHEA, probably proceeds via different pathways from those related to the adrenals or gonads. In fact, glial cells contain additional steroid-metabolizing enzymes that transform the classical steroid hormones into a variety of compounds[64–66].

Experimental evidence suggests that the effects of DHEA and DHEAS on the CNS occur directly through specific binding to the γ-aminobutyric acid-A ($GABA_A$) receptor, thus blocking in a dose-dependent manner the GABA-induced chloride transport or current in synaptoneurosomes and neurons, with an increase of neuronal excitability[64]. Moreover, a potentiating effect of DHEA on *N*-methyl-D-aspartate (NMDA) and sigma receptors has been reported in rat brain[63].

However, at present, it is unknown whether changes of circulating DHEA(S) levels or DHEA(S) treatment can directly affect CNS function. In experimental animals, DHEA treatment induced a memory-enhancing effect[65]. *In vitro* studies suggest a neurotrophic effect on neurons and glial cells[66].

In addition, recent data obtained in 186 postmenopausal women have demonstrated that DHEA circulating levels decrease progressively and significantly during 12 months' treatment using various estrogen or estrogen-progestin molecules, regimens and routes of administration[67] (Figure 2). Interestingly, tibolone administration does not induce a reduction in DHEA circulating levels (unpublished data). Concerning allopregnanolone, a GABA-agonist neurosteroid, all the therapies, including tibolone, are associated with a significant increase in its level[67]. These data show that hormone replacement therapy is able to affect circulating levels of neurosteroids, offering new physiopathological models of study concerning the effect of estro-progestin therapies in the modulation of central function.

All the above data clearly support DHEA as a replacement therapy and a new choice in the spectrum of hormone treatments, and therefore the impact of DHEA(S) administration on endocrine and neuroendocrine milieu in postmenopausal women has been evaluated.

NEUROENDOCRINE AND ENDOCRINE EFFECTS OF DHEA(S) SUPPLEMENTATION

Clinical studies have demonstrated that drug-induced changes in circulating β-endorphin (the most important and biologically active endogenous opioid peptide, having behavioral, analgesic and thermoregulatory effects) may be considered a marker of neuroendocrine modulation[68,69]. In women, sex steroid hormone withdrawal, typical of the climacteric and the postmenopause, modifies the neuroendocrine equilibrium by impairing the synthesis and function of several neuroactive transmitters. Regarding the opiatergic system, a decrease in plasma β-endorphin levels occurs in the postmenopause[70],

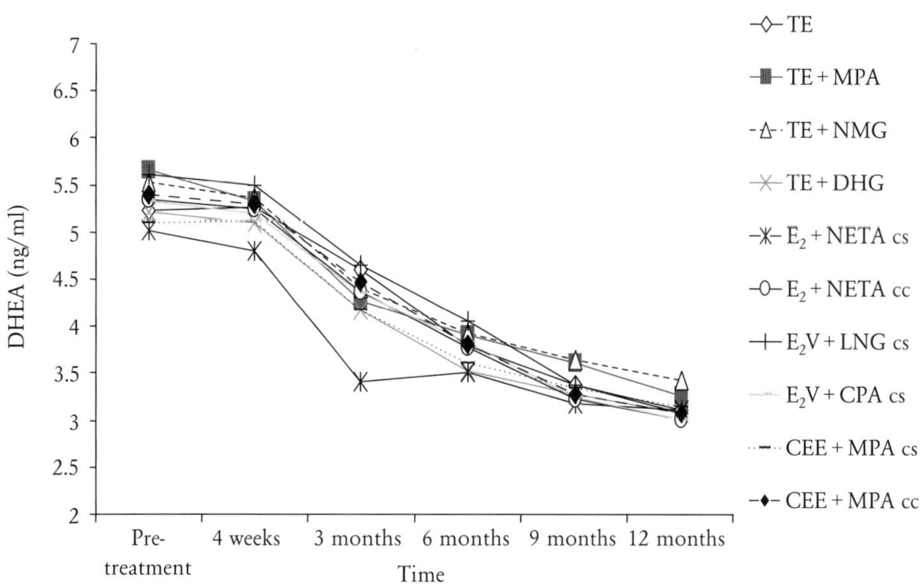

Figure 2 Dehydroepiandrosterone (DHEA) circulating levels in response to 12 months' treatment using various estrogen or estrogen-progestin molecules, regimens and routes of administration. TE, transdermal estradiol; MPA, medroxyprogesterone acetate; NMG, nomegestrol; DHG, dihydrogesterone; E_2, estradiol; NETA, norethisterone acetate; E_2V, estradiol valerate; LNG, levonorgestrel; CPA, cyproterone acetate; CEE, conjugated equine estrogens; cs, continuous sequential scheme; cc, continuous combined scheme

and it has been suggested that this modification plays a key role in the mechanism of hot flush and sweating occurrence[71]. Moreover, the decrease of β-endorphin levels may also be involved in the pathogenesis of mood, behavior and nociceptive disturbances during the postmenopausal period[72,73].

Experimental and clinical studies have shown that β-endorphin synthesis and release are modulated by noradrenaline, dopamine, serotonin, acetylcholine, GABA and corticotropin-releasing factor (CRF)[74,75]. Bolus administration of naloxone, an opioid receptor antagonist, and clonidine, an α_2-presynaptic receptor agonist, increases plasma β-endorphin levels in fertile women. In the postmenopause, a lack of response of β-endorphin to clonidine and naloxone occurs, and this finding suggests an impairment of adrenergic and opiatergic receptors in modulating β-endorphin release in postmenopausal women[76]. The fact that hormone replacement therapy (HRT) restores basal plasma β-endorphin levels and responses to clonidine and naloxone tests similar to those of fertile women demonstrates these neuroendocrine tests to be a valid tool for evaluation of neuroendocrine function in postmenopausal women undergoing HRT[77] (Figure 3).

Three months of DHEAS supplementation (50 mg/day) in postmenopausal women has been demonstrated to improve the Kuppermann score, together with restoration of the β-endorphin response to naloxone, clonidine and fluoxetine tests, similar to that with estrogen administration. These neuroendocrine data, together with the observation that DHEA administration induced an improvement in psychological and physical well-being in postmenopausal women[19,20]

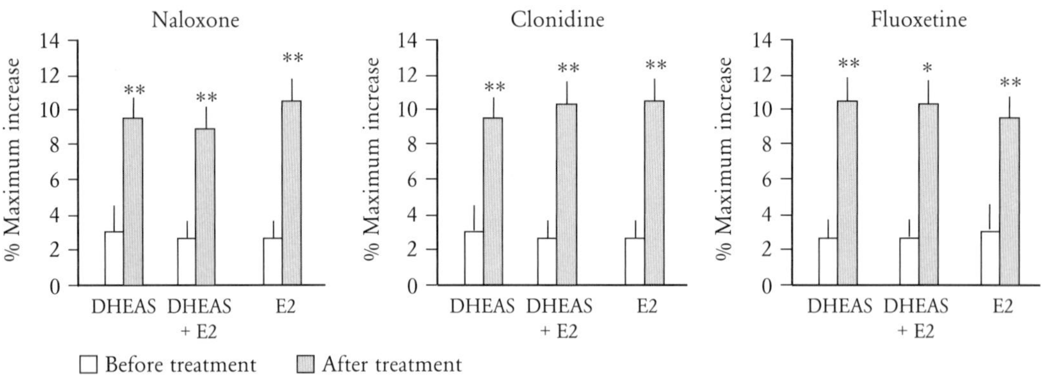

Figure 3 β-Endorphin response to naloxone, clonidine and fluoxetine tests before and after dehydroepiandrosterone sulfate (DHEAS) and/or estradiol (E_2) treatment. $p < 0.001$, significant difference compared with before treatment

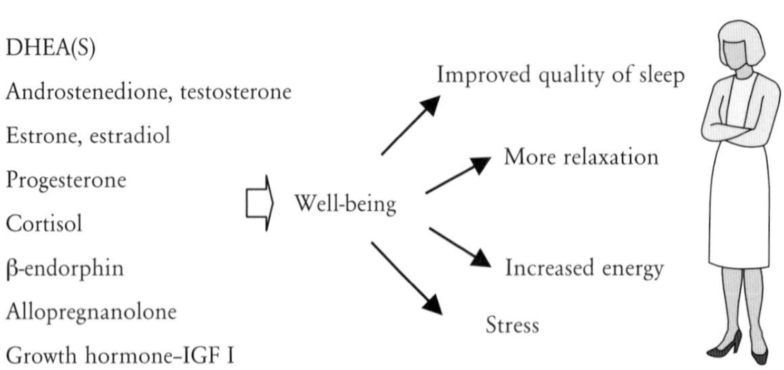

Figure 4 Dehydroepiandrosterone (DHEA) administration in postmenopausal women improves psychological and physical well-being. DHEA(S), DHEA (sulfate); IGF-I, insulin-like growth factor-I

(Figure 4), suggest that DHEAS and/or its active metabolites act as a modulator of CNS function[78].

In addition, an evaluation of endocrine parameters demonstrated that oral DHEA supplementation at the dose of 50 mg daily for 6 months in postmenopausal women induced physiological and supraphysiological modifications in the steroid milieu and adrenal function. In particular, DHEA treatment produced estrogen levels superimposable on those induced by transdermal patches, while the Δ^4-androgens (androstenedione, testosterone and DHT) increased to supraphysiological levels[79]. By analyzing the response to ACTH stimulus after dexamethasone suppression in these patients, it has been concluded that DHEA administration determines a greater response of Δ^5- and Δ^4-androgens and a blunted response of cortisol to ACTH. Therefore, it has been hypothesized that DHEA might enhance some adrenal pathways that lead to the production of Δ^5- and Δ^4-androgens, reducing cortisol biosynthetic pathways[79].

On the basis of the previously reported results, DHEA has been administered at lower doses (25 mg daily, orally) for 12 months in early- and late-postmenopausal women. DHEA, DHEAS, androstenedione, testosterone, DHT, estrone, estradiol, progesterone, 17OH-progesterone, allopregnanolone, β-endorphin and growth hormone levels increased progressively and significantly during the 12 months of treatment, reaching levels similar to those observed in fertile women, without significant differences between the two groups. While testosterone exhibited slightly supraphysiological levels after 1 year of therapy, SHBG levels did not show significant modification. In contrast, cortisol and gonadotropin levels decreased progressively in all groups. These data indicate that DHEA supplementation induces a dose-related modulation of endocrine and neuroendocrine parameters, and a low dose (25 mg/day) is more effective in restoring physiological levels (unpublished data). On the other hand, 12 months of 25-mg/day DHEA therapy did not change endometrial thickness. This observation might be ascribed to the absence at the endometrial level of the specific enzymes responsible for the conversion of DHEA to estrogens, and/or to the DHEA-induced increase in progesterone concentrations. Therefore, the effect of DHEA at the endometrial level seems to be similar to that induced by a continuous combined therapy.

In conclusion, DHEA is active as a prehormone, inducing modifications that counteract the phenomena occurring during the menopause and aging. The use of low doses of DHEA is effective in modulating positively the endocrine and neuroendocrine milieu. The beneficial effects of DHEA on quality of life and in reverting some aging processes may be related to these DHEA-induced changes, with an increase in anxiolytic (allopregnanolone and β-endorphin), anabolic (androstenedione, testosterone, DHT) and estrogenic molecules, and a favorable blunting of cortisol levels.

Also, growth hormone-insulin-like growth factor-I (IGF-I) levels are positively modulated by DHEA therapy. With DHEA administration, there is an increase in growth hormone and IGF-I levels similar to that with estro-progestin regimens. Finally, DHEA did not change endometrial thickness in these patients (unpublished data).

All the above data clearly support a putative role of DHEA supplementation as replacement therapy for the postmenopause and/or adrenopause.

CONCLUSIONS

Androgens play a fundamental role in female physiopathology. The age-related decline in the production of ovarian and adrenal androgens may significantly affect women's health and well-being. Androgen replacement therapy should be a primary choice, especially in younger women with either premature ovarian failure or surgically induced menopause, suffering loss of well-being, fatigue and loss of libido, which are not modified by estrogen therapy.

Among androgens, Δ^5-androgens such as DHEA(S) may be considered a new choice to treat women with androgen-deficiency syndrome and/or postmenopausal women. Our data indicate a positive impact of DHEA(S) administration on the endocrine and neuroendocrine systems. In particular, DHEA is active as a prehormone, inducing modifications which may counteract the negative phenomena related to the menopause and aging. The use of low doses positively modulates the endocrine and neuroendocrine milieu, avoiding the side-effects of a higher dosage. In addition, the positive effect on the Kuppermann score, with no changes of endometrial thickness, suggests that DHEA administration may be considered as a possible replacement treatment for postmenopausal women.

References

1. Kirschner MA, Bardin CW. Androgen production and metabolism in normal and virilized women. *Metabolism* 1972;21:667–88
2. Judd HL, Bardin CW. Serum androstenedione and testosterone levels during the menstrual cycle. *J Clin Endocrinol Metab* 1973;36:475–81
3. Dunn JF, Nisula BC, Rodbard D. Transport of steroid hormones. Binding of 21 endogenous steroids to both testosterone-binding globulin and corticosteroid-binding globulin in human serum. *J Clin Endocrinol Metab* 1981;53:58–68
4. Parker LN, Odell WD. Control of adrenal androgen secretion. *Endocr Rev* 1980;4:392–410
5. Yamaji T, Ibayashi H. Serum dehydroepiandrosterone sulphate in normal and pathological conditions. *J Clin Endocrinol Metab* 1969; 29:273–8
6. Vitukaitis JL, Dale SL, Melbi JC. Role of ACTH in the secretion of free DHA and its sulphate ester in man. *J Clin Endocrinol Metab* 1969;29: 1443–7
7. Varmeulen A, Ando S. Prolactin and adrenal androgen secretion. *Clin Endocrinol* 1978;8:295–303
8. Parker LN, Eugene J, Farber D, Lifrale E, Lai M, Juler G. Dissociation of adrenal androgen and cortisol levels in acute stress. *Horm Metab Res* 1985;17:209–12
9. Parker LN, Levin ER, Lifrat ET. Evidence for adrenocortical adaptation to severe illness. *J Clin Endocrinol Metab* 1985;60:947–52
10. Zumoff B, Walsh B, Katz J. Subnormal serum dehydroepiandrosterone to cortisol ratio in anorexia nervosa: a second hormone parameter of ontogenic regression. *J Clin Endocrinol Metab* 1983;56:668–72
11. Zummoff B, Rosenfeld RS, Strain GW. Sex differences in the 24-hour mean plasma concentrations of dehydroisoandrosterone (DHA) and dehydroisoandrosterone sulfate (DHAS) and the DHA to DHAS ratio in normal adults. *J Clin Endocrinol Metab* 1980;51:331–4
12. Longscope C, Franz C, Morello C, Baker K, Johnston CC Jr. Steroid and gonadotropin levels in women during the perimenopausal years. *Maturitas* 1986;8:189–96
13. Rannevik G, Jeppsson S, Johnell O. A longitudinal study of the perimenopausal transition. Altered profiles of steroid and pituitary hormones, SHBG and bone mineral density. *Maturitas* 1995; 21:103–13
14. Burger HG, Dudley EC, Hopper DL. The endocrinology of the menopausal transition: a cross-sectional study of a population-based sample. *J Clin Endocrinol Metab* 1995;80:3537–45
15. Judd HL. Hormonal dynamics associated with the menopause. *Clin Obstet Gynecol* 1976;19:775–88
16. Hopper BR, Yen SSC. Circulating concentrations of dehydroepiandrosterone and dehydroepiandrosterone sulphate during puberty. *J Clin Endocrinol Metab* 1975;40:458–61
17. Liu CH, Laughlin GA, Fischer UG, Yen SSC. Marked attenuation of ultradian and circadian rhythms of dehydroepiandrosterone in postmenopausal women: evidence for a reduced 17,20-desmolase enzymatic activity. *J Clin Endocrinol Metab* 1990;71:900–6
18. Couch RM, Muller J, Winter JSD. Regulation of the activities of 17-hydroxylase and 17,20-desmolase in the human adrenal cortex: kinetic analysis and inhibition by endogenous steroids. *J Clin Endocrinol Metab* 1986;63:613–18
19. Mortola JF, Yen SSC. The effects of oral dehydroepiandrosterone on endocrine-metabolic parameters in postmenopausal women. *J Clin Endocrinol Metab* 1990;71:696–704
20. Morales AJ, Nolan JJ, Nelson JC, Yen SSC. Effects of replacement dose of dehydroepiandrosterone in men and women of advancing age. *J Clin Endocrinol Metab* 1994;78:1360–7
21. Davis SR, Burger HG. Androgens and the postmenopausal woman. *J Clin Endocrinol Metab* 1996; 81:2759–63
22. Utian WH. The true clinical features of postmenopausal oophorectomy and their response to estrogen replacement therapy. *South Afr Med J* 1972;46:732–7
23. Campbell S, Whitehead M. Oestrogen therapy and the menopausal syndrome. *Clin Obstet Gynecol* 1977;4:31–47

24. Studd JWW, Chakavarti S, Oram D. The climacteric. *Clin Obstet Gynecol* 1977;4:3–29
25. Studd JWW, Collins WP, Chakavarti S. Estradiol and testosterone implants in the treatment of psychosexual problems in postmenopausal women. *Br J Obstet Gynaecol* 1988;84:314–15
26. Sherwin BB, Gelfand MM, Brender W. Androgen enhances sexual motivation in females: a prospective, crossover study of sex steroid administration in surgical menopause. *Psychosom Med* 1985; 47:339–51
27. Burger HG, Hailes J, Menelaus M. The management of persistent symptoms with estradiol-testosterone implants: clinical, lipid and hormonal results. *Maturitas* 1984;6:351–8
28. Burger HG, Hailes J, Nelson J, Menelaus M. Effects of combined implants of estradiol and testosterone on libido in postmenopausal women. *Br Med J* 1987;294:936–7
29. Davis SR, McCloud P, Strauss BJC, Burger HG. Testosterone enhances estradiol's effects on postmenopausal bone density and sexuality. *Maturitas* 1995;21:227–36
30. Davis S. The therapeutic use of androgens in women. *J Steroid Biochem Mol Biol* 1999;69:177–84
31. Davis S. Androgen replacement in women: a commentary. *J Clin Endocrinol Metab* 1999;84:1886–91
32. Barrett-Connor E, Khaw K, Yen SSC. A prospective study of DS mortality and cardiovascular disease. *N Engl J Med* 1986;315:1519–24
33. Helzlsouer KJ, Gordon GB, Alberg A, Bush TL, Comstock GW. Relationship of prediagnostic serum levels of DHEA and DS to the risk of developing premenopausal breast cancer. *Cancer Res* 1992;52:1–4
34. Bulbrook RD, Hayward JL, Spicer CC. Relation between urinary androgen and corticoid secretion excretion and subsequent breast cancer. *Lancet* 1975;2:395–8
35. Thoman ML, Weigle WO. The cellular and subcellular bases of immunosenescence. *Adv Immunol* 1989;46:221–61
36. Berr C, Lafont S, Debuire B, Dartigues J-F, Baulieu EE. Relationship of dehydroepiandrosterone sulphate in the elderly functional and mental status, and short-term mortality: a French community-based study. *Proc Natl Acad Sci USA* 1996;93:13410–15
37. Coleman DL, Leiter EH, Schwizer RW. Therapeutic effects of dehydroepiandrosterone in diabetic mice. *Diabetes* 1982;31:830–3
38. Coleman DL, Schwizer RW, Leiter EH. Effect of genetic background on the therapeutic effects of dehydroepiandrosterone (DHEA) in diabetes-obesity mutant and aged normal mice. *Diabetes* 1984;33:26–33
39. Yen TY, Allan JA, Pearson DV, Acton JM. Prevention of obesity in A^{vy}/a mice by dehydroepiandrosterone. *Lipids* 1977;12:409–13
40. Gordon GB, Bush DE, Weisman HF. Reduction of atherosclerosis by administration of dehydroepiandrosterone. A study in hypercholesterolemic New Zealand White rabbits with aortic intimal injury. *J Clin Invest* 1988;82:712–20
41. Schwartz AG. Inhibition of spontaneous breast cancer formation in female C3H (A^{vy}/a) mice by long-term treatment with dehydroepiandrosterone. *Cancer Res* 1979;39:1129–31
42. Shantz LM, Talav P, Gordon GB. Mechanism of inhibition of growth of 3T3-L1 fibroblasts and their differentiation to adipocytes by dehydroepiandrosterone and related steroids: role of glucose-6-phosphate dehydrogenase. *Proc Natl Acad Sci USA* 1989;86:3852–6
43. Blauer KL, Poth M, Rogers WM, Bernton EW. Dehydroepiandrosterone antagonizes the suppressive effects of dexamethasone on lymphocyte proliferation. *Endocrinology* 1991;129:3174–9
44. May M, Holmes E, Rogers W, Poth M. Protection from glucocorticoid induced thymic involution by dehydroepiandrosterone. *Life Sci* 1990;46: 1627–31
45. Nestler JE, Barlascini CO, Clore JN, Blackard WG. Dehydroepiandrosterone reduces serum low density lipoprotein levels and body fat but does not alter insulin sensitivity in normal men. *J Clin Endocrinol Metab* 1988;66:57–61
46. Usiskin KS, Butterworth S, Clore JN, *et al.* Lack of effect of DHEA in obese men. *Int J Obesity* 1990;14:457–63
47. Welle S, Jozefowicz R, Statt M. Failure of DHEA to influence energy and protein metabolism in humans. *J Clin Endocrinol Metab* 1990;71:1259–64
48. Young J, Couzinet B, Brailly S, Chanson P, Baulieu EE, Schaison G. Panhypopituitarism as a model to study the metabolism of dehydroepiandrosterone (DHEA) in humans. *J Clin Endocrinol Metab* 1997;82:2578–85
49. Taelman P, Kayman JM, Janssens X, Varmeulen A. Persistence of increased bone-resorption and possible role of dehydroepiandrosterone as a bone metabolism determinant in osteoporotic women in late menopause. *Maturitas* 1989;11:65–73
50. Nordin BEC, Robertson A, Seamark RF. The relation between calcium absorption, serum DHEA and vertebral mineral density in postmenopausal women. *J Clin Endocrinol Metab* 1985;60:651–7
51. Savvas M, Studd JWW, Fogelman I, Dooley M, Montgomenry J, Murby B. Skeletal effects of oral oestrogen compared with subcutaneous oestrogen and testosterone in postmenopausal women. *Br Med J* 1988;297:331–3
52. Wolf OT, Neumenn O, Helhammer DH, *et al.* Effects of a two-week physiological dehydroepiandrosterone substitution on cognitive performance and well-being in healthy elderly women and men. *J Clin Endocrinol Metab* 1997; 82:2363–7

53. Wolkowitz OM, Reus VI, Roberts E, *et al.* Dehydroepiandrosterone (DHEA) treatment of depression. *Biol Psychiatry* 1997;41:311–18
54. Simoncini T, Genazzani AR. Direct vascular effects of estrogens and selective estrogen receptor modulators. *Curr Opin Obstet Gynecol* 2000;12:181–7
55. Kleinert H, Wallerath T, Euchenhofer C, Ihrig-Biedert I, Li H, Forstermann U. Estrogens increase transcription of the human endothelial NO synthase gene: analysis of the transcription factors involved. *Hypertension* 1998;31:582–8
56. Simoncini T, Hafezi-Moghadam A, Brazil D, Ley K, Chin WW, Liao JK. Interaction of oestrogen receptor with the regulatory subunit of phosphatidylinositol-3-OH kinase. *Nature (London)* 2000;407:538–41
57. Hayashi T, Esaki T, Muto E, *et al.* Dehydroepiandrosterone retards atherosclerosis formation through its conversion to estrogen: the possible role of nitric oxide. *Arterioscler Thromb Vasc Biol* 2000;20:782–92
58. Liu D, Dillon JS. Dehydroepiandrosterone activates endothelial cell nitric-oxide synthase by a specific plasma membrane receptor coupled to $G\alpha_{i2,3}$. *J Biol Chem* 2002;277:21379–88
59. Liao JK. Endothelial nitric oxide and vascular inflammation. In Panza JA, Cannon ROI, eds. *Endothelium, Nitric Oxide and Atherosclerosis.* Armonk, NY: Futura Publishing Co., 1999:119–32
60. Simoncini T, Mannella P, Fornari L, Varone G, Caruso A, Genazzani AR. Dehydroepiandrosterone (DHEA) modulates endothelial nitric oxide synthesis via direct genomic and non-genomic mechanisms. *Endocrinology* 2003;in press
61. Majewska MD. Neurosteroids: endogenous bimodal modulators of the GABA-A receptor. Mechanism of action and physiological significance. *Prog Neurobiol* 1992;38:379–95
62. Corpechot C, Young J, Calvel M, *et al.* Neurosteroids: 3α-hydroxy-5α-pregnan-20-one and its precursors in the brain, plasma, and steroidogenic glands of male and female rats. *Endocrinology* 1993;133:1003–9
63. Mellon SH. Neurosteroids: biochemistry, modes of action, and clinical relevance. *J Clin Endocrinol Metab* 1994;78:1003–8
64. Majewska MD, Demirgoren S, Spivak CE, London ED. The neurosteroid DHEA is an allosteric antagonist of the $GABA_A$ receptor. *Brain Res* 1990;526:143–6
65. Myers ER, Sondheimer SJ, Freeman BW. Serum progesterone levels following vaginal administration of progesterone with different modes of administration. *Fertil Steril* 1987;47:71–5
66. Koninckx PR, Lauweryns JA, Cornillie FJ. The effects of a sequential oestradiol-valerate cyproterone acetate preparation on the endometrium during hormone replacement therapy. In Schneider HPG, Genazzani AR, eds. *A New Approach in the Treatment of Climateric Disorders.* Berlin: De Gruiter, 1992:37–53
67. Bernardi F, Pieri M, Stomati M, *et al.* Effect of different hormonal replacement therapies on circulating allopregnanolone and dehydroepiandrosterone levels in postmenopausal women. *Gynecol Endocrinol* 2003;17:65–77
68. Genazzani AR, Petraglia F, Cleva M, *et al.* Norgestimate increases pituitary and hypothalamic concentrations of immunoreactive β-endorphin. *Contraception* 1989;5:605–13
69. Genazzani AR, Petraglia F, Mercuri N, *et al.* Effect of steroid hormones and antihormones on hypothalamic β-endorphin concentrations in intact and castrated female rats. *J Endocrinol Invest* 1990;13:91–6
70. Petraglia F, Comitini G, Genazzani AR, *et al.* β-Endorphin in human reproduction. In Herz A, ed. *Opiods II.* Berlin: Springer-Verlag, 1993:763–80
71. Wiklund I, Helst J, Korlberg J. A new methodology for evaluating quality of life in postmenopausal women during transdermal estrogen replacement therapy. *Maturitas* 1992;14:211–24
72. Ortega E, Condras JL, Gonzales AR, *et al.* Effect of estrogen–progestin replacement therapy on plasma β-endorphin levels in menopausal women. *Biochem Mol Biol* 1993;29:831
73. Advis J, McConn S, Negro-Vilar A. Evidence that catecholaminergic and peptidergic (luteinizing hormone-releasing hormone) neurons in suprachiasmatic-medial preoptic, medial basal hypothalamus and median eminence are involved in estrogen negative feed back. *Endocrinology* 1980;107:892–902
74. Piva F, Limonta P, Dondi D, *et al.* Effects of steroids on the brain opioid system. *J Steroid Biochem Mol Biol* 1995;53:343–8
75. McEwen B. Steroid hormones are multifunctional messengers in the brain. *Trends Endocrinol Metab* 1991;12:62–7
76. Belaisch J, Eliakim V. Third generation progestagen. *Contraception* 1993;21:287–93
77. Stomati M, Bersi C, Rubino S, *et al.* Neuroendocrine effects of different oestradiol–progestin regimens in postmenopausal women. *Maturitas* 1997;28:127–35
78. Rubino S, Stomati M, Bersi C, *et al.* Neuroendocrine effect of a short-term treatment with DHEA in postmenopausal women. *Maturitas* 1998;28:251–7
79. Stomati M, Monteleone P, Casarosa E, *et al.* Six-month oral dehydroepiandrosterone supplementation in early and late postmenopause. *Gynecol Endocrinol* 2000;14:342–63

The perimenopause and depressive illness 17

P. J. Schmidt and D. R. Rubinow

INTRODUCTION

The focus of this chapter is the potential relationship between the onset of depression in women and the reproductive events of the perimenopause. The perimenopause is a time of considerable variability in reproductive function, which appears in some women to be associated with an increased susceptibility to depression. Elevated gonadotropin levels occur during the late perimenopause, with plasma follicle stimulating hormone (FSH) levels increasing in association with impaired ovarian function and decreased estradiol secretion. In contrast to the postmenopause, ovarian function may vary considerably in the perimenopause, with restoration of normal menstrual cycle function observed as frequently as the onset of menopause[1]. Moreover, during the perimenopause, levels of estradiol secretion may be reduced, normal or at times increased[2,3]. It is unclear, however, whether the variability in ovarian hormone secretion during the perimenopause has any causal role in the development of depression. Several questions are posed to highlight recent data suggesting that, in some women, perimenopausal reproductive events play a role in the onset of depression. Finally, recommendations for the evaluation and treatment of women with perimenopausal depression are presented.

PERIMENOPAUSAL DEPRESSION

What is the relationship between the onset of depression and the perimenopause?

Depressive symptoms

Although the postmenopause has not been associated with an increased risk for developing depression in women[4-8], depressive symptoms have been observed more frequently in perimenopausal women compared with postmenopausal women participating in some longitudinal, community-based studies[8,9].

Similarly, depressive-like symptoms have been evaluated in perimenopausal women attending gynecology clinics[10-13], with one study observing that up to 45% of the sample had high scores (consistent with clinically significant depression) on standardized rating scales for depression[13]. In two additional studies perimenopausal women were observed to report significantly more symptoms than postmenopausal women[11,12]. Thus, both clinic-based surveys and epidemiological studies suggest the relevance of the perimenopause in disturbances of mood in a substantial number of women.

Depressive syndromes

Community-based surveys of the prevalence of affective *syndromes* (conditions meeting standardized diagnostic criteria, such as major or minor depression) have observed patterns of morbidity consistent with those reported in the surveys examining mood *symptoms*. Several epidemiological studies examining gender- and age-related differences in the 6-month to 1-year prevalences of major depression reported the absence of an increase in the prevalence of major depression in women at midlife (age range approximately 45–55 years)[14,15]. The Study of Women's Health Across the Nation (SWAN)[16] employed a measure of 'psychological distress' as a proxy for the syndrome of depression by requiring that core depressive symptoms (sadness, anxiety and irritability) persist for at least 2 weeks. Similar to the studies of depressive symptoms, SWAN's initial cross-sectional survey observed that perimenopausal women reported significantly more psychological distress than either pre- or postmenopausal women (defined by self-reported menstrual cycle status)[16]. Moreover, the increased psychological distress appeared to be independent of the presence of vasomotor symptoms. These data, therefore, provide additional evidence supporting the role of the perimenopause but not the postmenopause in the development of mood disorders.

To date, only Hay and colleagues[13] have examined the prevalence rates of major and minor depression in endocrinologically confirmed perimenopausal women within a gynecological clinic-based setting. These investigators employed a structured diagnostic interview and reported that 37% of depressive episodes in this sample of women occurred during the period they defined as the perimenopause. The report by Hay and colleagues[13] confirms suggestions[11,12] that clinic samples contain a much larger proportion of perimenopausal women with clinically significant affective disorders than of postmenopausal women.

In summary, epidemiological studies examining the prevalence of both affective symptoms and syndromes have documented that the majority of postmenopausal women do not experience major depression associated with this phase of life. Nevertheless, several community-based and clinic-based surveys suggest that the perimenopause is relevant to the development of affective disorders[11,13,16], and that a substantial number of perimenopausal women do, in fact, experience clinically significant depression.

Is perimenopause-related depression associated with abnormal hormone secretion?

Cross-sectional studies

Hypothalamic-pituitary-ovarian axis While epidemiological studies have demonstrated associations between the perimenopause, hypoestrogenism and hot flushes in women, no similar relationship has been consistently identified between the menopausal transition and mood disorders[4,6,17,18]. None the less, several reports indirectly support a role for reproductive hormonal change during the perimenopause in depression: hormone replacement beneficially affects both hot flushes and mood in hypogonadal women[19-23]; and lower gonadotropin levels are observed in postmenopausal depressed women compared with asymptomatic comparison groups[24-27]. The observed improvement in depressive symptoms after hormone replacement suggests the contribution of hypoestrogenism to mood disturbances, permitting the speculation that depressed perimenopausal women are relatively more estrogen deficient than non-depressed perimenopausal women. Perimenopausal women with depressive symptoms have been reported to have lower plasma estrone (E_1) levels[28] than non-depressed perimenopausal women, and an association has been described between increased plasma FSH levels and depression[29]. In contrast, three studies of perimenopausal and postmenopausal women observed either no diagnosis-related differences in plasma estradiol (E_2) and FSH[30] or no correlation between plasma levels of estrogens or androgens and severity of depressive symptoms[31,32].

In a study of 21 women with their first episode of depression occurring during the perimenopause and 21 asymptomatic perimenopausal controls[33], we were unable to confirm previous reports of lower basal plasma levels of luteinizing hormone (LH)[24-27] or E_1[28] in perimenopausal and postmenopausal women with depression, compared with matched controls. Additionally, we observed no diagnosis-related differences in basal plasma levels of FSH, E_2, testosterone or free testosterone. Our data are consistent with those of Barrett-Connor and colleagues[31] and of Cawood and Bancroft[32], who found no correlation between mood symptoms and plasma levels of E_1, E_2 or testosterone.

Previous studies employing both high- and low-dose gonadotropin-releasing hormone (GnRH) stimulation have not demonstrated differences in hypothalamic-pituitary-ovarian (HPO) axis function in depression[34], nor have high-dose GnRH-stimulation studies shown differences in postmenopausal depressed subjects, compared with postmenopausal non-depressed controls[25].

Notwithstanding the limitations of basal hormonal measures, data suggest that depressed perimenopausal women are not distinguished from non-depressed perimenopausal women on the basis of abnormal ovarian hormone secretion.

Hypothalamic-pituitary-adrenal axis Age-related differences in the function of several physiological systems have been observed in both animals and humans. Some of these differences may occur coincidentally with the perimenopause, and, therefore, may potentially contribute to mood dysregulation at this time. Although postmenopausal women have been reported to exhibit increased stress-induced plasma norepinephrine levels compared with premenopausal women[8], only one previous study[28] reported elevated urinary cortisol levels in perimenopausal women reporting depressive symptoms compared with asymptomatic controls. No systematic study has been performed of hypothalamic-pituitary-adrenal (HPA) axis function in perimenopausal women with a depressive syndrome, and, therefore, the possibility of an interaction between perimenopause-related hormone changes and HPA axis function in perimenopausal depression remains to be clarified.

A role for the adrenal androgen dehydroepiandrosterone (DHEA) and its sulfated metabolite (DHEAS) in the regulation of mood state has also been suggested by both its effects on neural physiology[35-37] and its potential synthesis within the central nervous system[38,39] Moreover, in clinical trials, DHEA administration has been reported to improve mood in some[40-43], but not all, studies[44]. Finally, abnormalities of DHEA secretion have been observed in depressive disorders, with both increased and decreased levels observed relative to non-depressed controls[45-48]. DHEA's potential role in the onset of depression may be particularly relevant at midlife, given the declining levels of DHEA production that occur with aging and the accelerated decrease in DHEA levels reported in women, but not men, during midlife[49,50]. Plasma levels of DHEA and DHEAS decline progressively from the third decade at a rate of about 2–3% per year[51], reaching about 50% of peak levels during the fifth to sixth decades[52-54]. It is possible, therefore, that declining secretion (or abnormally low secretion) of DHEA may interact with perimenopause-related changes in ovarian function to trigger the onset of depression in some women. In fact, in perimenopausal and postmenopausal women, depression severity is inversely correlated with DHEA levels[31], while feelings of well-being are positively correlated with DHEAS levels[32]. We measured morning plasma levels of DHEA, DHEAS and cortisol in a separate sample of women with first onset of depression during the perimenopause and in non-depressed women matched for age and reproductive status. Depressed perimenopausal women had significantly lower levels of both plasma DHEA and DHEAS but not cortisol, compared with controls[33]. Our findings are similar to those of one previous study reporting lower salivary levels of DHEA in first-onset depression during adolescence, relative to an asymptomatic comparison group[45], and to those of three other studies reporting an association between low plasma DHEA or DHEAS levels and depressive symptoms (or feelings of well-being) in peri- and postmenopausal women[31,32] and elderly depressed subjects[47]. In contrast, our findings are in the opposite direction from those described by Heuser and colleagues[48], who reported elevated mean diurnal secretion of DHEA in depressed patients. However, the depressed subjects studied by Heuser[48] were also hypercortisolemic and of mixed age groups, and may have had prior depressive episodes. Our observation that DHEA secretion, but not adrenal glucocorticoid secretion, differed in depressed and non-depressed women suggests that depression during the perimenopause may be characterized by alterations in adrenal androgen activity, but not basal glucocorticoid activity, in contrast to depression occurring at other periods in life.

Longitudinal studies

The role of changes in ovarian steroids in the development of perimenopausal depression may require longitudinal studies that document the coincident onset of both endocrine evidence of perimenopausal reproductive function and behavioral evidence of depression. None the less, the oscillation between perimenopausal and premenopausal reproductive function that characterizes the perimenopause provides an opportunity to establish the temporal coincidence of perimenopausal reproductive function and depression.

We observed several women who presented to our clinic with depression and whose plasma FSH levels, obtained at each clinic visit, declined over a 6–8-week period of observation, concurrent with spontaneous improvements in mood symptoms. We were interested in systematically examining whether this putative relationship between normalization of ovarian function and mood could be generalized in our sample of women with perimenopausal depression. Consequently, we evaluated mood scores and plasma FSH levels serially over a 6-week screening phase in a larger group of women presenting to our clinic with perimenopausal depression. In the group of women ($n = 18$) whose Center for Epidemiologic Studies in Depression Scale (CES-D) scores decreased by ≥ 50%, we observed an incremental decline in FSH levels at each of the four clinic visits that paralleled the improvements in CES-D scores (Figure 1) (Daly, in press). In this study, we identified a subgroup of women with perimenopausal depression whose mood symptoms remitted spontaneously in association with a significant decline in gonadotropin levels (and a possible alteration in pituitary–ovarian function).

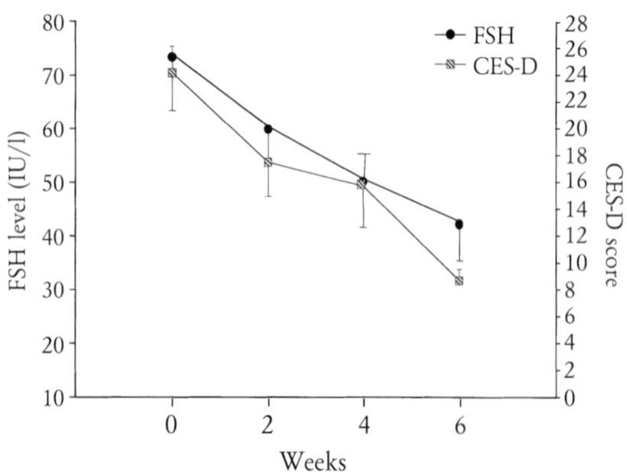

Figure 1 Concordant restoration of ovarian function and mood in women with perimenopausal depression ($n = 18$). Plasma follicle stimulating hormone (FSH) levels significantly decreased ($t_{17} = 2.6$, $p = 0.02$) in perimenopausal depressed women (defined by Center for Epidemiologic Studies in Depression Scale (CES-D) ≥ 15) whose scores on the CES-D scale improved by ≥ 50% over a 6-week follow-up. Reproduced with permission from *Am J Psychiatry*

Increased plasma FSH levels were not consistently associated with worsening CES-D scores, nor were increased CES-D scores associated with corresponding elevations in plasma FSH levels, whereas a more uniform relationship was observed between mood and plasma FSH level when either measure decreased. These data could suggest a threshold or ceiling of plasma FSH levels, below which differences may influence mood and above which there is little association between changes in measures of FSH and mood. In contrast to cross-sectional studies which suggest that perimenopausal depression is not associated with abnormalities of reproductive hormone function, longitudinal studies do in fact suggest that there may be a more direct relationship between alterations in pituitary–ovarian function and mood symptoms in these women.

What are the effects on mood of estradiol therapy in perimenopausal depression?

Perimenopausal depression is a condition defined by the onset of depression at middle age in association with the onset of menstrual cycle irregularity or amenorrhea. Perimenopausal reproductive status is confirmed by the presence of menstrual cycle irregularity (or amenorrhea of less than 1 year in duration) and hormonal evidence of ovarian dysfunction. This latter criterion has been operationalized to include either a single elevated plasma FSH level or more persistent elevations of plasma FSH levels (e.g. three out of four ≥ 14 IU/l)[55]. The *Diagnostic and Statistical Manual of Mental Disorders*, 4th edition, (DSM IV)[56] includes neither perimenopausal depression as a distinct mood disorder nor the perimenopause as a course specifier (as it does the postpartum period). Perimenopausal depression may not be distinguished from major depressive disorder on the basis of phenomenology, course, family or personal history of mood disorder. None the less, the relevance of changes in pituitary–ovarian function to depression during the perimenopause is suggested by evidence that estradiol therapy may have mood-enhancing effects, particularly in perimenopausal women with depression.

Controlled studies employing synthetic forms of estrogen in the treatment of depression have yielded mixed results. Estrogen has been reported to improve mood (albeit inconsistently)[57–59] in the following samples:

(1) Perimenopausal and postmenopausal women reporting depressive symptoms[21,60,61];

(2) Postmenopausal women with depression unresponsive to traditional antidepressant therapy[62];

(3) Non-depressed menopausal women not experiencing hot flushes[22].

We examined the therapeutic efficacy of estradiol replacement in 34 women (approximately half of whom had no prior history of depression) with perimenopausal depression under double-blind, placebo-controlled conditions[63]. After 3 weeks of estradiol, depression rating scale scores were significantly decreased compared with baseline scores, and significantly lower than scores in the women receiving placebo. A full or partial therapeutic response was seen in 80% of subjects on estradiol and in 22% of those on placebo, consistent with the observed effect size in a recent meta-analysis of studies examining estrogen's effects on mood[64]. The therapeutic response to estrogen was observed in both major and minor depression as well as in women with and without hot flushes. Finally, neither baseline nor post-treatment estradiol levels predicted therapeutic response. These data suggest that estrogen's effect on depression is not solely a product of its ability to reduce the distress of hot flushes.

Our findings are consistent with data from Montgomery and colleagues[21] and Saletu and associates[60] suggesting the beneficial effects of estrogen on mood in perimenopausal women reporting depressive symptoms. Two recent studies, by Soares and co-workers[65] and Morrison and colleagues (personal communication), have extended these observations. First, Soares and co-workers reported a significant and beneficial effect of estrogen replacement, compared with placebo, in women with perimenopause-related major depression (as defined by the Primary Care Evaluation of Mental Disorders (PRIME MD))[66], and, additionally, reported that baseline plasma estradiol levels did not predict response to estrogen treatment[65]. Second, Morrison and colleagues observed that estrogen was no more effective than placebo in postmenopausal depressed women, in contrast to previous results in perimenopausal women. These data emphasize that the stage of reproductive senescence may predict response to estrogen, as originally reported by Appleby and associates[67]. Thus, perimenopausal women who are undergoing changes in reproductive function may be more responsive to estrogen than postmenopausal women whose hormonal changes have long since stabilized.

CURRENT RECOMMENDATIONS

From both research and clinical perspectives, the assessment of perimenopause-related depression should include a careful history focused on several phenomena:

(1) The prominence of the affective and behavioral symptoms relative to somatic symptoms such as hot flushes or vaginal dryness;

(2) The presence of any past history of depression or hypomania, to compare the similarity of current symptoms with those of previous episodes;

(3) Possible comorbid or pre-existing medical or psychiatric conditions;

(4) The temporal relationship between the severity of mood symptoms and possible changes in menstrual cycle function (regular to irregular);

(5) The frequency of estrogen-sensitive somatic symptoms, such as hot flushes, that may predict the effectiveness of estrogen replacement in treating mood and behavioral symptoms;

(6) The current social and vocational context;

(7) Other symptoms that may impact on self-esteem and that may be responsive to estrogen replacement, such as urinary incontinence;

(8) Potential risk factors for osteoporosis which may suggest the potential benefit of estrogen replacement;

(9) The presence of contraindications to estrogen replacement, such as a personal or family history of breast cancer.

The differential diagnosis of perimenopause-related depression includes the following: dysphoria secondary to hot flush-induced dysomnia; depression secondary to adverse or stressful life events; and medical illness presenting as depression. Reproductive status may be characterized by serial plasma FSH or estradiol levels to confirm the presence of the perimenopause and to track improvements in mood if they occur in relation to changes in pituitary–ovarian hormone secretion.

In addition to the possible antidepressant efficacy of estrogen in perimenopausal depression, some but not all[68] studies have suggested that the response of peri- (Soares and colleagues, personal communication) and postmenopausal women[69,70] to some antidepressants (i.e. selective serotonin reuptake inhibitors) may be enhanced by the use of estrogen replacement. Consequently, if not otherwise contraindicated, estrogen augmentation may be of value in the treatment of perimenopausal depressed women who ostensibly are or who become antidepressant non-responders.

The decision to prescribe estradiol for perimenopausal depression must further be informed by associated risks and the availability of alternative treatments. The potential risks for cardiovascular morbidity and breast cancer after prolonged estrogen therapy appear to offset the benefits of estrogen therapy as a first-line treatment for depression[71]. Additionally, several adequate treatments for depression exist, and, therefore, the first-line medication for perimenopausal women presenting with depression is a traditional antidepressant such as a selective serotonin reuptake inhibitor. None the less, treatment of depression with estradiol may be considered under the following circumstances:

(1) As an alternative for the 50% or so of ambulatory depressed patients who fail to respond to a conventional, first-line intervention[72];

(2) In women who refuse to take psychotropic agents or who otherwise prefer treatment with estradiol;

(3) In women who will undertake treatment with estradiol for other acute symptoms (e.g. hot flushes) and who, therefore, could delay treatment with antidepressants until determining whether estradiol treatment is sufficient.

While estradiol treatment is no longer appropriate for prophylaxis, it is still reasonably prescribed for acute symptoms and syndromes, including depression. Finally, progestin may induce a dysphoric state in some women receiving estrogen therapy; however, progestin-induced dysphorias are not uniformly experienced in all women, nor are predictors of the dysphoric response known. Thus, progestins should not be contraindicated in the presence of an antidepressant response in a depressed perimenopausal woman.

CONCLUSIONS

The relationship between the onset of depressive illness and reproductive senescence has been a source of controversy. Those epidemiological and clinic-based studies that have distinguished between the perimenopause (a time of considerable variability in ovarian hormone secretion) and the postmenopause (a time when hormonal changes have long since stabilized) have suggested that, in some middle-aged women, the perimenopause is associated with an increased vulnerability to depression. Additional support for this suggestion is provided by double-blind, randomized controlled trials documenting the therapeutic efficacy of estradiol in perimenopausal depressed women, but not postmenopausal depressed women. Future studies should attempt to identify predictors of the therapeutic response to estradiol, the duration of estradiol's antidepressant effect and the role of estradiol withdrawal in the pathogenesis of perimenopausal depression.

References

1. Kaufert PA, Gilbert P, Tate R. Defining menopausal status: the impact of longitudinal data. *Maturitas* 1987;9:217-26
2. Santoro N, Brown JR, Adel T, *et al.* Characterization of reproductive hormonal dynamics in the perimenopause. *J Clin Endocrinol Metab* 1996;81: 1495-501
3. Burger HG, Dudley EC, Hopper JL, *et al.* The endocrinology of the menopausal transition: a cross-sectional study of a population-based sample. *J Clin Endocrinol Metab* 1995;80:3537-45
4. McKinlay JB, McKinlay SM, Brambilla D. The relative contributions of endocrine changes and social circumstances to depression in mid-aged women. *J Health Soc Behav* 1987;28:345-63
5. Kaufert PA, Gilbert P, Tate R. The Manitoba project: a re-examination of the link between menopause and depression. *Maturitas* 1992;14: 143-55
6. Avis NE, Brambilla D, McKinlay SM, *et al.* A longitudinal analysis of the association between menopause and depression: results from the Massachusetts Women's Health Study. *Ann Epidemiol* 1994;4:214-20
7. Matthews KA, Kuller LH, Wing RR, *et al.* Biobehavioral aspects of menopause: lessons from the healthy women study. *Exp Gerontol* 1994;29:337-42
8. Matthews KA. Myths and realities of the menopause. *Psychosom Med* 1992;54:1-9
9. Hunter M. The South-East England longitudinal study of the climacteric and postmenopause. *Maturitas* 1992;14:117-26
10. Anderson E, Hamburger S, Liu JH, *et al.* Characteristics of menopausal women seeking assistance. *Am J Obstet Gynecol* 1987;156:428-33
11. Stewart DE, Boydell K, Derzko C, *et al.* Psychologic distress during the menopausal years in women attending a menopause clinic. *Int J Psychiatry Med* 1992;22:213-20
12. Dennerstein L, Smith AMA, Morse C, *et al.* Menopausal symptoms in Australian women. *Med J Aust* 1993;159:232-6
13. Hay AG, Bancroft J, Johnstone EC. Affective symptoms in women attending a menopause clinic. *Br J Psychiatry* 1994;164:513-16
14. Weissman MM, Leaf PJ, Tischler GL, *et al.* Affective disorders in five United States communities. *Psychol Med* 1988;18:141-53
15. Kessler RC, McGonagle KA, Swartz M, *et al.* Sex and depression in the National Comorbidity Survey I: lifetime prevalence, chronicity and recurrence. *J Affect Disord* 1993;29:85-96
16. Bromberger JT, Meyer PM, Kravitz HM, *et al.* Psychologic distress and natural menopause: a multiethnic community study. *Am J Public Health* 2001;91:1435-42
17. Kaufert PA, Gilbert P, Hassard T. Researching the symptoms of menopause: an exercise in methodology. *Maturitas* 1988;10:117-31
18. Matthews KA, Wing RR, Kuller LH, *et al.* Influences of natural menopause on psychological characteristics and symptoms of middle-aged healthy women. *J Consult Clin Psychol* 1990;58: 345-51
19. Steingold KA, Laufer L, Chetkowski RJ, *et al.* Treatment of hot flashes with transdermal estradiol administration. *J Clin Endocrinol Metab* 1985;61: 627-32
20. Brincat M, Studd JWW, O'Dowd T, *et al.* Subcutaneous hormone implants for the control of climacteric symptoms: a prospective study. *Lancet* 1984;1:16-18
21. Montgomery JC, Brincat M, Tapp A, *et al.* Effect of oestrogen and testosterone implants on psychological disorders in the climacteric. *Lancet* 1987;1:297-9
22. Ditkoff EC, Crary WG, Cristo M, *et al.* Estrogen improves psychological function in asymptomatic postmenopausal women. *Obstet Gynecol* 1991;78: 991-5
23. Sherwin BB, Gelfand MM. Differential symptom response to parenteral estrogen and/or androgen administration in the surgical menopause. *Am J Obstet Gynecol* 1985;151:153-60
24. Brambilla F, Maggioni M, Ferrari E, *et al.* Tonic and dynamic gonadotropin secretion in depressive and normothymic phases of affective disorders. *Psychiatry Res* 1990;32:229-39
25. Amsterdam JD, Winokur A, Lucki I, *et al.* Neuroendocrine regulation in depressed postmenopausal women and healthy subjects. *Acta Psychiatr Scand* 1983;67:43-9
26. Altman N, Sachar EJ, Gruen PH, *et al.* Reduced plasma LH concentration in postmenopausal depressed women. *Psychosom Med* 1975;37:274-6
27. Guicheney P, Léger D, Barrat J, *et al.* Platelet serotonin content and plasma tryptophan in peri- and postmenopausal women: variations with plasma oestrogen levels and depressive symptoms. *Eur J Clin Invest* 1988;18:297-304
28. Ballinger S. Stress as a factor in lowered estrogen-levels in the early postmenopause. *Ann NY Acad Sci* 1990;592:95-113
29. Huerta R, Mena A, Malacara JM, *et al.* Symptoms at perimenopausal period: its association with attitudes toward sexuality, life-style, family function, and FSH levels. *Psychoneuroendocrinology* 1995; 20:135-48

30. Saletu B, Brandstatter N, Metka M, *et al.* Hormonal, syndromal and EEG mapping studies in menopausal syndrome patients with and without depression as compared with controls. *Maturitas* 1996;23:91–105
31. Barrett-Connor E, von Muhlen D, Laughlin GA, *et al.* Endogenous levels of dehydroepiandrosterone sulfate, but not other sex hormones, are associated with depressed mood in older women: the Rancho Bernardo study. *J Am Geriatr Soc* 1999; 47:685–91
32. Cawood EHH, Bancroft J. Steroid hormones, the menopause, sexuality and well-being of women. *Psychol Med* 1996;26:925–36
33. Schmidt PJ, Murphy JH, Haq N, *et al.* Basal plasma hormone levels in depressed perimenopausal women. *Psychoneuroendocrinology* 2002;27:907–20
34. Amsterdam JD, Maislin G, Rosenzweig M, *et al.* Gonadotropin (LH and FSH) response after submaximal GnRH stimulation in depressed premenopausal women and healthy controls. *Psychoneuroendocrinology* 1995;20:311–21
35. Majewska MD, Demirgören S, Spivak CE, *et al.* The neurosteroid dehydroepiandrosterone sulfate is an allosteric antagonist of the $GABA_A$ receptor. *Brain Res* 1990;526:143–6
36. Compagnone NA, Mellon SH. Dehydroepiandrosterone: a potential signalling molecule for neocortical organization during development. *Proc Natl Acad Sci USA* 1998;95:4678–83
37. Baulieu E-E, Robel P. Dehydroepiandrosterone (DHEA) and dehydroepiandrosterone sulfate (DHEAS) as neuroactive neurosteroids. *Proc Natl Acad Sci USA* 1998;95:4089–91
38. Robel P, Baulieu E-E. Neurosteroids, biosynthesis and function. *Trends Endocrinol Metab* 1994;5:1–8
39. Zwain IH, Yen SSC. Dehydroepiandrosterone: biosynthesis and metabolism in the brain. *Endocrinology* 1999;140:880–7
40. Morales AJ, Nolan JJ, Nelson JC, *et al.* Effects of replacement dose of dehydroepiandrosterone in men and women of advancing age. *J Clin Endocrinol Metab* 1994;78:1360–7
41. Wolkowitz OM, Reus VI, Keebler A, *et al.* Double-blind treatment of major depression with dehydroepiandrosterone. *Am J Psychiatry* 1999;156: 646–9
42. Wolkowitz OM, Reus VI, Roberts E, *et al.* Dehydroepiandrosterone (DHEA) treatment of depression. *Biol Psychiatry* 1997;41:311–18
43. Bloch M, Schmidt PJ, Danaceau MA, *et al.* Dehydroepiandrosterone treatment of mid-life dysthymia. *Biol Psychiatry* 1999;45:1533–41
44. Wolf OT, Neumann O, Hellhammer DH, *et al.* Effects of a two-week physiological dehydroepiandrosterone substitution on cognitive performance and well-being in healthy elderly women and men. *J Clin Endocrinol Metab* 1997;82: 2363–7
45. Goodyer IM, Herbert J, Altham PME, *et al.* Adrenal secretion during major depression in 8- to 16-year-olds, I. Altered diurnal rhythms in salivary cortisol and dehydroepiandrosterone (DHEA) at presentation. *Psychol Med* 1996;26: 245–56
46. Goodyer IM, Herbert J, Altham PME. Adrenal steroid secretion and major depression in 8- to 16-year-olds, III. Influence of cortisol/DHEA ratio at presentation on subsequent rates of disappointing life events and persistent major depression. *Psychol Med* 1998;28:265–73
47. Ferrari E, Locatelli M, Arcaini A, *et al.* Chronobiological study of some neuroendocrine features of major depression in elderly people. Presented at the *79th Annual Meeting of the Endocrine Society*, Minneapolis MN, June 1997:abstr
48. Heuser I, Deuschle M, Luppa P, *et al.* Increased diurnal plasma concentrations of dehydroepiandrosterone in depressed patients. *J Clin Endocrinol Metab* 1998;83:3130–3
49. Laughlin GA, Barrett-Connor E. Sexual dimorphism in the influence of advanced aging on adrenal hormone levels: the Rancho Bernardo study. *J Clin Endocrinol Metab* 2000;85:3561–8
50. Cumming DC, Rebar RW, Hopper BR, *et al.* Evidence for an influence of the ovary on circulating dehydroepiandrosterone sulfate levels. *J Clin Endocrinol Metab* 1982;54:1069–71
51. Gray A, Feldman HA, McKinlay JB, *et al.* Age, disease and changing sex hormone levels in middle-aged men: results of the Massachusetts male aging study. *J Clin Endocrinol Metab* 1991;73: 1016–23
52. Orentreich N, Brind JL, Rizer RL, *et al.* Age changes and sex differences in serum dehydroepiandrosterone sulfate concentrations throughout adulthood. *J Clin Endocrinol Metab* 1984;59:551–5
53. Orentreich N, Brind JL, Vogelman JH, *et al.* Long-term longitudinal measurements of plasma dehydroepiandrosterone sulfate in normal men. *J Clin Endocrinol Metab* 1992;75:1002–4
54. Belanger A, Candas B, Dupont A, *et al.* Changes in serum concentrations of conjugated and unconjugated steroids in 40- to 80-year-old men. *J Clin Endocrinol Metab* 1994;79:1086–90
55. Schmidt PJ, Rubinow DR. Mood and the perimenopause. *Contemp Ob/Gyn* 1994;39:68–75
56. American Psychiatric Association. *Diagnostic and Statistical Manual of Mental Disorders*, 4th edn. Washington, DC: American Psychiatric Press, 1994
57. Coope J. Is oestrogen therapy effective in the treatment of menopausal depression? *J R Coll Gen Pract* 1981;31:134–40
58. Campbell S. Double-blind psychometric studies on the effects of natural estrogens on postmenopausal women. In Campbell S, ed. *The Management of the Menopause and Postmenopausal Years*. Lancaster, UK: MTP Press, 1976:149–58

59. George GCW, Utian WH, Beumont PJV, *et al.* Effect of exogenous oestrogens on minor psychiatric symptoms in postmenopausal women. *S Afr Med J* 1973;47:2387–8
60. Saletu B, Brandstatter N, Metka M, *et al.* Double-blind, placebo-controlled, hormonal, syndromal and EEG mapping studies with transdermal oestradiol therapy in menopausal depression. *Psychopharmacology* 1995;122:321–9
61. Sherwin BB. Affective changes with estrogen and androgen replacement therapy in surgically menopausal women. *J Affect Disord* 1988;14:177–87
62. Klaiber EL, Broverman DM, Vogel W, *et al.* Estrogen therapy for severe persistent depressions in women. *Arch Gen Psychiatry* 1979;36:550–4
63. Schmidt PJ, Nieman L, Danaceau MA, *et al.* Estrogen replacement in perimenopause-related depression: a preliminary report. *Am J Obstet Gynecol* 2000;183:414–20
64. Zweifel JE, O'Brien WH. A meta-analysis of the effect of hormone replacement therapy upon depressed mood. *Psychoneuroendocrinology* 1997;22: 189–212
65. Soares CD, Almeida OP, Joffe H, *et al.* Efficacy of estradiol for the treatment of depressive disorders in perimenopausal women: a double-blind, randomized, placebo-controlled trial. *Arch Gen Psychiatry* 2001;58:529–34
66. Spitzer RL, Kroenke K, Linzer M, *et al.* Health-related quality of life in primary care patients with mental disorders: results from the PRIME-MD 1000 study. *J Am Med Assoc* 1995;274:1511–17
67. Appleby L, Montgomery J, Studd J. Oestrogens and affective disorders. In Studd J, ed. *Progress in Obstetrics and Gynaecology*. Edinburgh: Churchill Livingstone, 1981:289–302
68. Amsterdam J, Garcia-Espana F, Fawcett J, *et al.* Fluoxetine efficacy in menopausal women with and without estrogen replacement. *J Affect Disord* 1999; 55:11–17
69. Schneider LS, Small GW, Hamilton SH, *et al.* Estrogen replacement and response to fluoxetine in a multicenter geriatric depression trial. *Am J Geriatr Psychiatry* 1997;5:97–106
70. Schneider LS, Small GW, Clary CM. Estrogen replacement therapy and antidepressant response to sertraline in older depressed women. *Am J Geriatr Psychiatry* 2001;9:393–9
71. Writing Group for the Women's Health Initiative Investigators. Risks and benefits of estrogen plus progestin in healthy postmenopausal women: principal results from the Women's Health Initiative randomized controlled trial. *J Am Med Assoc* 2002;288:321–33
72. Fava M, Abraham M, Alpert J, *et al.* Gender differences in axis I comorbidity among depressed outpatients. *J Affect Disord* 1996;38:129–33

Depression in menopausal women 18

U. Halbreich and L. S. Kahn

INTRODUCTION

Kraeplin[1] suggested that menopausal or postmenopausal women may be subject to a specific severe form of depression, which he termed involutional melancholia. This entity was recognized by the *Diagnostic and Statistical Manual* of the American Psychiatric Association I and II (DSM I and II)[2], but was deleted from DSM III[3] and subsequent editions.

The reasons for exclusion of a specific menopausal form of depression from the American diagnostic nomenclature are several, and are not discussed here. However, one of the main reasons for the deletion is the demonstration that, during the menopause, women are not more depressed than during reproductive age. If anything, the opposite may be true.

PREVALENCE OF DEPRESSION IN WOMEN

Gender differences in the prevalence of depression have been consistently documented, with a preponderance of about 2 : 1 in women compared with men[4]. Initial large-scale epidemiological studies (see, for example, references 4–11) suggested that the gender difference is most pronounced during reproductive age, and the prevalence of depression is substantially decreased in menopausal women. A small increase in prevalence in women in their late 40s was suggested as being attributable to the perimenopause or the menopausal transition[6]. In older populations, the prevalence of depression was suggested to be actually higher among men[8].

The association of increased prevalence of depression in women of reproductive age, and increased prevalence in women compared with men in that age group, is further substantiated by reports that the gender difference emerges only during early to mid-adolescence[12–18], while prior to puberty the prevalence of depression is higher in boys[19,20].

PREVALENCE OF DEPRESSION DURING PERIMENOPAUSE (IN NORMAL WOMEN)

An association between perimenopause and mood was found in several cross-sectional studies[21–24].

Weissman and co-workers[6,25] suggested an increase in onset of major depressive disorders in women aged 45–50 years, which they attributed to the perimenopausal years. This suggestion is in concurrence with previous studies[26,27] reporting an increase in the prevalence of depression in women between the ages of 45 and 54, but not in men of the same age group. The perimenopause is also a time of increased vulnerability for bipolar patients, and Angst[28] reported an increase in the frequency of cycling in women during that period. Whether or not there is an increase in repeated episodes of unipolar depression during that time is still unclear, although it has been suggested[29–31]. The notion that depression during the perimenopause occurs more in women who are vulnerable is supported by reports of an association between the risk of development of perimenopausal depression and a history of postpartum depression and premenstrual dysphoria[30,32]. This association may be limited to treatment-seeking women (Hunter and colleagues[22] assessed only women in an ovarian screening clinic), or may be influenced by culture (Avis[33] found an association between recent symptoms and previous surgical menopause only in American and not in Canadian or Japanese women). Collins and Landgren[24] studied 1324 Swedish women aged 48 years who were more than 6 months from their last menses; therefore, many would have been perimenopausal. The association referred to above disappeared when vasomotor symptoms were controlled for.

Results of prospective studies were somewhat different. No association between onset of menopause and depression (using the Centre for Epidemiologic Studies Depression Scale (CES-D)) was found by Kaufert and colleagues[34] and Woods and Mitchell[32] in premenopausal women (at baseline). Natural menopause did not increase anxiety or depression[35].

No increase in depression from premenopause to postmenopause 1 year later was found by Holte[36] (with Goldberg's General Health Questionnaire), nor by Hällstrom and Samuelsson[37] in a 6-year follow-up. Both studied general populations.

The appearance of dysphoric symptoms only in vulnerable women might be implied by Kuh and colleagues[38] from their study of 1202 British women at age 47, compared with their status at age 36. Only a slight increase in irritability was reported at the perimenopause, and no symptoms were related to menopausal status. The prevalence of psychological symptoms was high in women post-hysterectomy or taking hormone replacement therapy (HRT), as well as in those with stress, anxiety and depression and related problems at age 36.

In a prospective study (27 months) of women during the perimenopausal transition[29], women who were depressed before the perimenopause, or who underwent a long perimenopausal period, and those who reported physical perimenopausal symptoms showed a high rate of depression, but others did not.

No prospective increase of depression during the perimenopause was found by Hunter[39].

Some attribute mood disorders during the perimenopause to perimenopausal symptoms such as hot flushes, insomnia, night sweats and tiredness[33].

The impression that perimenopausal women experience more depression may be due to psychosocial factors and not necessarily the menopause *per se*. Such factors include stressful life events, changes in social network[40], death of a parent, changing relationships with children[21], separation, divorce or death of spouse[41], negative expectations or attitudes towards the menopause and aging[38,42,43] or general poor health[32]. Vulnerability to a report of depression during the menopause is associated with reports of depression before the menopause[29,38,39], and menstrual cycle- or reproductive-related disorders, especially premenstrual syndrome (PMS)[24,30,32,44], dysmenorrhea[24] and postpartum depression[30,32].

The importance of psychosocial factors in the onset of symptoms during the menopausal transition is underscored by reports of a decreased rate of complaints by women in non-Western societies, where women improve their status in society when they reach the menopause by becoming equal to men and/or attaining life status, compared with younger women[45,46].

Lock and Kaufert[47–49] surveyed 1225 Japanese women between 45 and 55 years of age about symptoms corresponding to the menopause, and compared the results with those from similarly structured studies undertaken in the USA[50] and Canada[34]. Only 10.3% of Japanese menopausal women reported feeling blue/depressed, compared with 23.4% of Canadian and 35.9% of American women ($p < 0.01$).

PREVALENCE OF DEPRESSION DURING MENOPAUSE

In most cross-sectional studies, no association between the menopause and depression was found[34,37,41,42,51–54] (for review see references 33, 55 and 56). No association with previous stress, lability of mood, irritability, anxiety and individual depressive symptoms was found, either[22,38,43,51,57,58].

This assumption of decreased prevalence of depression in menopausal women has been supported by a recent British epidemiological study of 9792 subjects, aged 16–67 years, which compared prevalence of depression among men and women younger and older than 55 years of age[59]. However, early dissenters from this hypothesis[60], who reported that the preponderance of depression in women is not diminished after the menopause, may be supported by a more recent article[61] stating that the gender difference may increase after middle age.

Based on a Canadian study of 16 650 men and women, Cairney and Wade[18] reported that, between ages 15 and 54, the odds ratio for depressed women compared with men was 2.24: 9.0% 12-month prevalence in women, and 4.2% in men. The prevalence decreased in both men (1.9%) and women (3.9%) over age 55, but the odds ratio stayed the same: 2.13. Interestingly, HRT did not significantly influence rate of depression. Women who had HRT in the month prior to the study had slightly higher rates of depression (odds ratio 1.24, not significant). This study did not distinguish between different HRT modalities, nor did it account for cohort effect, which may suggest an increase in the prevalence of depression in recent birth cohorts for both men and women[62,63]. For some reason, the authors did not give a breakdown of ages, and only the cut-off before and after age 55 is presented.

A preponderance of menopausal women developing depression was reported by Green and colleagues[64] and by Stallones and associates[65]. A different epidemiological picture emerges from the recent large (38 434 men and 40 024 women) European epidemiological community study carried out by Angst and co-workers[66]. Rates of major depression as well as minor depression (subthreshold, only 2–4 reported symptoms out of nine) were not found to decrease substantially during the menopause, and until age 75 years and older the gender difference was maintained. As previously reported, there was a slight increase in prevalence in the age group 45–54 years, but that slight increase was similar in women and men.

PREVALENCE OF DYSTHYMIA DURING MENOPAUSE

New onset of dysthymic disorder is relatively rare during the menopause[67–69], and may be a residue of a major depressive episode, or follow a psychosocial stressor such as illness or separation[70].

Symptoms

Compared with early-onset dysthymic disorder, during the menopause there are no atypical symptoms[71]: mood reactivity, weight gain and/or increased appetite, leaden paralysis and long-standing hypersensitivity to interpersonal rejection. Dysthymia with onset during the menopause has been reported not to be associated with personality disorders[72], but with medical illnesses or physical impairment.

In Finnish women over 60 years of age, 22.9% had dysthymia, but the age of onset was in later life[73]. This is similar to the results of Devanand and colleagues[68] and Kirby and associates[70] who also reported a later age of onset in elderly dysthymia.

Because, to our knowledge, 'late onset' dysthymic disorder is reported with a cut-off age of 21 years, at one end of the scale, and over 60 years, at the other, it is still unclear whether younger postmenopausal women, i.e. those 50–60 years of age, actually have a lesser prevalence of dysthymic disorder.

PREVALENCE OF BIPOLAR DISORDERS (VERSUS UNIPOLAR)

The prevalence of bipolar disorders was reported in an Italian study of 525 out-patients with major depressive disorder episodes[74], of whom two-thirds were women (no separate analysis was done for women). While the prevalence of unipolar depression among these patients was higher in patients older than 50 (67.0%), compared with those younger than 50 years (46.5%), the prevalence of bipolar II (BP II) was less in the older group (32.9% vs. 53.4%). Atypical features were significantly less common among BP II and unipolar patients over 50, compared with those younger than 50 years. This is in contrast to dysthymic patients in other studies. The age-related decrease in BP II may be a cohort effect (younger generations might be more likely to have bipolar disorders compared with older generations[75]).

Late-onset (> 50 years), late-life BP II patients were only 19.3% of late-life BP II patients, suggesting that the likelihood of new-onset BP II disorder following age 50 may be rather low.

Mania in late life[6]

In a small group (22 women) of peri- and postmenopausal women with bipolar disorder[77], only two women reported onset of the first bipolar episode during the perimenopause, and another three (BP I) during or after the perimenopause. Only one woman (age 46) reported having her first episode 6 years after the menopause. However, 7/8 women who had not used HRT reported peri- or postmenopausal worsening of bipolar symptoms, including depression, irritability, hypomania or mania, and only 3/12 women taking HRT reported a worsening course of mood disorders. Six women of the total group reported more frequent cycling (unclear whether or not they were taking HRT).

ESTROGEN AND DEPRESSION IN POSTMENOPAUSAL WOMEN

Estrogen has been shown to have an impact on many brain processes that are putatively associated with depression and anxiety disorders. Therefore, it might be assumed that a state of hypogonadism, as during the menopause, would be associated with higher rates of depression and other mood disorders. Surveys of the prevalence of such disorders in menopausal women demonstrate that clearly this is not so.

This is supported by studies in which both mood and hormonal levels were concurrently measured. No association between estrogen levels in postmenopausal women and mood was found[58,78,79]. Ballinger and colleagues[79] also did not find any association between luteinizing hormone (LH) and follicle stimulating hormone (FSH) levels and major depression.

An association between low levels of estradiol and depressive symptoms was reported[80]; this association may be affected by progesterone. While progesterone may decrease the effect of estrogen, androgens might potentiate it[81–85].

ESTROGEN EFFECTS ON DYSPHORIC SYMPTOMS DURING MENOPAUSE

Until recently, most studies of depressed perimenopausal women also included postmenopausal women, and the distinction was not completely clear (for review see reference 86)[87–91]. Only a few studies were limited to perimenopausal women[88,92,93]. Beneficial effects of estrone sulfate, estradiol and estradiol plus testosterone were reported. It is still unclear whether the improvement is maintained over periods longer than 4 months[90]. Two recent, randomized, placebo-controlled double-blind studies support the efficacy of transdermal estradiol as an antidepressant for perimenopausal women[92,93]. It appears that transdermal estradiol may be more efficacious than conjugated equine estrogen and estrone sulfate for the treatment of dysphoric symptoms and depressive disorders in perimenopausal women.

This situation may be somewhat different in menopausal women. Here there is probably a need to distinguish between surgically induced menopause and naturally occurring menopause.

Despite two early negative trials of treatment of dysphoric symptoms in surgically induced menopause, with estrone sulfate[94] and conjugated estrogens[95], it seems that estrogen is efficacious as treatment of dysphoric symptoms in this situation. Positive effects on psychological functions were reported with conjugated estrogens[96] given to asymptomatic women. Similar results were demonstrated with ethinylestradiol and estradiol valerate[97]. The possible effects of estradiol valerate are probably enhanced by the addition of testosterone enanthate[98]. Testosterone alone also has a robust effect, but may cause more behavioral adverse effects, such as increased aggression and irritability.

While estrogens are probably effective for increasing well-being and elevation of dysphoric mood, it is still unclear whether estrogen by itself would be an effective antidepressant in surgically menopausal women with major depressive disorder.

In women who have undergone menopause naturally, estrogens were shown to increase well-being and quality of life and decrease mild dysphoric symptoms[96,99–103]. Transdermal estradiol is probably more efficacious for these effects, compared with other preparations, although this is still not completely determined because some of the studies included perimenopausal women.

The addition of testosterone to estrogen probably improves libido, sense of well-being and dysphoric mood[85].

EFFICACY OF ESTROGEN AS SOLE ANTIDEPRESSANT IN POSTMENOPAUSAL WOMEN

Considering the serotoninergic agonist and norepinephrine agonist effects of estrogen, it would be attractive to attempt the application of estrogen as an antidepressant, especially in depressed people who may have low endogenous levels of estrogen, as is the case with postmenopausal women. However, so far, research is quite disappointing.

The effect of estrogen and HRT as antidepressant treatment of women with major depressive disorder (MDD) is still unclear[104–106], despite some positive reports[107].

Ripley and colleagues[108] were unable to show any antidepressant effects of estrogens. Schneider and associates[109] demonstrated that 4 weeks of estrogen treatment was not efficacious as an antidepressant for ten women with severe depression. Estrogen did induce an enhanced sense of well-being, however, in ten non-depressed women. Shortly thereafter, Klaiber and co-workers[110] reported a placebo-controlled trial of 15–25 mg/day conjugated equine estrogen (CEE) in a small group of treatment-resistant depressed 'postmenopausal' women, in whom a statistically significant improvement of depression with estrogen was demonstrated. Hamilton Depression Scale (HAM-D) improved from 31 to 22, and 6/23 women taking estrogen were in remission, compared with none of the 18 taking placebo. However, only eight women in this study were postmenopausal, and age was not related to improvement. More recently, transdermal estradiol (50 μg/day) was reported not to be superior to placebo[111]; however, the placebo effect in the study was relatively high. A somewhat positive effect of CEE (0.625 mg/day) was reported in a small group ($n = 12$) of postmenopausal women with MDD[107].

To our knowledge, there are still no published recent large-scale studies of the use of estrogen alone for treatment of MDD in postmenopausal women.

AUGMENTATION OF CONVENTIONAL ANTIDEPRESSANTS WITH ESTROGEN

The same rationale for the use of estrogen as an antidepressant is also valid for its use as an adjunct or augmentation therapy to antidepressants. Earlier reports of the supplementation of tricyclic antidepressants (TCAs) with estrogen were quite disappointing. Initially, estrogen in high doses (1.25–3.75 mg/day CEE) was added to norepinephrine reuptake inhibitors as imipramine[112], and was not found to be efficacious. Furthermore, in vulnerable women it may have induced rapid mood cycling when added to TCAs[113]. A small prospective study was prematurely discontinued because, even though some positive therapeutic effects were observed, estrogen also augmented cholinergic adverse effects that were intolerable[114].

With the advent of large-scale clinical trials of selective serotonin reuptake inhibitors (SSRIs), some women who were included in these trials were already taking estrogen replacement therapy (ERT) with and without progestins. Therefore, the opportunity to compare the responses of women with and without ERT was presented. In a *post hoc* analysis, it has been reported[115] that 31 women who received 20 mg/day fluoxetine and ERT had better improvement of the severity of their symptoms (40.1% decrease in the HAM-D), compared with 41 women who received placebo plus ERT (17.0% improvement). Interestingly, in that study there was no difference between placebo and fluoxetine (improvement 30.4% and 36.1%, respectively) among elderly women who did not receive ERT. The authors speculated that elderly women (over 65 years) who did not receive ERT would respond less to SSRIs, which indeed is not the case. ERT was not controlled in that reportedly positive study. The same group[116] also analyzed data on sertraline with a similar *post hoc* approach. Among women who completed the study, more women who were taking ERT (in addition to sertraline) responded according to Clinical Global Impressions Scale (CGI), compared with those who did not receive ERT (96% vs. 73%). When severity was assessed (with HAM-D), no difference was found.

The doubtful results are underscored by the report of Amsterdam and colleagues[117] that 45 women with MDD and over 45 years of age who received fluoxetine and HRT did not have a better response than 132 women who did not receive HRT. They also did not have a better response when compared with 396 women younger than 45 years and 262 men. Furthermore, Meier survival analysis to week 26 demonstrated a non-significant ($p < 0.06$) trend for greater relapse in women over 45 years of age on ERT, compared with those in the other treatment groups. As was the case with the previous studies, ERT was not controlled, and different estrogen–progestin combinations were taken for various periods of time.

A somewhat different approach was adopted by Joffe and colleagues[118] when 30–45 mg/day mirtazapine, which is a serotoninergic agonist and α_2-antagonist, was given in an open trial with no placebo to 22 women aged 40–61 years who were peri- or postmenopausal and receiving ERT. It is reported that full remission was achieved in 14/16 completers. However, subjects responded better to mirtazapine whether or not the depression preceded ERT or regardless of menopausal status, and with no influence of HRT preparation (with and without medroxyprogesterone).

Considering the strong theoretical rationale for an augmentation of efficacy of SSRIs and norepinephrine agonists with estrogen, two issues are important: first, the results of actual analyses are quite disappointing; and second, so far there are no prospective, adequately designed published studies to support or dispute that hypothesis.

The interaction between menopause and depression may be bidirectional. It has been demonstrated[119] that early menopause (before 40 years of age) may be associated with severe MDD (relative risk of 1.9). Therefore, it is of interest whether and how lifetime history of MDD may lead to early menopause, and not only whether menopause may be associated with the increased vulnerability to depression.

While the current data still cast doubt on the efficacy of estrogen as an antidepressant or as an augmentation therapy in depressed women, there is more support to the long-term notion that estrogen as well as some related hormones improve mood and well-being of non-depressed menopausal women. Three months of treatment with CEE 0.625 mg/day with either 2.5 or 5 mg medroxyprogesterone acetate (MPA) improved mood as measured with the Beck Depression Inventory (BDI). Simultaneously, they increased tritiated imipramine binding on the women's platelets. A similar effect was induced by tibolone, but not in the control group who received alendronate. Indeed, the improved mood was attributed by the authors[120] to improved serotoninergic functioning.

The dose, preparation and combination of HRT probably influences its effects on mood[86,121,122]. Especially, addition of the progestin may decrease the beneficial effects of estrogen[82,123].

The importance of the progestin applied, as well as central nervous system (CNS) activities other than that of serotonin, is demonstrated by a report[124] that estrogen valerate improved SCL-90 scales of depression and anxiety in normal non-depressed postmenopausal women. Biphasic addition of the progestin cyproterone acetate (CPA) further improved these complaints, as well as caused improvement in somatization, obsessive compulsive disorder (OCD) and interpersonal sensitivity. Furthermore, when the sulpiride stimulation test was applied as a test of blockade of the dopaminergic system, the group who received estrogen plus CPA had higher prolactin response, indicating an increased dopaminergic blockade and suggesting an association between improvement of mood symptoms and enhanced restoration of the dopaminergic system, while estrogen by itself did not induce it.

CONCLUSION

Despite earlier assumptions, at present there is no support for an increased rate of depression in postmenopausal women. If anything, there might be some decrease of depression in older women. There is no proof of the efficacy of estrogen as a sole antidepressant, nor any proof of its ability to augment the efficacy of selective serotonin reuptake inhibitors. The role of progestins is still unclear.

Hormone replacement therapy enhances the well-being and libido of healthy postmenopausal women and probably selectively improves cognitive functions; however, even this has recently been challenged. A clear distinction should be made between postmenopausal life and the perimenopause, or the menopausal transition period during which estrogen is effective as an antidepressant, probably owing to its homeostatic and stabilizing effects.

References

1. Kraepelin E. *Lehrbuch der Psychiatrie.* New York: MacMillan, 1907
2. American Psychiatric Association. *DSM-II: Diagnostic and Statistical Manual of Mental Disorders*, 2nd edn. Washington, DC: American Psychiatric Press, 1968
3. American Psychiatric Association. *DSM-III: Diagnostic and Statistical Manual of Mental Disorders*, 3rd edn. Washington, DC: American Psychiatric Press, 1980
4. Weissman MM, Myers JK. Affective disorders in a US urban community: the use of research diagnostic criteria in an epidemiological survey. *Arch Gen Psychiatry* 1978;35:1304–11
5. Weissman MM, Leaf PJ, Bruce ML, *et al.* The epidemiology of dysthymia in five communities: rates, risks, comorbidity, and treatment. *Am J Psychiatry* 1988;145:815–19
6. Weissman MM, Bland RC, Canino GJ, *et al.* Cross-national epidemiology of major depression and bipolar disorder. *J Am Med Assoc* 1996; 276:293–9
7. Robins LN, Regier DA. *Psychiatric Disorders in America: The Epidemiologic Catchment Study.* New York: Free Press, 1991
8. Bland RC, Newman SC, Orn H. Period prevalence of psychiatric disorders in Edmonton. *Acta Psychiatr Scand Suppl* 1988;338:33–42
9. Wells JE, Bushnell JA, Hornblow AR, *et al.* Christchurch Psychiatric Epidemiology Study, Part I: Methodology and lifetime prevalence for specific psychiatric disorders. *Aust NZ J Psychiatry* 1989;23:315–26
10. Leon AC, Klerman GL, Wickramaratne P. Continuing female predominance in depressive illness. *Am J Public Health* 1993;83:754–7
11. Kessler RC, DuPont RL, Berglund P, *et al.* Impairment in pure and comorbid generalized anxiety disorder and major depression at 12 months in two national surveys. *Am J Psychiatry* 1999;156: 1915–23
12. Nolen-Hoeksema S, Girgus JS. The emergence of gender differences in depression during adolescence. *Psychol Bull* 1994;115:424–43
13. Cairney J. Gender differences in the prevalence of depression among Canadian adolescents. *Can J Public Health* 1998;89:181–2
14. Allgood-Merron B, Lewinsohn PM, Hyman H. Sex difference and adolescent depression. *J Abnorm Psychol* 1990;99:55–63
15. Kandel DB, Davies M. Adult sequelae of adolescent depressive symptoms. *Arch Gen Psychiatry* 1986;43:255–62
16. Petersen AC, Sarigiani PA, Kennedy RE. Adolescent depression: why more girls? *J Youth Adolesc* 1991;20:247–71
17. Hankin BL, Abramson LY, Moffitt TE, *et al.* Development of depression from preadolescence to young adulthood: emerging gender differences in a 10-year longitudinal study. *J Abnorm Psychol* 1998;107:128–40
18. Cairney J, Wade TJ. The influence of age on gender differences in depression: further population-based evidence on the relationship between menopause and the sex difference in depression. *Soc Psychiatry Psychiatr Epidemiol* 2002;37:401–8
19. Nolen-Hoeksema S, Girgus JS, Seligman ME. Sex differences in depression and explanatory style in children. *J Youth Adolesc* 1991;20:2333–45
20. Anderson JC, Williams S, McGee R, *et al.* DSM-III disorders in preadolescent children. Prevalence in a large sample from the general population. *Arch Gen Psychiatry* 1987;44:69–76
21. Ballinger SE. Psychosocial stress and symptoms of menopause: a comparative study of menopause clinic patients and non-patients. *Maturitas* 1985; 7:315–27
22. Hunter M, Battersby R, Whitehead M. Relationships between psychological symptoms, somatic complaints and menopausal status. *Maturitas* 1986;8:217–28
23. Avis NE, Kaufert PA, Lock M, *et al.* The evolution of menopausal symptoms. *Baillierés Clin Endocrinol Metab* 1993;7:17–32
24. Collins A, Landgren BM. Reproductive health, use of estrogen and experience of symptoms in

perimenopausal women: a population-based study. *Maturitas* 1994;20:101–11
25. Weissman MW. Epidemiology of major depression in women. Women and the controversies in hormone replacement therapy. Presented at the *American Psychiatric Association Meeting*, New York, May 1996
26. Bebbington P, Hurry J, Tennant C. Epidemiology of mental disorders in Camberwell. *Psychol Med* 1981;11:576–9
27. Eagles JM, Whalley LJ. Ageing and affective disorders: the age at first onset of affective disorders in Scotland, 1969–1978. *Br J Psychiatry* 1985;147: 180–7
28. Angst J. The course of depressive disorders. II. Typology of bipolar manic-depressive illness. *Arch Psychiatr Nervankr* 1978;226:65–72
29. Avis NE, Brambilla D, McKinlay SM, *et al.* A longitudinal analysis of the association between menopause and depression. Results from the Massachusetts Women's Health Study. *Ann Epidemiol* 1994;4:214–20
30. Stewart DE, Boydell KM. Psychologic distress during menopause: associations across the reproductive life cycle. *Int J Psychiatry Med* 1993;23: 157–62
31. Stewart DE, Boydell K, Derzko C, *et al.* Psychologic distress during the menopausal years in women attending a menopause clinic. *Int J Psychiatry Med* 1992;22:213–20
32. Woods NF, Mitchell ES. Patterns of depressed mood in midlife women; observations from the Seattle Midlife Women's Health Study. *Res Nurs Health* 1996;19:111–23
33. Avis NE. Sexual behavior in aging women. In Hof PR, Mobbs CV, eds. *Functional Neurobiology of Aging*. San Diego: Academic Press, 2001:749–60
34. Kaufert PA, Gilbert P, Tate R. The Manitoba Project: a re-examination of the link between menopause and depression. *Maturitas* 1992;14: 143–55
35. Matthews KA, Wing RR, Kuller LH, *et al.* Influences of natural menopause on psychological characteristics and symptoms of middle-aged healthy women. *J Consult Clin Psychol* 1990;58: 345–51
36. Holte A. Influences of natural menopause on health complaints: a prospective study of healthy Norwegian women. *Maturitas* 1992;14: 127–41
37. Hällstrom T, Samuelsson S. Mental health in the climacteric. The longitudinal study of women in Gothenburg. *Acta Obstet Gynecol Scand Suppl* 1985; 130:13–18
38. Kuh DL, Wadsworth M, Hardy R. Women's health in midlife: the influence of the menopause, social factors and health in earlier life. *Br J Obstet Gynaecol* 1997;104:923–33
39. Hunter MS. Psychological and somatic experience of the menopause: a prospective study. *Psychosom Med* 1990;52:357–67
40. Greene JG, Cooke DJ. Life stress and symptoms at the climacterium. *Br J Psychiatry* 1980;136:486–91
41. McKinlay JB, McKinlay SM, Brambilla D. The relative contributions of endocrine changes and social circumstances to depression in mid-aged women. *J Health Soc Behav* 1987;28:345–63
42. Dennerstein L, Smith AM, Morse C, *et al.* Menopausal symptoms in Australian women. *Med J Aust* 1993;159:232–6
43. Holte A, Mikkelsen A. Psychosocial determinants of climacteric complaints. *Maturitas* 1991;13: 205–15
44. Dennerstein L, Dudley EC, Hopper JL, *et al.* Sexuality, hormones and the menopausal transition. *Maturitas* 1997;26:83–93
45. Arnim-Baas A. Befindlichkeit von Frauen im Klimakterium. In Rosemeier HP, ed. *Personlichkeit, Berufstaigkeit und Beschwerdebild*. Berlin: Quintessenz Verlags, 1995
46. Banger M. Affective syndrome during perimenopause. *Maturitas* 2002;41:S13–18
47. Lock M, Kaufert P. Menopause, local biologies, and cultures of aging. *Am J Hum Biol* 2001;13: 494–504
48. Lock M. Menopause: lessons from anthropology. *Psychosom Med* 1998;60:410–19
49. Locke M. *Encounters with Aging: Mythologies of Menopause in Japan and North America*. Berkeley: University of California Press, 1993
50. Avis NE, McKinlay SM. A longitudinal analysis of women's attitudes toward the menopause: results from the Massachusetts Women's Health Study. *Maturitas* 1991;13:65–79
51. Porter M, Penney GC, Russell D, *et al.* A population based survey of women's experience of the menopause. *Br J Obstet Gynaecol* 1996;103:1025–8
52. Woods NF, Mitchell ES. Pathways to depressed mood for midlife women: observations from the Seattle Midlife Women's Health Study. *Res Nurs Health* 1997;20:119–29
53. Gath D, Osborn M, Bungay G, *et al.* Psychiatric disorder and gynaecological symptoms in middle aged women: a community survey. *Br Med J Clin Res Ed* 1987;294:213–18
54. Dennerstein L, Smith AM, Morse C. Psychological well-being, mid-life and the menopause. *Maturitas* 1994;20:1–11
55. Pearlstein T, Rosen K, Stone AB. Mood disorders and menopause. *Endocrinol Metab Clin North Am* 1997;26:279–94
56. Nicol-Smith L. Causality, menopause, and depression: a critical review of the literature. *Br Med J* 1996;313:1229–32
57. Ballinger CB. Psychiatric morbidity and the menopause: clinical features. *Br Med J* 1976;1: 1183–5

58. Cawood EH, Bancroft J. Steroid hormones, the menopause, sexuality and well-being of women. *Psychol Med* 1996;26:925–36
59. Bebbington PE, Dunn G, Jenkins R, *et al.* The influence of age and sex on the prevalence of depressive conditions: report from the National Survey of Psychiatric Morbidity. *Psychol Med* 1998;28:9–19
60. Jorm AF. Sex and age differences in depression: a quantitative synthesis of published research. *Aust NZ J Psychiatry* 1987;21:46–53
61. Mirowsky J. Age and the gender gap in depression. *J Health Soc Behav* 1996;37:362–80
62. Kessler RC, McGonagle KA, Swartz M, *et al.* Sex and depression in the National Comorbidity Survey. I: Lifetime prevalence, chronicity and recurrence. *J Affect Disord* 1993;29:85–96
63. Kessler RC, McGonagle KA, Nelson CB, *et al.* Sex and depression in the National Comorbidity Survey. II: Cohort effects. *J Affect Disord* 1994; 30:15–26
64. Green BH, Copeland JR, Dewey ME, *et al.* Risk factors for depression in elderly people: a prospective study. *Acta Psychiatr Scand* 1992;86:213–17
65. Stallones L, Marx MB, Garrity TF. Prevalence and correlates of depressive symptoms among older US adults. *Am J Prev Med* 1990;6:295–303
66. Angst J, Gamma A, Gastpar M, *et al.* Gender differences in depression. Epidemiological findings from the European DEPRES I and II studies. *Eur Arch Psychiatry Clin Neurosci* 2002;252:201–9
67. Kocsis JH. Geriatric dysthymia. *J Clin Psychiatry* 1998;59:13–15
68. Devanand DP, Nobler MS, Singer T, *et al.* Is dysthymia a different disorder in the elderly? *Am J Psychiatry* 1994;151:1592–9
69. Gwirtsman HE, Blehar MC, McCullough JP Jr, *et al.* Standardized assessment of dysthymia: report of a National Institute of Mental Health conference. *Psychopharmacol Bull* 1997;33:3–11
70. Kirby M, Bruce I, Coakley D, *et al.* Dysthymia among the community-dwelling elderly. *Int J Geriatr Psychiatry* 1999;14:440–5
71. Barzega G, Maina G, Venturello S, *et al.* Dysthymic disorder: clinical characteristics in relation to age at onset. *J Affect Disord* 2001;66: 39–46
72. Bellino S, Patria L, Ziero S, *et al.* Clinical features of dysthymia and age: a clinical investigation. *Psychiatry Res* 2001;103:219–28
73. Kivela SL, Pahkala K. Dysthymic disorder in the aged in the community. *Soc Psychiatry Psychiatr Epidemiol* 1989;1989:77–83
74. Benazzi F. Female depression before and after menopause. *Psychother Psychosom* 2000;69:280–3
75. Goodwin FK, Jamison KR. *Manic-Depressive Illness*. New York: Oxford University Press, 1990
76. Young RC, Klerman GL. Mania in late life: focus on age at onset. *Am J Psychiatry* 1992;149:867–76
77. Freeman MP, Smith KW, Freeman SA, *et al.* The impact of reproductive events on the course of bipolar disorder in women. *J Clin Psychiatr* 2002; 63:284–7
78. Chakravarti S, Collins WP, Thom MH, *et al.* Relation between plasma hormone profiles, symptoms, and response to oestrogen treatment in women approaching the menopause. *Br Med J* 1979;1:983–5
79. Ballinger CB, Browning MC, Smith AH. Hormone profiles and psychological symptoms in perimenopausal women. *Maturitas* 1987;9: 235–51
80. De Lignieres B, Basdevant A, Thomas G, *et al.* Biological effects of estradiol-17β in postmenopausal women: oral versus percutaneous administration. *J Clin Endocrinol Metab* 1986;62:536–41
81. Sarrel PM. Psychosexual effects of menopause: role of androgens. *Am J Obstet Gynecol* 1999;180: S319–24
82. Zweifel JE, O'Brien WH. A meta-analysis of the effect of hormone replacement therapy upon depressed mood. *Psychoneuroendocrinology* 1997;22: 189–212
83. Smith RN, Studd JW. Recent advances in hormone replacement therapy. *Br J Hosp Med* 1993;49:799–808
84. Sands R, Studd J. Exogenous androgens in postmenopausal women. *Am J Med* 1995;98:76S–9S
85. Genazzani AR, Bernardi F, Stomati M, *et al.* Δ^5-Androgen replacement therapy: a new piece of the mosaic. In Genazzani AR, ed. *Hormone Replacement Therapy and the Brain*. London, UK: Parthenon Publishing, 2003:131
86. Halbreich U, Kahn LS. Role of estrogen in the aetiology and treatment of mood disorders. *CNS Drugs* 2001;15:797–817
87. Coope J, Thomson JM, Poller L. Effects of 'natural oestrogen' replacement therapy on menopausal symptoms and blood clotting. *Br Med J* 1975;4:139–43
88. Coope J. Is oestrogen therapy effective in the treatment of menopausal depression. *J R Coll Gen Pract* 1981;31:134–40
89. Aylward M, Holly F, Parker RI. An evaluation of clinical response to piperazineoestronesulphate ('Harmogen') in menopausal patients. *Curr Med Res Opin* 1974;2:417
90. Montgomery JC, Appleby L, Brincat M, *et al.* Effect of oestrogen and testosterone implants on psychological disorders in the climacteric. *Lancet* 1987;1:297–9
91. Strickler RC, Borth R, Cecutti A, *et al.* The role of oestrogen replacement in the climacteric syndrome. *Psychol Med* 1977;7:631–9
92. Schmidt PJ, Nieman L, Danaceau MA, *et al.* Estrogen replacement in perimenopause-related depression: a preliminary report. *Am J Obstet Gynecol* 2000;183:414–20

93. Soares CN, Almeida OP, Joffe H, *et al.* Efficacy of estradiol for the treatment of depressive disorders in perimenopausal women: a double-blind, randomized, placebo-controlled trial. *Arch Gen Psychiatry* 2001;58:529–34
94. Coppen A, Bishop M, Beard RJ. Effects of piperazine oestrone sulphate on plasma tryptophan, oestrogens, gonadotrophins and psychological functioning in women following hysterectomy. *Curr Med Res Opin* 1977;4:29–36
95. George GCW, Utian WH, Beumont PJV, *et al.* Effect of exogenous oestrogens on minor psychiatric symptoms in postmenopausal women. *S Afr Med J* 1973;47:2387–8
96. Ditkoff EC, Crary WG, Cristo M, *et al.* Estrogen improves psychological function in asymptomatic postmenopausal women. *Obstet Gynecol* 1991; 78:991–5
97. Sherwin BB, Gelfand MM. Sex steroids and affect in the surgical menopause: a double-blind, crossover study. *Psychoneuroendocrinology* 1985;10: 325–35
98. Sherwin BB, Gelfand MM, Brender W. Androgen enhances sexual motivation in females: a prospective, crossover study of sex steroid administration in the surgical menopause. *Psychosom Med* 1985; 47:339–51
99. Palinkas LA, Barrett-Connor E. Estrogen use and depressive symptoms in postmenopausal women. *Obstet Gynecol* 1992;80:30–6
100. Brincat M, Studd JW, O'Dow W, *et al.* Subcutaneous hormone implants for the control of climacteric symptoms. *Lancet* 1984;1:16–18
101. Derman RJ, Dawood MY, Stone S. Quality of life during sequential hormone replacement therapy – a placebo-controlled study. *Int J Fertil Menopausal Stud* 1995;40:73–8
102. Fedor-Freybergh P. The influence of oestrogen on the wellbeing and mental performance in climacteric and postmenopausal women. *Acta Obstet Gynecol Scand* 1977;64:1–91
103. Wiklund I, Karlberg J, Mattson L. Quality of life of menopausal women on a regimen of transdermal estradiol therapy: a double-blind placebo-controlled study. *Am J Obstet Gynecol* 1993;168: 824–30
104. Saletu B, Brandstatter N, Metkam M, *et al.* Double-blind, placebo-controlled, hormonal, syndromal and EEG mapping studies with trandermal oestradiol therapy in menopasual depression. *Psychopharmacology* 1995;122:321–9
105. Campbell S, Whitehead M. Oestrogen therapy and the menopausal syndrome. *Clin Obset Gynaecol* 1977;4:31–47
106. Campbell S. Double blind psychometric studies on the effects of natural estrogens on postmenopausal women. In Campbell S, ed. *The Management of Menopause and Postmenopausal Years.* Lancaster, UK: MTP Press, 1976:149–58
107. Carranza-Lira S, Valentino-Figueroa ML. Estrogen therapy for depression in postmenopausal women. *Int J Gynaecol Obstet* 1999; 65:35–8
108. Ripley HS, Short E, Papanicolaou GN. The effect of treatment of depression in the menopause with estrogenic hormone. *Am J Psychiatry* 1940;96: 905–15
109. Schneider MA, Brotherton PL, Hailes J. The effect of exogenous oestrogens on depression in menopausal women. *Med J Aust* 1977;2:162–3
110. Klaiber EL, Broverman DM, Vogel W, *et al.* Estrogen therapy for severe persistent depressions in women. *Arch Gen Psychiatry* 1979;36:550–4
111. Saletu B, Brandstatter N, Metka M, *et al.* Hormonal, syndromal and EEG mapping studies in menopausal syndrome patients with and without depression as compared with controls. *Maturitas* 1996;23:91–105
112. Shapira B, Oppenheim G, Zohar J, *et al.* Lack of efficacy of estrogen supplementation to imipramine in resistant female depressives. *Biol Psychiatry* 1985;20:576–9
113. Oppenheim G. Estrogen in the treatment of depression: neuropharmacological mechanisms. *Biol Psychiatry* 1983;18:721–5
114. Prange AJ, Wilson IC, Breese GR, *et al.* Hormonal alterations of imipramine response: a review. In Sachar E, ed. *Hormones, Behavior and Psychopathology.* New York: Raven Press, 1976:41–67
115. Schneider LS, Small GW, Hamilton SH, *et al.* Estrogen replacement and response to fluoxetine in a multicenter geriatric depression trial. Fluoxetine Collaborative Study Group. *Am J Geriatr Psychiatry* 1997;5:97–106
116. Schneider LS, Small GW, Clary CM. Estrogen replacement therapy and antidepressant response to sertraline in older depressed women. *Am J Geriatr Psychiatry* 2001;9:393–9
117. Amsterdam J, Garcia-Espana F, Fawcett J, *et al.* Fluoxetine efficacy in menopausal women with and without estrogen replacement. *J Affect Disord* 1999;55:11–17
118. Jaffe H, Groninger H, Soares C, Nonacs R, Cohen LS. An open trial of mirtazapine in menopausal women with depression unresponsive to estrogen replacement therapy. *J Womens Health Gend Based Med* 2001;10:999–1004
119. Harlow BL, Cramer DW, Annis KM. Association of medically treated depression and age at natural menopause. *Am J Epidemiol* 1995;141:1170–6
120. Bukulmez O, Al A, Gurdal H, *et al.* Short-term effects of three continuous hormone replacement therapy regimens on platelet tritiated imipramine binding and mood scores: a prospective randomized trial. *Fertil Steril* 2001;75:737–43
121. Halbreich U. Role of estrogen in postmenopausal depression. *Neurology* 1997;48:S16–19

122. Birkhauser M. Depression, menopause and estrogens: is there a correlation? *Maturitas* 2002; 41:S3–8
123. Backstrom T. Symptoms related to the menopause and sex steroid treatments. *Ciba Foundation Symp* 1995;191:171–86
124. Paoletti AM, Floris S, Mannias M, *et al.* Evidence that cyproterone acetate improves psychological symptoms and enhances the activity of the dopaminergic system in postmenopause. *J Clin Endocrinol Metab* 2001;86:608–12

Gender differences in anxiety disorders: the role of female hormones

19

M. Mauri, A. Calderone and V. Camilleri

INTRODUCTION

Epidemiological studies have demonstrated that there is a significant gender difference in the incidence of psychiatric disorders. It has been suggested that the hormonal profile has a crucial role in the development of these disorders, particularly anxiety and mood disorders. In the literature, mood disorders have received more attention than anxiety disorders. This chapter investigates the role of anxiety disorders in women and their comorbidity with mood disorders.

Attention is focused on gender differences in central nervous system development and in gender features of psychiatric disorders, and the conclusion is reached that, since women and men are genetically very similar, the hormonal profile plays an important role in provoking these differences. The reciprocal role of neurotransmitters and sex hormones in mood and anxiety disorders is also reviewed, as well as the occurrence of anxiety disorders in the female life cycle, particularly in the menopause.

EPIDEMIOLOGY OF PSYCHIATRIC DISORDERS

Several studies have reported high rates of major depression, agoraphobia and simple phobia in women, and high rates of alcohol abuse, substance abuse and antisocial personality disorder in men. These results have been confirmed in various settings (Tables 1-4 and Figure 1). In particular, the incidence of social phobia is 2% in the general population, and 70% of those affected are women; uncomplicated panic disorder has an incidence of 20/1000 in the case of women and 8/1000 in the case of men; agoraphobia with or without panic attacks has an incidence of 8% in women and 3% in men; generalized anxiety in the community has an incidence of 1-2% among men and 2-5% among women; and post-traumatic stress disorder affected 31% of women and 19% of men exposed to a major trauma[9].

GENDER DIFFERENCES IN CNS DEVELOPMENT AND PSYCHIATRIC DISORDERS

Differences between men and women are determined by genes, societal norms, gender roles, social class and, last but not least, sex hormones. In particular, sex hormones play a very important role in the development and maintenance of the central nervous system (CNS). Women and men are genetically very similar, except that different hormones enter the brain at different times and with different tempos, encouraging some brain cells to sprout more than others at time periods

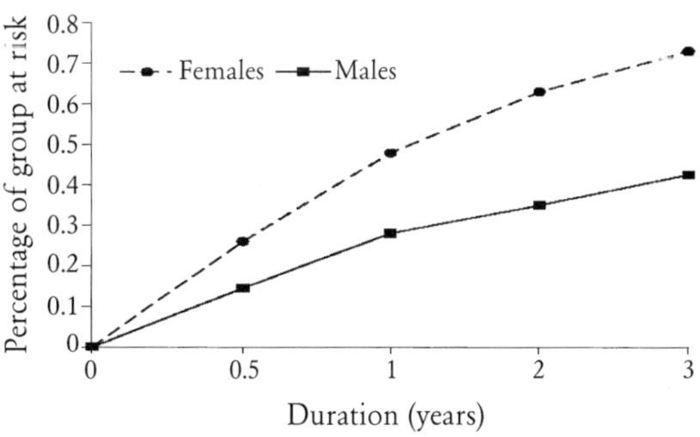

Figure 1 Symptom recurrence in men and women with panic and agoraphobia. Likelihood of symptom recurrence based upon Kaplan-Meier survival analysis. Difference between men and women was significant according to Wilcoxon log-rank test = 7.70, df = 1, $p = 0.006$. Number of men at risk was 49 at 6 months, 40 at 1 year, 29 at 2 years and 10 at 3 years (see reference 8 for full report)

Table 1 Canadian study: 1-year prevalence (%) of psychiatric disorders by gender. Adapted from reference 1

Disorder	*Male*	*Female*	*Total*
Anxiety disorders			
Social phobia	5.4	7.9	6.7
Simple phobia	4.1	8.9	6.4
Agoraphobia	0.7	2.5	1.6
Panic disorder	–	1.5	1.1
Generalized anxiety disorder	0.9	1.2	1.1
One or more anxiety disorders	8.9	15.5	12.2
Affective disorders			
Major depressive episode	2.8	5.4	4.1
Dysthymia	–	0.8	0.8
Manic disorder	–	0.6	0.6
One or more affective disorders	3.2	5.9	4.5
Bulimia	–	1.0	0.5
Substance use disorders			
Alcohol abuse/dependence	7.1	1.8	4.4
Marijuana abuse/dependence	1.7	0.4	1.1
Other substance abuse/dependence	–	–	0.5
One or more substance abuse/dependence	8.2	2.1	5.2
Antisocial behaviors			
Antisocial personality	2.9	0.5	1.7
Adult antisocial behavior	0.5	–	0.5
One or more antisocial behaviors	3.9	0.6	2.2
One or more disorders	17.9	19.4	18.6
One disorder only	13.2	15.1	14.2
Two or more disorders	4.6	4.3	4.5

Missing value means numbers were too small to be reported

critical to brain development. Follicle stimulating hormone (FSH) is found in the pituitary glands of both sexes by fetal week 10, and its concentration increases dramatically, but only in females, between weeks 12 and 20.

During sexual maturity, the hormonal levels of women fluctuate cyclically over a much larger range, compared with those of men. At the menopause, ovarian secretion shuts down.

In men, the testes continue to produce testosterone, which is partly converted to estradiol in the brain, but at an increasingly slower rate. In very old age, the brain hormonal environment is once again similar in the two sexes. These differences in hormonal profile during the life cycle are implicated in a sex differentiation of the brain. In fact, men have larger cerebral volume, and women more cerebral blood flow and a larger corpus callosum.

NEUROTRANSMITTERS AND SEX HORMONES IN MOOD AND ANXIETY DISORDERS

There is an epidemiological association between mood disorders and the reproductive years in women, the most important reproductive events being puberty, pregnancy and menopause that are related to premenstrual syndrome, postpartum affective disorders and menopausal/perimenopausal depressive syndromes. The neuroendocrine rhythmicity related to female reproduction is vulnerable to change, and is sensitive to psychosocial, environmental and physiological factors. The control of mood and behaviors involves many different neurotransmitter systems, including glutamate, γ-aminobutyric acid (GABA), acetylcholine, serotonin, dopamine, noradrenaline and

Table 2 National Comorbidity Studies: 1-year prevalence (%) of University of Michigan Revision of the Composit International Diagnostic Interview/Diagnostic and Statistical Manual-III (revised) disorders by gender. Adapted from reference 2

Disorder	*Male*	*Female*	*Total*
Anxiety disorders			
Panic disorder	1.3	3.2	2.3
Agoraphobia*	1.7	3.8	2.8
Social phobia	6.6	9.1	7.9
Simple phobia	4.4	13.2	8.8
Generalized anxiety disorder	2.0	4.3	3.1
Any anxiety disorder	11.8	22.6	17.2
Affective disorders			
Major depressive episode	7.7	12.9	10.3
Manic episode	1.4	1.3	1.3
Dysthymia	2.1	3.0	2.5
Any affective disorder	8.5	14.1	11.3
Substance use disorders			
Alcohol abuse	3.4	1.6	2.5
Alcohol dependence	10.7	3.7	7.2
Drug abuse	1.3	0.3	0.8
Drug dependence	3.8	1.9	2.8
Any substance abuse/dependence	16.1	6.6	11.3
Other disorders			
Antisocial personality	–	–	–
Non-affective psychosis	0.5	0.6	0.5
Any NCS disorder	27.7	31.2	29.5

*Without panic disorder; missing value means numbers were too small to be reported; NCS, National Comorbidity Study

neuropeptides. The precise relationship between estrogens and progesterone and serotoninergic function has yet to be fully delineated. None the less, many investigators have suggested that the neuromodulatory effect of estrogens may contribute to a greater risk for depression and anxiety in women, and might point the way to effective hormonal treatments for mood disorders in female patients. These reproductive-related mood and anxiety syndromes could be used as models for the proposed differential vulnerability of subpopulations of women to normal changes in hormonal levels during the premenstrual, postpartum and perimenopausal periods[10,11].

Steroid hormones can modulate neuronal transmission by a variety of mechanisms. They may affect the synthesis and release of neurotransmitters, as well as the expression of receptors and membrane plasticity and permeability. It has been suggested that steroid hormone receptors function as general transcription factors to achieve integration of neural information in the CNS[12]. Steroid hormones are believed to act primarily by a classical genomic mechanism through intracellular receptors to modulate transcription and protein synthesis. This mechanism involves the binding of the steroid to a cytoplasmic or nuclear receptor. Recently, it has been shown that steroids can also produce rapid effects on electrical excitability and synaptic function through a direct membrane mechanism, such as ligand-gated ion channels, G-proteins and neurotransmitter transporters[13]. This short-term (seconds to minutes) effect of steroids may occur through binding to the cell membrane, binding to membrane receptors or modulation of ion channels, by direct activation of a second-messenger system[14] or by activation of receptors such as cytokines and dopamine[15]. Topical application of estrogen or progesterone to nervous tissue has been shown to result in a rapid change in membrane potential, and sex steroids can affect membrane fluidity thereby modifying

Table 3 Netherlands study: 1-year prevalence (%) of Diagnostic and Statistical Manual-III (revised) disorders by gender. Adapted from reference 3

Disorder	*Male*	*Female*	*Total*
Anxiety disorders	8.3	16.6	19.3
Panic disorder	1.1	3.4	3.8
Agoraphobia*	0.9	2.2	3.4
Simple phobia	4.1	10.1	10.1
Social phobia	3.5	6.1	7.8
Generalized anxiety disorder	0.8	1.5	2.3
Obsessive-compulsive disorder	0.5	0.4	0.9
Affective disorders	5.7	9.7	7.6
Major depressive disorder	4.1	7.5	5.8
Dysthymia	1.4	3.2	2.3
Bipolar disorder	1.1	1.1	1.1
Schizophrenia	0.2	0.2	0.2
Substance use disorders	14.1	3.5	8.9
Substance abuse disorders	7.8	1.9	4.9
Alcohol abuse	7.3	1.8	4.6
Drug abuse	0.6	0.3	0.5
Substance dependence disorders	6.7	1.7	4.3
Alcohol dependence	6.1	1.1	3.7
Drug dependence	1.0	0.7	0.8
Eating disorders	0.2	0.6	0.4
Anorexia nervosa	0.0	0.0	0.0
Bulimia nervosa	0.2	0.6	0.4
One or more DSM-III-R diagnoses	23.5	23.6	23.2

*Without panic disorder; DSM-III-R, Diagnostic and Statistical Manual-III (revised)

Table 4 Prevalence rates for panic and agoraphobia (%)

Study	*Men*	*Women*
National Comorbidity Survey[2] (n = 8098)		
Panic	2.0	5.0
Agoraphobia	3.5	7.0
Epidemiology Catchment Area Study[4] (n = 18 572)		
Panic	1.0	2.1
Agoraphobia	2.9	7.7
Taiwan Psychiatric Epidemiological Project[5] (n = 5005) (metropolitan Taipai)		
Panic	1.2	2.8
Agoraphobia	3.5	14.6
Edmonton[6] (n = 3258)		
Panic	0.6	2.1
Agoraphobia	3.5	7.0
Munich Follow-Up Study[7] (n = 483)		
Panic	1.7	2.9
Agoraphobia	2.9	8.3

ion transport or receptor function[16]. Estrogen has been described as a serotonin, noradrenaline and acetylcholine agonist; it also modulates dopamine receptors. Estrogen and progesterone receptors have been identified in multiple regions of the brain, incuding the amygdala, hippocampus, cingulated cortex, midbrain raphe nucleus and central gray matter. Female hormones exert a wide range of actions on different neurons including serotoninergic, noradrenergic, GABA-ergic, dopaminergic and anticholinergic neurons.

Estrogens play an important role in various aspects of neurotransmission, in particular those related to serotonin and dopamine. In fact, these female hormones influence the synthesis, the receptor number and binding and the synaptic transmission of serotonin, and they might determine an augmentation effect on serotoninergic global activity. Estrogens may block or inhibit dopamine activity, and have an antidopaminergic effect[17]. These data may explain later onset of schizophrenia in women and the more benign course than in men.

It is also well known that neurotransmitters are strongly implicated in the development of anxiety disorders.

Data suggest that there is a relationship between anxiety disorders and levels of catecholamine. Norepinephrine release in the brain is an important part of the stress response[18]. Noradrenergic neurons in the locus ceruleus are activated in association with fear and anxiety states[19,20], and limbic and cortical regions innervated by these neurons are thought to be involved in the elaboration of adaptive responses to stress. Exposure to chronic stress results in a potentiation of norepinephrine release with subsequent stressors[18], and a relationship between this metabolic response and increased panic or anxiety has been found[21].

Acute stress increases dopamine release and metabolism in several specific brain areas[22]. However, the dopamine innervation of the prefrontal cortex appears to be particularly vulnerable to stress. Stress can enhance dopamine release and metabolism also in other areas receiving dopaminergic innervation, provided that stress is of high intensity or long duration. Thus, medial prefrontal cortex dopaminergic innervation is preferentially activated by stress, compared with the mesolimbic and nigrostriatal systems, and mesolimbic dopaminergic innervation appears to be more sensitive to stress than striatal innervation.

The effect of stress activating serotonin turnover may stimulate systems that have both anxiogenic and anxiolytic pathways within the forebrain[23]. A primary distinction in the qualitative effects of serotonin may be between the dorsal and the median raphe nuclei, the two midbrain nuclei that produce most of the forebrain serotonin. Serotoninergic innervation of the amygdala and the hippocampus by the dorsal raphe is believed to mediate anxiogenic effects via serotonin or 5-hydroxytryptamine-2 (5-HT_2) receptors. In contrast, the median raphe innervation of hippocampal 5-HT_{1A} receptors seems to facilitate the disconnection of previously learned association with aversive events, or to suppress the formation of new association, thus providing a resilience to adverse events[23]. Chronic stress increases the number of cortical 5-HT_2 receptors and reduces hippocampal 5-HT_{1A} receptors[24].

Endogenous benzodiazepines also play an important role in stress response and anxiety[25]. Benzodiazepine receptors are present throughout the brain, particularly in the cortical gray matter; benzodiazepines enhance and prolong the synaptic action of the inhibitory neurotransmitter GABA. The administration of inverse agonists of benzodiazepine receptors, such as β-carboline 3-carboxylic acid ethyl ester, results in behavioral and biological effects similar to those seen in anxiety and stress, including increases in heart rate, blood pressure, plasma cortisol and catecholamines. These effects are blocked by the administration of a benzodiazepine or pretreatment with benzodiazepine antagonist flumazenil.

The relationship between the hormonal profile and anxiety disorders has been demonstrated by recent studies. In particular, all steroids modulate the $GABA_A$-benzodiazepine receptor with progesterone metabolites acting as agonists and, therefore, as anxiolytics. In addition, estrogens have been shown to up-regulate the $GABA_A$-benzodiazepine receptor. It is possible that the cyclical withdrawal of progesterone and estrogen 'kindles' neuronal systems, and promotes anxiety states by mechanisms similar to those which have been implicated in the provocation of perimenstrual epilepsy.

In summary, there is some indication that women become more anxious during times of relatively low levels of circulating estrogens and progesterone[9,26].

ANXIETY DISORDERS AND HORMONAL REPRODUCTIVE EVENTS

A correlation between psychiatric disorders and hormonal reproductive events, considering only anxiety disorders, is widely accepted. These include the premenstrual syndrome, postpartum anxiety disorder and perimenopausal anxiety syndrome, in addition to panic attacks associated with placental abruption and, finally, panic disorder induced by oral contraceptives.

Moreover, menopausal depression appears to occur as a consequence of a pre-existing anxiety disorder, or some menopausal symptoms are unrecognized panic symptoms. In fact, there is a broad symptomatological overlapping between the two conditions (hot flushes, palpitations, insomnia, etc.). In addition, in early menopause, the incidence of alcohol use is high, and anxiety disorders are the most frequent disorders related to substance abuse. Alcohol use could be self-treatment of an unrecognized or subthreshold anxiety symptomatology[9].

However, there are still some open questions:

(1) Is there a real increase of anxiety and affective disorders in the menopause?

(2) Could the menopause act as a trigger for a subthreshold symptomatology?

(3) Could menopausal depression really be a consequence of an anxiety disorder?

(4) Are some menopausal symptoms unrecognized panic symptoms?

(5) Does hormone replacement therapy (HRT) prevent anxiety disorder development in the menopause?

(6) The distribution of anxiety and depressive disorders is different between males and females: what is the impact of female hormones on these differences?

(7) Is HRT effective only on menopausal symptoms, or might HRT be efficacious also for the treatment of anxiety symptoms related to specific hormonal mechanisms?

References

1. Offord DR, Boyle MH, Campbell D, *et al.* One-year prevalence of psychiatric disorder in Ontarians 15 to 64 years of age. *Can J Psychiatry* 1996;41:559–63
2. Kessler RC, McGonagle KA, Khao S, *et al.* Lifetime and 12-month prevalence of DSM-III-R psychiatric disorders in the United States: results from the National Comorbidity Survey. *Arch Gen Psychiatry* 1994;51:8–19
3. Bijl RV, De Graaf R, Ravelli A, Smit F, Vollebergh WA. Gender and age-specific first incidence of DSM-III-R psychiatric disorders in the general population. Results from the Netherlands Mental Health Survey and Incidence Study (NEMESIS). *Soc Psychiatry Psychiatr Epidemiol* 2002;37:372–9
4. Bijl RV, Ravelli A, van Zessen G. Prevalence of psychiatric disorder in the general population: results of The Netherlands Mental Health Survey and Incidence Study (NEMESIS). *Soc Psychiatry Psychiatr Epidemiol* 1998;33:587–95
5. Hwu HG, Yeh EK, Chang LY. Prevalence of psychiatric disorders in Taiwan defined by the Chinese Diagnostic Interview Schedule. *Acta Psychiatr Scand* 1989;79:136–47
6. Thompson AH, Bland RC, Orn HT. Relationship and chronology of depression, agaraphobia, and panic disorder in the general population. *J Nerv Ment Dis* 1989;177:456–63

7. Wittchen HU, Essau CA, von Zerssen D, Krieg JC, Zaudig M. Lifetime and six-month prevalence of mental disorders in the Munich follow-up study. *Eur Arch Psychiatry Clin Neurosci* 1992;241:247–58
8. *J Am Med Women's Assoc* 1998;53:
9. Seeman MV. Psychopathology in women and men: focus on female hormones. *Am J Psychiatry* 1997; 154:12
10. Joffe H, Cohen LS. Estrogen, serotonin, and mood disturbance: where is the therapeutic bridge? *Biol Psychiatry* 1998;44:798–811
11. Rapkin AJ. The clinical nature and formal diagnosis of premenstrual, postpartum, and perimenopausal affective disorders. *Curr Psychiatry Rep* 2002;4:419–28
12. Mani SK, Blaustein JD, O'Malley BV. Progesterone receptor function from a behavioural perspective. *Horm Behav* 1997;31:244–55
13. Wong M, Thompson TL, Moss RL. Nongenomic actions of estrogen in the brain: physiological significance and cellular mechanism. *Crit Rev Neurobiol* 1996;10:189–203
14. Moss RL, Gu Q, Wong M. Estrogen: nontranscriptional signalling pathway. *Recent Prog Horm Res* 1997;52:33–68, discussion 68–9
15. Brann DW, Hendry LB, Mahesh VB. Emerging diversities in the mechanism of action of steroid hormones. *J Steroid Biochem Mol Biol* 1995;52: 113–33
16. Maggi A, Perez J. Role of female gonadal hormones in the CNS: clinical and experimental aspects. *Life Sci* 1985;37:893–906
17. Xie JX, Liu B. Effect of estrogen on dopamine release evoked by electric stimulation of central amygdaloid nucleus. *Sheng Li Xue Bao* 2001;53: 170–4
18. Bremner JD, Kristal JH, Southwick SM, Charney D. Noradrenergic mechanism in stress and anxiety, I: Preclinical studies. *Synapse* 1996;23:28–38
19. Abercrombie ED, Jacobs BL. Single-unit response of noradrenergic neurons in the locus ceruleus of freely moving cats. *J Neurosci* 1987;7:2837–43
20. Redmond DE. Studies of the nucleus ceruleus in monkeys and hypotheses for neuropsychopharmacology. In Meltzer HY, ed. New York: Raven, 1987:967–75
21. Bremner JD, Innis RB, Ng CK. Positron emission tomography measurement of cerebral metabolic correlates of yohimbine administration. *Arch Gen Psychiatry* 1997;54:246–54
22. Thierry AM, Pirot S, Gioanni Y, Glowinski J. Dopamine function in the prefrontal cortex. *Adv Pharmacol* 1998;42:717–20
23. Graeff FG. Role of 5-HT in defensive behaviour and anxiety. *Rev Neurosci* 1993;4:181–211
24. Mendelson SD, McEwen BS. Autoradiographic analyses of the effects of restraint-induced stress on 5-HT1A and 5-HT1B receptors. *Neuroendocrinology* 1991;54:454–61
25. Guidotti A, Baraldi M, Leon A, Costa E. Benzodiazepines: a tool to explore the biochemical and neurophysiological basis of anxiety. *Federation Proc* 1990;39:1039–42
26. Toriizuka K, Mizowaki M, Hanawa T. Menopause and anxiety: focus on steroidal hormones and GABA-A receptor. *Nippon Yakurigaku Zasshi* 2000; 115:21–8

Schizophrenia, menopause and estrogen replacement therapy: a review

20

A. Riecher-Rössler

WHAT IS SCHIZOPHRENIA?

Schizophrenia is still one of the most serious psychiatric disorders. With a lifetime prevalence of almost 1%, it is one of the world's leading causes of chronic disability. The symptomatology can be divided into 'positive' and 'negative' symptoms. Positive symptoms include delusions, hallucinations and thought disorders. Negative or deficit symptoms include cognitive defects, emotional defects and deficits in energy, language and contact.

In about one-third of all cases, the course of the illness is benign with almost complete remission after an acute phase with mainly positive symptoms. However, two-thirds of all cases suffer from a chronic recurrent course. Acute psychotic phases are predominated by positive symptoms, but usually resolve within days or weeks under adequate treatment. After this acute phase, patients are often left with chronic negative symptoms, which sometimes do not respond very well to treatment and can be a major impediment for rehabilitation and reintegration.

The etiology of schizophrenia is still not fully understood and might be multifactorial. It has even been hypothesized that schizophrenia consists of a group of disorders with different etiologies. Genetic predisposition is undoubtedly the major risk factor for at least a subgroup of these psychoses. Pre- and perinatal complications are also discussed. The main hypothesis today regards schizophrenia as a neurodevelopmental disorder with a disturbance of neuronal circuits in the brain and a neurotransmitter dysbalance, especially during the acute psychotic episodes.

Neuroleptic medication is aimed at normalizing neurotransmission, by influencing especially the dopaminergic, but also the serotonergic and other systems. Neuroleptic medication is used for the treatment of acute psychotic episodes, but also for relapse prevention. Many patients take such medication for several years or even decades.

Today, we know that estrogens can modulate neurotransmission and also influence other brain functions in a way that makes them very interesting for schizophrenia research, not only concerning potential pathogenetic mechanisms, but also concerning therapeutic implications.

ESTROGENS: A PROTECTIVE FACTOR IN SCHIZOPHRENIA?

Historical findings

As long ago as the beginning of the last century, psychiatrists recognized the possible association between schizophrenia and estrogens (for review see reference 1). On the one hand, early clinicians such as Kraepelin[2] or Kretschmer[3] described signs of *chronic* 'hypoestrogenism' in women with schizophrenia. On the other hand, there have long existed observations indicating an association between estrogen blood levels and *acute* psychotic symptomatology.

Krafft-Ebing[4] was among the first to describe women becoming psychotic before or during menstruation, i.e. when blood levels of estrogen are relatively low. Kraepelin[2] even created a separate diagnostic category, labelled 'menstrual psychosis'. Kretschmer[3] reported cases where the outbreak of schizophrenia had a temporal relationship with 'surgery of ovaries, pregnancy, delivery and puerperium'. Finally, Manfred Bleuler[5] noted that late-onset schizophrenia with onset after age 40 years was much more frequent in women than in men, a finding he attributed to the 'loss of ovarian function' starting at around that age.

Basic research findings

Research of the past two decades has confirmed many of the historical observations concerning a protective effect of estrogens in schizophrenia. And even more important, *basic research* has made important contributions towards explaining possible modes of action.

To begin with, identification of estrogen receptors in the limbic system has led to the assumption that estrogens not only play a role in the modulation of endocrine functions, but also must have a 'neuromodulating function' (for review see reference 1). In the early 1980s, it was observed that the effect of estrogens in laboratory animals was in some respects similar to that of neuroleptics. Estrogens can, for example, enhance neuroleptic-induced catalepsy and reduce amphetamine- and apomorphine-induced behavioral changes such as stereotypies[6-9]. It has also been shown that estrogens can modulate the sensitivity and number of dopamine receptors[10-12].

Today, we know that estrogens produce many other effects. They not only improve cerebral blood flow and glucose metabolism[13], but also promote neuronal sprouting, and are therefore regarded as neuroprotective. Their modes of action include the classical genomic ones as well as involve non-genomic, rapid interactions, which explains the different latencies of effects. They modulate monoaminergic neurotransmission and can thereby influence our mood and cognition, and appear to have specific and significant effects not only on dopamine but also on serotonin, γ-aminobutyric acid (GABA) and acetylcholine[14-21], to such a degree that they have even been called 'nature's psychoprotectant'[22].

Epidemiological findings

In addition, *epidemiological* studies of sex differences in schizophrenic disorders suggest that the physiologically high estradiol production in young fertile women contributes to the later age of onset in women compared with men, and also to the better course of the disease, especially in young women.

Various epidemiological studies show that in women, the disease on average begins 4-5 years later than in men (age 20-24 in men, 25-29 in women)[23-25], and, even more interesting, women also exhibit an additional smaller peak after age 45. We postulated that estrogens raise the vulnerability threshold for the outbreak of the disease. According to this hypothesis, women are, to some extent, protected against schizophrenia between puberty and the menopause by their relatively high gonadal estrogen production during this time. Then, around age 45, several years before the menopause sets in (currently at a mean age of 51.4 years), estrogen production begins to fall[26]. Thus, women lose the protection of estrogens, which could account for their second peak of illness onset after age 45.

Puberty and schizophrenia

Cohen and colleagues[27] have recently shown that late puberty is associated with an early onset of schizophrenia. This also indicates that physiological estrogens may play a role in delaying the outbreak of the disease. Well in line with this, we have shown in another study (see below) that women with schizophrenia have their menarche on average at a higher age than do healthy controls.

Menstrual cycle and schizophrenia

Clinically, psychotic symptomatology has been shown to grow worse pre- or perimenstrually, i.e. in the low estrogen phase of the cycle[28-32]. In our own *clinical study*, we examined 32 acutely admitted women with schizophrenia who gave a history of regular menstrual cycles, and we saw a significant excess of admissions during the perimenstrual low estrogen phase of the cycle. Furthermore, during the hospital stay of the 32 women, a significant association emerged between estradiol levels and psychiatric symptomatology: it seemed to improve when estradiol levels rose, and vice versa.

Well in line with our findings, Hallonquist and colleagues[33] observed lower psychopathology scores in women with schizophrenia during the mid-luteal phase compared with the early follicular phase of the menstrual cycle. They concluded that estrogens may act as 'endogenous neuroleptics'.

Therapeutic response and physiological estrogen levels

Seeman[34] noted that women with schizophrenia in the fertile age group of 20–40 years, i.e. the time of highest ovarian estradiol production, need lower doses of neuroleptics than do men of comparable age or older women, even when body weight is controlled. In collaboration with Gattaz and associates[35] in a further study, we found evidence of a superior therapeutic response in schizophrenic in-patients admitted during perimenstruation, i.e. the low estrogen phase of their cycle. To achieve the same degree of remission as found in patients admitted during intermenstruation (the high estrogen phase), these women needed lower doses of neuroleptics and shorter treatment. We speculated that the better therapeutic response of the low-estrogen admission group may have been related to increasing levels of circulating estradiol just after admission.

Menopause and schizophrenia

One of the most interesting influences, however, is that of the menopause. As stated above, the risk of falling ill around the age of menopause is significantly increased for women.

In a study of a large representative population of 392 first-admitted patients[36,37], we were able to show that the incidence of schizophrenia in the age group 40–60 years was about double in women, compared with men. First admission for schizophrenia after age 40 occurred in only 10% of all men with schizophrenia, but in about 21% of all women with this diagnosis. The yearly incidence rate in women over age 40 was 8.9 per 100 000, whereas it was only 4.2 per 100 000 in men[37].

In addition, we discovered a very interesting new finding as regards the symptomatology and disease course of these late-onset women. *Men with onset over age 40* show significantly milder symptoms and spend less time in hospital than do early-onset patients, whereas late-onset women suffer from a disease that is almost as severe as that of patients who fall ill early in life[37].

On explanation for this could again be the estrogen effect: if illness onset of women with a relatively high underlying vulnerability is delayed by estrogens, this high vulnerability is 'unmasked' by the loss of this estrogen protection around the time of the menopause. These women, thus, are not only more frequently represented in the late-onset group, they also have more severe symptoms and a worse course of illness.

Well in line with this are the results of long-term schizophrenia studies which have shown that the course of schizophrenia in women tends to deteriorate during the peri- and postmenopause (for review see references 1 and 38).

Influences of estrogen excess and withdrawal

During pregnancy, when estrogen levels are about 200-fold higher than normal, chronic psychoses seem to improve[39], but there is a 20-fold excess of psychosis after delivery[40], when estrogen levels suddenly drop to normal. Psychoses associated with other forms of estrogen withdrawal such as post-abortion, removal of a hydatiform mole, cessation of oral contraceptives, clomiphene and tamoxifen administration (both estrogen receptor antagonists) and gonadrenalin agonist administration (blocking pituitary stimulation of endogenous estrogen secretion) have also been described[41].

Intervention studies

Also, *intervention studies* have been done. They have a very long tradition. As early as the 1940s, Manfred Bleuler[5] reported the first unsystematic trials using a combination of ovarian and pituitary hormones. Mall[42,43], a German psychiatrist in charge of a large hospital, examined 167 women suffering from schizophrenia with respect to estrogen excretion in a 24-h urine sample, basal temperature and vaginal cytology. Based on his findings, he divided the psychoses into two groups: hypofollicular and hyperfollicular. In the former group, he replaced estrogens and found that 'hypofollicular psychosis can be healed relatively easily by this substitution therapy'. Unfortunately, Mall does not give many details about these interesting studies.

Several contemporary investigators have now reported promising results using estrogen as a *therapeutic* agent. Kulkarni and co-workers[44,45] found that schizophrenic women receiving estradiol as an adjunct to neuroleptic treatment showed more rapid improvement in psychotic symptoms than women receiving neuroleptics alone.

Similar effects were noted by Lindamer and colleagues[46] in a case report of a postmenopausal women. Also, in 2001, Lindamer and associates[47] studied a community sample of postmenopausal women with schizophrenia. Twenty-four women received hormone replacement therapy (HRT); twenty-eight women had never received such therapy. Interestingly, the users of HRT needed a relatively lower average dose of antipsychotic medication and suffered from less severe negative symptoms. Jeste and colleagues[48] report 'encouraging' results using estrogen 'augmentation' of antipsychotics in an ongoing study of postmenopausal women with schizophrenia.

Ahokas and co-workers[49] demonstrated positive effects of estrogen substitution in two women with postpartum psychosis, and Sichel and associates[50] noted a prophylactic effect concerning this disorder.

HYPOESTROGENISM IN WOMEN WITH SCHIZOPHRENIA

Historical findings

Early workers also reported *chronic* 'hypoestrogenism' in some women with schizophrenia. Kraepelin[2] and Kretschmer[3], for example, observed physical signs and other anatomical abnormalities indicating 'insufficient functioning of the sexual glands' with 'hypoestrogenism'. In the 1930s, studies analyzing estrogen levels in the blood and urine confirmed these observations. Researchers found decreased blood levels of estrogen in most of the schizophrenic in-patients they examined (for reviews see references 1 and 51). At that time, neuroleptic therapy had not yet been introduced, so the observed abnormalities cannot be interpreted as side-effects of drug treatment.

In later decades, studies showed that the gonadotropins, follicle stimulating hormone (FSH) and luteinizing hormone (LH), are low in women with schizophrenia, compared with controls. Many authors also reported irregular cycles in these women (for review see reference 1). All these disturbances can possibly be attributed to a gonadal dysfunction with insufficient estrogen production from the ovaries.

Recent findings

Recently, there have been several studies confirming the earlier findings of disturbed gonadal function and hypoestrogenism in schizophrenic women[1,32,44,52-62]. They describe menstrual irregularities and reduced estradiol, progesterone and gonadotropin (FSH, LH) blood levels throughout the menstrual cycle, as well as anovulation in the majority of women with schizophrenia. Reduced fertility is also reported.

In our study of 32 acutely admitted schizophrenic women (referred to above), many women with schizophrenia had failed to qualify for the study because of menstrual irregularities. But even the 32 women who gave a history of regular menstrual cycles and were therefore included in our study showed many signs of severely disturbed gonadal function[32,52]. Compared with the 29 controls, they not only showed a greater variation in their cycle length, as observed on the ward, but they also had significantly lower estradiol and progesterone blood levels throughout their menstrual cycle. Fifty-six per cent presumably suffered from anovulation, which is a much higher proportion than in the control patients, where anovulation was suspected in only 19%[52].

The reasons for these disturbances seem to be multifold. Partly, they are probably a consequence of stress- and/or neuroleptic-induced hyperprolactinemia, which is know to suppress gonadal function[63]. But these do not seem to be the only causes. Thus, other psychiatric disorders accompanied by similar 'stress' do not show the same disturbances, or at least not to the same degree[52,58]. Furthermore, hypoestrogenism was observed long before the introduction of neuroleptics.

For theoretical reasons and also historically, an interesting question is whether gonadal dysfunction with estrogen deficiency is a state (acute psychosis) or a trait (vulnerability to psychosis) marker. To address this question we investigated women aged 18–45 years from the large representative population of first-admitted schizophrenia patients referred to above. Forty-four women took part and were compared with 33 age-matched healthy women from the general population, randomly recruited with the help of the residential registration office. The comparison was based on a retrospective interview addressing potential indicators of pre-existing chronic gonadal dysfunction with estrogen deficiency[64]. Patients were explicitly asked about disturbance *before* the onset of the first mental changes. The results were most interesting. Women with schizophrenia could be differentiated from controls by several factors: their menarche had occurred at a later age, and they had more often suffered from loss of hair, mid-cycle bleeding, light bleeding and hirsutism. There was also a tendency towards more infertility in the patients. All these findings are well in line with a potential early hormonal imbalance, at least in a subgroup of patients.

ESTROGEN INFLUENCE ON 'ACCOMPANYING' SYMPTOMATOLOGY IN SCHIZOPHRENIA

Further interesting results with potential implications for schizophrenia come from other areas of research (see also other chapters in this volume).

Thus, physiological estrogens as well as HRT might have stress-protective potencies[65,66]. This means that estrogens could possibly buffer against stress, which is a well known trigger for the outbreak of and also relapses in psychoses.

Also, estrogen's positive effects on cognition (for review see references 67 and 68) could be meaningful for the therapy of schizophrenia[69], as minor cognitive deficits are often one of the main obstacles for rehabilitation in the post-acute phase of the disease.

Further psychopathology of schizophrenia patients such as depression and aggressive and suicidal behavior might also be ameliorated by estrogens, as implied by estrogen's effects on affective symptoms (for review see references 68 and 70), especially postpartum depression[71,72] and postmenopausal depression[73–75], bipolar disorder[76], and aggressive[77,78] and suicidal behavior[36,79].

CONCLUSIONS: CONSEQUENCES FOR RESEARCH AND CLINIC

The presumed estrogen deficiency in women with schizophrenia and also the presumed protective effects of estrogens concerning this disorder could have important consequences for prophylaxis and therapy. However, further research is needed before broad clinical recommendations can be made.

One recommendation could be *hormonal replacement* with estrogens for women with schizophrenia *during and after the perimenopause* as an augmentation strategy, an adjunct to neuroleptic medication. The dose of neuroleptics would be reduced and corresponding side-effects minimized. To replace estrogens in these women would at least attenuate perimenopausal complaints, which can contribute to a general deterioration of the mental state and, in vulnerable women, potentially provoke a psychotic episode. Estrogen replacement therapy for women of this age group has been recommended for many reasons, for example prophylaxis of osteoporosis, and also improvement of cognitive function and possibly also delay of Alzheimer's dementia[80,81]. Further research into schizophrenia as an *additional* indication is urgently needed.

Research should also be carried out into the best mode of HRT for psychiatric patients. Progestogens are usually added to estrogens to prevent endometrial cancer, but can antagonize the positive effects of estrogens with respect to mental state[82,83]. Furthermore, we have to consider other risks of hormone therapy such as breast cancer or cardiovascular disease for certain combinations[81,84].

As an alternative to conventional HRT, compounds with more specific and potent estrogenic activity in the brain as opposed to other tissues should be searched for[85,86]. This would not only minimize side-effects of hormonal therapy, but may also allow new therapeutic strategies in men. Possible candidates are the selective estrogen receptor modulators (SERMs), whose agonist or antagonist properties depend on the target tissue. The effects of the so-far existing SERMs on the brain, however, remain to be clarified. Raloxifene, for example, seems to exert its main effects on bone, although there are recent data suggesting that it also acts on various brain receptors[83]. Also, the synthetic steroid tibolone seems to cause less endometrial proliferation. But its effects on the central nervous system are still not clear, apart from the observation that it seems to have an androgenic effect and to increase β-endorphin levels with improvement of mood and libido[87]. Further studies of the brain effects of SERMs and other estrogenic compounds (e.g. phytoestrogens, xenoestrogens, dehydroepiandrosterone) are urgently needed.

In women suffering from frequent perimenstrual psychotic *relapses, 'cycle-modulated' neuroleptic therapy* could be tried. If this is not possible, and/or contraception is needed at the same time, *monophasic contraceptive pills could be taken continuously* (i.e. without intervals) to maintain a constant serum level of estrogens[82]. However, systemic progestogens should be avoided as far as possible. Research into the best regimen is also needed here.

As there is growing evidence for disturbed gonadal function in schizophrenia, *estrogens and the gonadal axis should in the future be more seriously considered.* History-taking should always include questions regarding menstrual irregularities, amenorrhea, loss of libido, anorgasmia, infertility and galactorrhea. If there are any clinical suggestions of estrogen deficiency, prolactin and estrogen levels should be tested.

Hyperprolactinemia can theoretically be caused by the disease itself and the accompanying stress, but also by neuroleptic treatment, and can lead to secondary suppression of physiological estrogen production. This means that many women with schizophrenia who take narcoleptics over years suffer from a partially *'iatrogenic early menopause'*, with all its short-term and potentially serious long-term consequences, i.e. osteoporosis, enhanced cardiovascular risk and cognitive disturbances.

In the case of neuroleptic-induced hyperprolactinemia with secondary *estrogen deficiency*, medication should be switched to atypical neuroleptics causing little or no hyperprolactinemia (e.g. clozapine, quetiapine, olanzapine). If this is not possible or hypoestrogenism persists, estrogens need to be added as an adjunct to standard neuroleptic medication.

The issue of *contraception* should always be taken into account. Thus, with the change to atypical neuroleptics which do not produce hyperprolactinemia, the menstrual cycle is normalized and fertility is regained, with a high risk of unplanned pregnancy. Women with schizophrenia may not wish to be mothers and, as well, the new neuroleptics may have unknown teratogenic potential. Therefore, when changing to an atypical neuroleptic, contraception counselling involving a gynecologist should be initiated.

In summary, there are emerging hopes that estrogens as neuro- and psychoprotective adjunctive therapy may in the future complement the traditional drug therapies in schizophrenia. But it must be emphasized that most strategies are still being researched. Especially before using estrogens as an adjunct therapy in *younger* women without proven estrogen deficiency, results of larger controlled studies are needed.

Other strategies, however, should even now be part of standard clinical care[88]. These include examination of the gonadal axis with therapeutic consequences, if indicated. Regarding estrogen substitute as well as replacement therapy, it must be stressed that the decision should always be made on the basis of an individual risk-benefit assessment[80,84], and with close co-operation between psychiatrist and gynecologist.

For future research, there arise many questions, not only regarding new therapeutic strategies and compounds, but also regarding some so-far not well explained disturbances of estrogens and the hypothalamic-pituitary-gonadal axis in women with schizophrenia. Further research into this area could hopefully even contribute to understanding the pathogenesis of this disease, at least in a subgroup of women.

References

1. Riecher-Rössler A, Häfner H. Schizophrenia and oestrogens - is there an association? *Eur Arch Psychiatry Clin Neurosci* 1993;242:323-8
2. Kraepelin E. *Psychiatrie*, 8th edn. Leipzig: Barth, 1909
3. Kretschmer E. *Körperbau und Charakter. Untersuchungen zum Konstitutionsproblem und zur Lehre von den Temperamenten*, 25th edn. Berlin: Springer, 1921
4. Krafft-Ebing G. Untersuchungen über Irresein zur Zeit der Menstruation: ein klinischer Beitrag zur Lehre vom periodischen Irresein. *Arch Psychiatry* 1896;8:65-107
5. Bleuler M. Die spätschizophrenen Krankheitsbilder. *Neurology* 1943;15:259-90
6. Gordon JH, Borison RL, Diamond BL. Modulation of dopamine receptors sensitivity by estrogen. *Biol Psychiatry* 1980;15:389-96
7. Hruska RE, Silbergeld EK. Estrogen treatment enhances dopamine receptor sensitivity in the rat striatum. *Eur J Pharmacol* 1980;61:397-400
8. Di Paolo T, Payet P, Labrie F. Effect of chronic estradiol and haloperidol treatment on striatal dopamine receptors. *Eur J Pharmacol* 1981;73:105-6
9. Nicoletti F, Ferrara N, Patti F, *et al.* Influence of sex steroids and prolactin on haloperidol-induced catalepsy. *Brain Res* 1983;279:352-8
10. Koller WC, Weiner WJ, Klawans HL, *et al.* Influence of female sex hormones on neuroleptic-induced behavioral super-sensitivity. *Neuropharmacology* 1980;19:387-91
11. Gordon JH, Diamond BL. Antagonism of dopamine supersensitivity by estrogen: neurochemical studies in an animal model of tardive dyskinesia. *Biol Psychiatry* 1981;16:365-71
12. Bédard P, Boucher R, Daigle M, *et al.* Similar effect of estradiol and haloperidol on experimental tardive dyskinesia in monkeys. *Psychoneuroendocrinology* 1984;9:375-9
13. Rasgon NL, Small GW, Siddarth P, *et al.* Estrogen use and brain metabolic change in older adults. A preliminary report. *Psychiatry Res: Neuroimaging Section* 2001;107:11-18
14. Fink G, Sumner BEH. Estrogen and mental state. *Nature (London)* 1996;383:306
15. McEwen BS, Alves SE, Bulloch K, *et al.* Clinically relevant basic science studies of gender differences and sex hormone effects. *Psychopharmacol Bull* 1998;34:251-9
16. Stahl SM. Basic psychopharmacology of antidepressants, part 2: estrogen as an adjunct to antidepressant treatment. *J Clin Psychiatry* 1998; 59(Suppl 4):15-24
17. Stahl SM. Why drugs and hormones may interact in psychiatric disorders. *J Clin Psychiatry* 2001;62: 225-6
18. Stahl SM. Effects of estrogen on the central nervous system. *J Clin Psychiatry* 2001;62:317-18
19. De Battista C, Lawrence Smith D, Schatzberg AF. Modulation of monoamine neurotransmitters by estrogen: clinical implications. *Rev Psychiatry* 1999; 18:137-66
20. Garcia-Segura LM, Azcoitia I, DonCarlos LL. Neuroprotection by estradiol. *Prog Neurobiol* 2001; 63:29-60
21. Kuhl H. Einfluss von Oestrogenen und Gestagenen auf das Zentralnervensystem. In Kuhl H, ed. *Sexualhormone und Psyche.* Stuttgart: Thieme, 2002: 9-17
22. Fink G, Sumner BEH, Rosie R, *et al.* Estrogen control of central neurotransmission: effect on mood, mental state, and memory. *Cell Mol Neurobiol* 1996;16:325-44
23. Riecher A, Maurer K, Löffler W, *et al.* Gender differences in age at onset and course of schizophrenic disorders. In Häfner H, Gattaz WF, eds. *Search for the Causes of Schizophrenia.* Berlin: Springer, 1990; 14-33
24. Häfner H, Behrens S, De Vry J, *et al.* Warum erkraken Frauen später an Schizophrenie? Erhöhung der Vulnerabilitätsschwelle durch Oestrogen. *Nervenheilkunde* 1991;10:154-63
25. Häfner H, Behrens S, De Vry J, *et al.* An animal model for the effects of estradiol on dopamine-mediated behavior: implications for sex differences in schizophrenia. *Psychiatry Res* 1991;38:125-34
26. Labhart A. *Klinik der inneren Sekretion.* Berlin: Springer, 1978
27. Cohen RZ, Seeman MV, Gotowiec A, *et al.* Earlier puberty as a predictor of later onset of schizophrenia in women. *Am J Psychiatry* 1999;156: 1059-64
28. Endo M, Daiguji M, Asano Y, *et al.* Periodic psychosis recurring in association with menstrual cycle. *J Clin Psychiatry* 1978;39:456-66
29. Glick J, Stewart D. A new drug treatment for premenstrual exacerbation of schizophrenia. *Compr Psychiatry* 1980;21:281-7
30. Gerada C, Reveley A. Schizophreniform psychosis associated with the menstrual cycle. *Br J Psychiatry* 1988;152:700-2
31. Riecher-Rössler A, Häfner H, Dütsch-Strobel A, *et al.* Further evidence for a specific role of estradiol in schizophrenia. *Biol Psychiatry* 1994;36:492-4
32. Riecher-Rössler A, Häfner H, Stumbaum M, *et al.* Can estradiol modulate schizophrenic symptomatology? *Schizophr Bull* 1994;20:203-14
33. Hallonquist JD, Seeman MV, Lang M, *et al.* Variation in symptom severity over the menstrual cycle of schizophrenics. *Biol Psychiatry* 1993;33: 207-9

34. Seeman MV. Interaction of sex, age and neuroleptic dose. *Compr Psychiatry* 1983;24:125-8
35. Gattaz WF, Vogel P, Riecher-Rössler A, *et al.* Influence of the menstrual cycle phase on the therapeutic response in schizophrenia. *Biol Psychiatry* 1994;36:137-9
36. Riecher-Rössler A. *Die Spätschizophrenie - eine valide Entität? Eine empirische Studie zu Risikofaktoren, Krankheitsbild und Verlauf.* Thesis, Universität Heidelberg-Mannheim, 1994
37. Riecher-Rössler A, Löffler W, Munk-Jorgensen P. What do we really know about late-onset schizophrenia? *Eur Arch Psychiatry Clin Neurosci* 1997; 247:195-208
38. Riecher-Rössler A, Rössler W. The course of schizophrenic psychoses: what do we really know? A selective review from an epidemiological perspective. *Eur Arch Psychiatry Clin Neurosci* 1998;248:189-202
39. Chang SS, Renshaw DC. Psychosis and pregnancy. *Compr Ther* 1986;12:36-41
40. Kendell RE, Chalmers JC, Platz C. Epidemiology of puerperal psychoses. *Br J Psychiatry* 1987;150: 662-73
41. Mahé V, Dumaine A. Oestrogen withdrawal associated psychoses. *Acta Psychiatr Scand* 2001; 104:323-31
42. Mall G. Neuere Ergebnisse der Psycho-Endokrinologie. *Aerztliche Praxis* 1959;XI:1357-60
43. Mall G. Diagnostik und Therapie ovarieller Psychosen. *Zentralbl Neurol Psychiatrie* 1960;155: 250
44. Kulkarni J, de Castella A, Smith D, *et al.* A clinical trial of the effects of estrogen in acutely psychotic women. *Schizophr Res* 1996;20:247-52
45. Kulkarni J, Riedel A, de Castella AR, *et al.* Estrogen - a potential treatment for schizophrenia. *Schizophr Res* 2001;48:137-44
46. Lindamer LA, Lohr JB, Harris MJ, *et al.* Gender, estrogen, and schizophrenia. *Psychopharmacol Bull* 1997;33:221-8
47. Lindamer LA, Buse DC, Lohr JB, *et al.* Hormone replacement therapy in postmenopausal women with schizophrenia: positive effect on negative symptoms? *Biol Psychiatry* 2001;49:47-51
48. Jeste DV, Lindamer LA, Lacro JP. Gender differences in late-life schizophrenia and its treatment. Presented at the *American Psychiatric Association's 2001 Annual Meeting*, 2001:310(abstr)
49. Ahokas A, Aito M, Turtianen S. Association between oestradiol and puerperal psychosis. *Acta Psychiatr Scand* 2000;101:167-70
50. Sichel DA, Cohen LS, Robertson LM, *et al.* Prophylactic estrogen in recurrent postpartum affective disorders. *Biol Psychiatry* 1995;38:814-18
51. Diczfalusy E, Lauritzen C. Psychiatrische und neurologische Erkrankungen. In Diczfalusy E, Lauritzen C, eds. *Oestrogene beim Menschen.* Berlin: Springer, 1961:461-2
52. Riecher-Rössler A, Häfner H, Dütsch-Strobel A, *et al.* Gonadal function and its influence on psychopathology. A comparison of schizophrenic and non-schizophrenic female inpatients. *Arch Women's Ment Health* 1998;1:15-26
53. Bergemann N, Mundt C, Resch F, *et al.* On the hypoestrogen hypothesis in female schizophrenia: preliminary results. *Schizophr Res* 1996;18:158
54. Bergermann N. Psychotrope Effekte der Hormonsubstititionstherapie. In Riecher-Rössler A, Rohde A, eds. *Psychische Erkrankungen bei Frauen - Für eine geschlechtersensible Psychiatrie und Psychotherapie.* Basel: Karger, 2001:138-64
55. Choi SH, Kang SB, Joe SH. Changes in premenstrual symptoms in women with schizophrenia: a prospective study. *Psychosom Med* 2001; 6:822-9
56. Hoff AL, Kremen WA, Wieneke MH, *et al.* Association of estrogen levels with neuropsychological performance in women with schizophrenia. *Am J Psychiatry* 2001;158:1134-9
57. Huber TJ. Hormonspiegel bei Frauen mit schizophrenen Erkrankungen. In Riecher-Rössler A, Rohde A, eds. *Psychische Erkrankungen bei Frauen - Für eine geschlechtersensible Psychiatrie und Psychotherapie.* Basel: Karger, 2001:165-9
58. Huber TJ, Rollnik J, Wilhelms J, *et al.* Estradiol levels in psychotic disorders. *Psychoneuroendocrinology* 2001;26:27-35
59. Bergemann N, Parzer P, Nagi I, *et al.* Acute psychiatric admission and menstrual cycle phase in women with schizophrenia. *Arch Women's Ment Health* 2002;5:119-26
60. Canuso CM, Goldstein JM, Wojcik J, *et al.* Antipsychotic medication, prolactin elevation, and ovarian function in women with schizophrenia and schizoaffective disorder. *Psychiatry Res* 2002; 111:11-20
61. Smith S, Wheeler MJ, Murray R, *et al.* The effects of antipsychotic-induced hyperprolactinaemia on the hypothalamic-pituitary-gonadal axis. *J Clin Psychopharmacol* 2002;22:109-14
62. Zhang-Wong J, Seeman MV. Antipsychotic drugs, menstrual regularity, and osteoporosis risk. *Arch Women's Ment Health* 2002;5:93-8
63. Maguire GA. Prolactin elevation with antipsychotic medications: mechanisms of action and clinical consequences. *J Clin Psychiatry* 2002;63 (Suppl 4):56-62
64. Schepp A. *Pilotstudie zur Frage eines überdauernden relativen Hypoöstrogenismus bei schizophrenen Frauen.* Inaugural dissertation, Universität Heidelberg-Mannheim, 1997
65. Carlson LE, Sherwin BB. Relatiopnship among cortisol (CRT), dehydroepiandrosterone-sulfate (DHEAS), and memory in a longitudinal study of healthy elderly men and women. *Neurobiol Aging* 1999;20:315-24

66. Wolf OT, Schommer NC, Hellhamer DH, *et al.* The relationship between stress induced cortisol levels and memory differs between men and women. *Psychoneuroendocrinology* 2001;26:711-20
67. Hogervorst E, Williams J, Budge M, *et al.* The nature of the effect of female gonadal hormone replacement therapy on cognitive function in post-menopausal women: a metaanalysis. *Neuroscience* 2000;101:485-512
68. Oesterlund MK. The role of estrogens in neuropsychiatric disorders. *Curr Opin Psychiatry* 2002;15: 307-12
69. Ehrenreich H, Heyer A, Siren AL. Future perspectives of gender hormones in neuroprotection. *Eur Psychiatry* 2002;17(Suppl 1):42S(abstr)
70. Kahn L, Halbreich U. Estrogen's effect on depression. In Bergemann N, Riecher-Rössler A, eds. *Estrogen Effects in Psychiatric Disorders.* Vienna: Springer, 2003:in press
71. Ahokas A, Kaukoranta J, Wahlbeck K, *et al.* Estrogen deficiency in severe postpartum depression: successful treatment with sublingual physiologic 17β-estradiol: a preliminary study. *J Clin Psychiatry* 2001;62:332-6
72. Lawrie TA, Herxheimer A, Dalton K. Oestrogens and progestogens for preventing and treating postnatal depression (Cochrane Review). *Cochrane Library*, Issue 3. Oxford: Update Software, 2001
73. Zweifel JE, O'Brien WH. A meta-analysis of the effect of hormone replacement therapy upon depressed mood. *Psychoneuroendocrinology* 1997;22: 189-212
74. de Noaves Soares C, Almeida OP, Joffe H, *et al.* Efficacy of estradiol for the treatment of depressive disorders in perimenopausal women. *Arch Gen Psychiatry* 2001;58:529-34
75. Schmidt PJ, Nieman L, Danaceau MA, *et al.* Estrogen replacement in perimenopause-related depression: a preliminary report. *Am J Obstet Gynecol* 2000;183:414-20
76. Freeman MP, Wosnitzer Smith K, Freeman SA, *et al.* The impact of reproductive events on the course of bipolar disorder in women. *J Clin Psychiatry* 2002;63:284-7
77. Carlson LE, Sherwin BB, Chertkow MH. Relationship between mood and estradiol (E2) levels in Alzheimer's disease (AD) patients. *J Gerontol B Psychol Sci Soc Sci* 2000;55:P47-53
78. Kyomen HH, Hennen J, Gottlieb GL, *et al.* Estrogen therapy and noncognitive psychiatric signs and symptoms in elderly patients with dementia. *Am J Psychiatry* 2002;259:1225-7
79. Riecher-Rössler A. Oestrogene und Schizophrenie - Patientinnen an der Schnittstelle zwischen Psychiatrie und Gynäkologie. *Geburtsh Frauenheilk* 2002;62:429-35
80. North American Menopause Society. A decision tree for the use of estrogen replacement therapy or hormone replacement therapy in postmenopausal women: consensus opinion of the North American Menopause Society. *Menopause* 2000;7:76-86
81. Barrett-Connor E, Stuenkel CA. Hormone replacement therapy (HRT): risks and benefits. *Int J Epidemiol* 2001;30:423-6
82. Braendle W, Breckwoldt M, Kuhl H, *et al.* Sexualhormone und Psyche - Ergebnisse des 2. Interdisziplinären Frankfurter Gesprächs zur Kontrazeption. *Frauenarzt* 2001;42:154-60
83. Cyr M, Calon F, Morissette M, *et al.* Estrogenic modulation of brain activity: implications for schizophrenia and Parkinson's disease. *J Psychiatry Neurosci* 2002;27:12-27
84. Writing Group for the Women's Health Initiative Investigators. Risks and benefits of estrogen plus progestin in healthy postmenopausal women. *J Am Med Assoc* 2002;288:321-33
85. Halbreich U. The spectrum of estrogens, estrogen agonists and SERMs. *Int J Neuropsychopharmacol* 2002;5(Suppl 1):S12(abstr)
86. Riecher-Rössler A. Estrogen effects in schizophrenia and their potential therapeutic implications - a review. *Arch Women's Ment Health* 2002;5:111-18
87. Davis SR. The effects of tibolone on mood and libido. *Menopause* 2002;9:162-70
88. Grigoriadis S, Seeman MV. The role of estrogen in schizophrenia: implications for schizophrenia practice guidelines for women. *Can J Psychiatry* 2002;47:437-42

Unsolved and controversial issues regarding neuroprotection by estrogen 21

I. Azcoitia, I. Ciriza, D. Garcia-Ovejero, P. Mendez, A. Sierra, S. Veiga, F. Naftolin and L. M. Garcia-Segura

INTRODUCTION: ESTRADIOL AND BRAIN FUNCTION

Estradiol regulates the development of brain areas involved in the control of neuroendocrine function and behaviors related to reproduction, inducing structural and functional sex differences in brain tissue[1,2]. In addition, estradiol acts on the adult brain to regulate acutely the hypothalamic-pituitary-gonadal axis and reproductive behavior[3-7]. Furthermore, estradiol acts in brain areas that are not considered to be involved in the control of neuroendocrine events or reproductive function[8,9]. At the same time, a new view of estradiol as a trophic factor for neurons and glial cells has emerged[10,11]. Acting via estrogen receptors (α and β), estradiol regulates gene expression, neuronal survival and neuronal differentiation in the brain in a way that is not very different from that exerted by neurotrophins and classical growth factors[12,13].

Receptors for estradiol are nuclear transcription factors that regulate the expression of specific genes. These receptors are expressed in different brain areas, primarily, but not exclusively, in neurons[14-19]. In addition, estradiol activates the signalling pathways of tyrosine kinase receptors, such as neurotrophin receptors and insulin-like growth factor-I receptor[11,13,20,21]. The mechanisms involved in the rapid activation by estradiol of these membrane-associated signalling pathways remain to be elucidated, and may be associated with new membrane forms of estrogen receptors or with transient association of classical estrogen receptors with specific membrane compartments[22,23].

ESTRADIOL IS NEUROPROTECTIVE IN ANIMAL MODELS

It is known that decreasing levels of estradiol after the menopause are associated with the progression of neurodegenerative disorders, increased depressive symptoms and other psychological disturbances. The potential benefits of estrogen for brain function are supported by experimental data in animal models that provide convincing evidence of the neuroprotective properties of estradiol[10,24-26]. The hormone has been shown to protect brain neurons *in vivo* and *in vitro* from a large variety of stressors, neurotoxins and deleterious conditions, including serum or growth factor deprivation, anoxia, excitotoxicity and oxidative damage[10,24-26]. Estradiol is also neuroprotective in experimental models of Parkinson's disease and forebrain ischemia[27-31].

IS ESTRADIOL NEUROPROTECTIVE IN THE HUMAN BRAIN?

While basic studies in animals clearly indicate that estradiol is neuroprotective, the situation is not so clear when information collected from human studies is analyzed. The effect of hormone replacement therapy (HRT) in memory and verbal performances of postmenopausal women has been assessed in various manners, and some results suggest that HRT may increase cognitive function[32-36]. For example, in the Baltimore Longitudinal Study of Aging, non-demented postmenopausal women receiving hormone therapy performed better on tests of verbal and visual memory compared with never-treated women, in samples in which both groups of women were comparable with respect to educational attainment, general medical health and performance on a test of verbal knowledge[34]. HRT may also be an effective treatment of depression for perimenopausal women[37], and in postmenopausal women may reduce negative symptoms in schizophrenia[38], decrease the risk of stroke[39], reduce the motor disability associated with Parkinson's disease[40] and improve cognition in Alzheimer's disease[41]. However, the evidence for a protective effect of estrogen in the human brain is not without controversy. Indeed, several studies show that estrogen replacement therapy has no positive effect on neurodegenerative diseases or stroke, and other studies suggest that HRT may have a negative impact on cognition in postmenopausal women with Alzheimer's disease[42]. Therefore, there is an apparent discrepancy between the potent neuroprotective effect of estradiol in animal models and the high variability of results in human studies.

One potential source for the discrepancies in the results of different studies is that there is a considerable variation in the exact hormonal composition and pattern of administration in HRT in humans. Usually, a mixture of natural or synthetic estrogens and progestins is administered. Various hormonal compositions and differences in the age of onset and duration of treatment may alter the effects of HRT on the human brain. However, there are other possible explanations for the different effects of estradiol in the brains of animals and humans. Most studies in animal models use young adult rodents submitted to various forms of brain injury. Very little is known about the effects of estradiol in the brains of old animals. Neuroprotective effects of estradiol may be impaired in the aged brain, because aging may affect the expression of estrogen receptors and estrogen receptor coactivators[43–45]. Therefore, estrogen receptor signalling may be very different in young and old brains, and, in consequence, the effects of estradiol in the brains of young animals may not be predictive of the effects of the same molecules in aged human brains.

In addition to changes in estrogen receptor expression and signalling, there is at least another good reason to explain why neuroprotective effects of estradiol may be reduced in the aged brain; other substances that may be necessary for the effects of the hormone may also be depleted by aging. These may include growth factors, neuromodulators and neurotransmitters and their receptors. Insulin-like growth factor-I (IGF-I) is a growth factor involved in the actions of estradiol is insulin-like growth factor-I (IGF-I). Several studies have shown that the actions of estrogen and IGF-I in the brain are interdependent. This interdependence between estrogen and IGF-I, or between estrogen receptors and IGF-I receptors, has been documented for neuronal differentiation, synaptic plasticity and neuroprotection[46]. Plasma levels of IGF-I decrease with aging, and the treatment of old rats with IGF-I ameliorates several age-related deficits in the brain[47,48]. Since brain IGF-I and IGF-I receptor levels are affected by aging[49], the effect of estrogen receptor activation may be very different in young and old brains because aging decreases the availability of this key synergist. The limited evidence available from studies with old animals that have assessed the neurological actions of estradiol is still inconclusive. It has been shown that estradiol protects the brains of middle-aged rats (9–12 months) from middle cerebral artery occlusion[50]. However, other studies suggest that synaptic plasticity in response to estrogen is abolished in the brains of old rats[51]. More studies are needed to determine to what extent estradiol is neuroprotective in old animals.

THERAPEUTIC PERSPECTIVES

We are still a long way from being able to design rational protocols for HRT to protect the brain from aging. More studies to understand the mechanisms of action of estradiol in the aging brain are necessary. We need more information on the interaction of estrogen and progesterone with other neuronal survival factors that are affected by the aging process. Moreover, HRT may be protective against some types of damage but deleterious in the case of other types of brain insult. Alternative strategies to HRT that may be clinically more effective should be experimentally tested.

Neuroprotective effects of estradiol in animal models depend, at least in part, on the activation of estrogen receptors[10]. Therefore, estrogen receptors are good candidates for pharmacological targeting aimed to prevent neurological diseases. However, before the therapeutic assessment of selective estrogen receptor modulators (SERMs) as neuroprotectants, it is essential to learn much more about the expression and regulation of estrogen receptors and their cofactors in the aging brain, and also about the impact of aging on the convergence of estrogen receptor signalling with other signalling pathways.

It may also be useful to exploit the endogenous capacity of the brain to synthesize estradiol. Different types of brain lesions in both male and female animals result in the induction in the injured tissue of aromatase, the enzyme that catalyzes the formation of estradiol from testosterone. The enzyme is induced in reactive astrocytes located near neurodegenerative foci, and this induction is accompanied by an increased capacity of the injured brain to synthesize estrogen[52]. Studies using specific aromatase inhibitors infused in the rat brain as well as aromatase knock-out mice combined with estrogen replacement indicate that the induction of brain aromatase after a brain lesion is neuroprotective and reduces neuronal death. Furthermore, it has been shown that this neuroprotective effect of aromatase is specifically mediated by the formation of estradiol[53]. Since aromatase is neuroprotective, this enzyme is a possible target for therapeutic approaches. We need more information on the levels of expression of aromatase in the aged human brain, since a potential mechanism to increase estrogen levels locally in the brain is to change the expression or the activity of this enzyme specifically in the nervous system. The aromatase gene is under the control of different tissue-specific promoters[54], and it is conceivable that it will be possible to develop specific drugs that will enhance the expression of this enzyme in the brain but not in other tissues.

ACKNOWLEDGEMENTS

We acknowledge support from the Commission of the European Communities, specific RTD program 'Quality of Life and Management of Living Resources', QLK6-CT-2000-00179, and Ministerio de Ciencia y Tecnología, Spain, SAF 2002-00652.

References

1. Arnold AP, Gorski RA. Gonadal steroid induction of structural sex differences in the central nervous system. *Annu Rev Neurosci* 1984;7:413–42
2. Breedlove SM, Arnold AP. Hormonal control of a developing neuromuscular system. I. Complete demasculinization of the male rat spinal nucleus of the bulbocavernosus using the anti-androgen flutamide. *J Neurosci* 1983;3:417–23
3. Gomez DM, Newman SW. Medial nucleus of the amygdala in the adult Syrian hamster: a quantitative Golgi analysis of gonadal hormonal regulation of neuronal morphology. *Anat Rec* 1991;231: 498–509
4. Naftolin F, Mor G, Horvath TL, *et al.* Synaptic remodeling in the arcuate nucleus during the estrous cycle is induced by estrogen and precedes the preovulatory gonadotropin surge. *Endocrinology* 1996;137:5576–80
5. Olmos G, Naftolin F, Perez J, Tranque PA, Garcia-Segura LM. Synaptic remodeling in the rat arcuate nucleus during the estrous cycle. *Neuroscience* 1989;32:663–7
6. Russell JA, Douglas AJ, Ingram CD. Brain preparations for maternity – adaptive changes in behavioral and neuroendocrine systems during pregnancy and lactation. An overview. *Prog Brain Res* 2001;133:1–38
7. Swaab DF, Chung WC, Kruijver FP, Hofman MA, Ishunina TA. Structural and functional sex differences in the human hypothalamus. *Horm Behav* 2001;40:93–8
8. Chowen JA, Azcoitia I, Cardona-Gomez GP, Garcia-Segura LM. Sex steroids and the brain: lessons from animal studies. *J Pediatr Endocrinol Metab* 2000;13:1045–66

9. Woolley CS, McEwen BS. Estradiol mediates fluctuation in hippocampal synapse density during the estrous cycle in the adult rat. *J Neurosci* 1992; 12:2549–54
10. Garcia-Segura LM, Azcoitia I, DonCarlos LL. Neuroprotection by estradiol. *Prog Neurobiol* 2001; 63:29–60
11. Toran-Allerand CD, Singh M, Setalo G. Novel mechanisms of estrogen action in the brain: new players in an old story. *Front Neuroendocrinol* 1999; 20:97–121
12. Azcoitia I, Sierra A, Garcia-Segura LM. Neuroprotective effects of estradiol in the adult rat hippocampus: interaction with insulin-like growth factor-I signalling. *J Neurosci Res* 1999;58: 815–22
13. Bi R, Broutman G, Foy MR, Thompson RF, Baudry M. The tyrosine kinase and mitogen-activated protein kinase pathways mediate multiple effects of estrogen in hippocampus. *Proc Natl Acad Sci USA* 2000;97:3602–7
14. DonCarlos LL, Greene GL, Morrell JI. Estrogen plus progesterone increases progestin receptor immunoreactivity in the brain of ovariectomized guinea pigs. *Neuroendocrinology* 1989;50:613–23
15. DonCarlos LL, Monroy E, Morrell JI. Distribution of estrogen receptor-immunoreactive cells in the forebrain of the female guinea pig. *J Comp Neurol* 1991;305:591–612
16. Greco B, Allegretto EA, Tetel MJ, Blaustein JD. Coexpression of ER β with ER α and progestin receptor proteins in the female rat forebrain: effects of estradiol treatment. *Endocrinology* 2001; 142:5172–81
17. McAbee MD, DonCarlos LL. Ontogeny of region-specific sex differences in androgen receptor messenger ribonucleic acid expression in the rat forebrain. *Endocrinology* 1998;139:1738–45
18. Shughrue PJ, Lane MV, Merchenthaler I. Comparative distribution of estrogen receptor-α and -β mRNA in the rat central nervous system. *J Comp Neurol* 1997;388:507–25
19. Simerly RB. Distribution and regulation of steroid hormone receptor gene expression in the central nervous system. *Adv Neurol* 1993;59:207–26
20. Garcia-Segura LM, Cardona-Gomez GP, Chowen JA, Azcoitia I. Insulin-like growth factor-I receptors and estrogen receptors interact in the promotion of neuronal survival and neuroprotection. *J Neurocytol* 2000;29:425–37
21. Singh M, Setalo G, Guan X, Warren M, Toran-Allerand CD. Estrogen-induced activation of mitogen-activated protein kinase in cerebral cortical explants: convergence of estrogen and neurotrophin signaling pathways. *J Neurosci* 1999;19: 1179–88
22. Singh M, Setalo G, Guan X, Frail DE, Toran-Allerand CD. Estrogen-induced activation of the mitogen-activated protein kinase cascade in the cerebral cortex of estrogen receptor-α knock-out mice. *J Neurosci* 2000;20:1694–700
23. Mendez P, Azcoitia I, Garcia-Segura LM. Estrogen receptor α forms estrogen-dependent multimolecular complexes with insulin-like growth factor receptor and phosphatidylinositol 3-kinase in the adult rat brain. *Mol Brain Res* 2003;112:170–6
24. Green PS, Simpkins JW. Neuroprotective effects of estrogens: potential mechanisms of action. *Int J Dev Neurosci* 2000;18:347–58
25. Lee SJ, McEwen BS. Neurotrophic and neuroprotective actions of estrogens and their therapeutic implications. *Annu Rev Pharmacol Toxicol* 2001;41:569–91
26. Wise PM, Dubal DB, Wilson ME, Rau SW, Liu Y. Estrogens: trophic and protective factors in the adult brain. *Front Neuroendocrinol* 2001;22:33–66
27. Grandbois M, Morissette M, Callier S, Di Paolo T. Ovarian steroids and raloxifene prevent MPTP-induced dopamine depletion in mice. *Neuroreport* 2000;11:343–6
28. Leranth C, Roth RH, Elsworth JD, Naftolin F, Horvath TL, Redmond DE. Estrogen is essential for maintaining nigrostriatal dopamine neurons in primates: implications for Parkinson's disease and memory. *J Neurosci* 2000;20:8604–9
29. Sawada M, Alkayed NJ, Goto S, *et al.* Estrogen receptor antagonist ICI 182 780 exacerbates ischemic injury in female mouse. *J Cereb Blood Flow Metab* 2000;20:112–18
30. Stein DG. Brain damage, sex hormones and recovery: a new role for progesterone and estrogen? *Trends Neurosci* 2001;24:386–91
31. Wise PM, Dubal DB. Estradiol protects against ischemic brain injury in middle-aged rats. *Biol Reprod* 2000;63:982–5
32. Hogervorst E, Williams J, Budge M, Riedel W, Jolles J. The nature of the effect of female gonadal hormone replacement therapy on cognitive function in postmenopausal women: a meta-analysis. *Neuroscience* 2000;101:485–512
33. Mulnard RA, Cotman CW, Kawas C, *et al.* Estrogen replacement therapy for treatment of mild to moderate Alzheimer disease: a randomized controlled trial. Alzheimer's Disease Cooperative Study. *J Am Med Assoc* 2000;283:1007–15
34. Resnick SM, Maki PM. Effects of hormone replacement therapy on cognitive and brain aging. *Ann NY Acad Sci* 2001;949:203–14
35. Saunders-Pullman R, Gordon-Elliott J, Parides M, Fahn S, Saunders HR, Bressman S. The effect of estrogen replacement on early Parkinson's disease. *Neurology* 1999;52:1417–21
36. Sherwin BB. Can estrogen keep you smart? Evidence from clinical studies. *J Psychiatry Neurosci* 1999;24:315–21
37. Birkhauser M. Depression, menopause and estrogens: is there a correlation? *Maturitas* 2002; 41(Suppl 1):3–8

38. Stevens JR. Schizophrenia: reproductive hormones and the brain. *Am J Psychiatry* 2002;159:713–19
39. Paganini-Hill A. Estrogen replacement therapy and stroke. *Prog Cardiovasc Dis* 1995;38:223–42
40. Cyr M, Calon F, Morissette M, Di Paolo T. Estrogenic modulation of brain activity: implications for schizophrenia and Parkinson's disease. *J Psychiatry Neurosci* 2002;27:12–27
41. Henderson VW, Paganini-Hill A, Miller BL, *et al.* Estrogen for Alzheimer's disease in women: randomized, double-blind, placebo-controlled trial. *Neurology* 2000;54:295–301
42. Shaywitz BA, Shaywitz SE. Estrogen and Alzheimer disease: plausible theory, negative clinical trial. *J Am Med Assoc* 2000;283:1055–6
43. Adams MM, Fink SE, Shah RA, *et al.* Estrogen and aging affect the subcellular distribution of estrogen receptor-α in the hippocampus of female rats. *J Neurosci* 2002;22:3608–14
44. Jezierski MK, Sohrabji F. Neurotrophin expression in the reproductively senescent forebrain is refractory to estrogen stimulation. *Neurobiol Aging* 2001;22:309–19
45. Matsumoto A, Prins GS. Androgenic regulation of expression of androgen receptor protein in the perineal motoneurons of aged male rats. *J Comp Neurol* 2002;443:383–7
46. Cardona-Gomez GP, Mendez P, DonCarlos LL, Azcoitia I, Garcia-Segura LM. Interactions of estrogens and insulin-like growth factor-I in the brain: implications for neuroprotection. *Brain Res Rev* 2001;37:320–34
47. Lichtenwalner RJ, Forbes ME, Bennett SA, Lynch CD, Sonntag WE, Riddle DR. Intracerebroventricular infusion of insulin-like growth factor-I ameliorates the age-related decline in hippocampal neurogenesis. *Neuroscience* 2001;107:603–13
48. Lynch CD, Lyons D, Khan A, Bennett SA, Sonntag WE. Insulin-like growth factor-1 selectively increases glucose utilization in brains of aged animals. *Endocrinology* 2001;142:506–9
49. Sonntag WE, Lynch CD, Bennett SA, *et al.* Alterations in insulin-like growth factor-1 gene and protein expression and type 1 insulin-like growth factor receptors in the brains of ageing rats. *Neuroscience* 1999;88:269–79
50. Dubal DB, Wise PM. Neuroprotective effects of estradiol in middle-aged female rats. *Endocrinology* 2001;142:43–8
51. Adams MM, Shah RA, Janssen WG, Morrison JH. Different modes of hippocampal plasticity in response to estrogen in young and aged female rats. *Proc Natl Acad Sci USA* 2001;98:8071–6
52. Garcia-Segura LM, Wozniak A, Azcoitia I, Rodriguez JR, Hutchison RE, Hutchison JB. Aromatase expression by astrocytes after brain injury: implications for local estrogen formation in brain repair. *Neuroscience* 1999;89:567–78
53. Azcoitia I, Sierra A, Veiga S, Honda S, Harada N, Garcia-Segura LM. Brain aromatase is neuroprotective. *J Neurobiol* 2001;47:318–29
54. Honda S, Harada N, Abe-Dohmae S, Takagi Y. Identification of *cis*-acting elements in the proximal promoter region for brain-specific exon 1 of the mouse aromatase gene. *Mol Brain Res* 1999; 66:122–32

Sex hormone receptor polymorphisms and cognitive impairment in older men and women

22

K. Yaffe

INTRODUCTION

Alzheimer's disease (AD) is the most common form of dementia, affecting over four million Americans currently, with a likely increase in prevalence over the next few decades[1]. Several genes associated with familial and sporadic AD have been identified, but it is estimated that approximately 50% of genetic factors remain unidentified[2]. Recently, genetic research has focused on identifying common population polymorphism loci, such as apolipoprotein E (ApoE) and α_1-antichymotrypsin, that are associated with an increased susceptibility to AD. This chapter addresses the evidence that sex hormone receptor gene variants or polymorphisms may be associated with risk of AD and cognitive decline in older men and women.

SEX HORMONES MAY HAVE A MAJOR ROLE IN PREVENTING COGNITIVE DECLINE

Sex hormones may modulate cognitive decline in older men and women. Estrogen receptors (ERs) ERα and ERβ are located throughout the brain, especially in areas involved in learning and memory such as the hippocampus and amygdala[3], and the enzymes necessary for sex steroid biosynthesis have been identified in these same regions[4]. Indeed, ovariectomized ERα knock-out mice have impaired performance on a hippocampal-dependent cognitive task that is reversed with estradiol administration[5]. The abundant localization of the ERβ in human hippocampus supports a role for this receptor in cognition as well[6,7]. The density of ERβ has been reported to be increased in the brains of patients with AD, compared with elderly controls[6]. Androgen receptors (ARs) tend to colocalize with ERs and are found primarily in the thalamus, hippocampus and cerebral cortex[8]. In postmenopausal women, the primary source of estradiol is from conversion (via aromatase) of androgens. Aromatase is present throughout the body and the central nervous system, including the temporal and frontal lobes[9]. Thus, both estrogens and androgens are present and synthesized in the brain, and may play an important role in cognition.

Mechanisms by which sex hormones could improve cognition and prevent decline remain unknown, but several have been suggested. One is the modulation of neurotransmitters, particularly seen with estrogen's enhancement of acetylcholine activity[10,11]. In mice, testosterone supplementation also improves age-related cognitive impairment[12]. Estrogen and testosterone stimulate axonal sprouting and dendritic spine formation in adult rat CA1 hippocampal pyramidal neurons[13,14], and this may be a mechanism for sex hormone protection, as neuronal loss in the hippocampal CA1 region is found in patients with AD and cognitive decline. In addition, estradiol may be neuroprotective, limiting oxidative stress injury, and both estradiol and testosterone treatments protect neuronal cells from the toxicity of Alzheimer-type β-amyloid[15,16] and reduce the generation of β-amyloid in neurons[17,18]. Estradiol and testosterone thus may reduce the risk of cognitive decline through a variety of mechanisms.

ERα GENE POLYMORPHISMS AND RISK OF ALZHEIMER'S DISEASE AND COGNITIVE DECLINE

The ERα gene polymorphism is a possible candidate for AD susceptibility in sporadic AD. Several studies have shown that estrogen therapy improves cognitive function or prevents AD in elderly women[19-22], and women have a slightly higher age-adjusted risk of developing AD compared with men, possibly mediated by ApoE genotype[23]. The gene for the ERα has several single nucleotide polymorphisms (SNPs), the PvuII, XbaI and B variants, that may be associated with receptor expression and function[24,25]. While controversial, differences in ERα polymorphism frequencies have been demonstrated in several diseases including breast cancer, osteoporosis and endometriosis[26-28]. Recently, several case-control studies[2,29,30], but not all[25], have found an increased frequency of the PvuII and XbaI polymorphisms (polymorphic sites that are in linkage disequilibrium) in patients with AD, compared with controls. Furthermore, a recent case-control study reported a synergistic effect of ERα CA repeat polymorphism and ERα PvuII and XbaI polymorphisms on risk of developing AD in white elders[31].

As part of a prospective cohort study, we recently investigated the association between ERα polymorphisms, cognitive test performance and risk of cognitive impairment and dementia in community-dwelling older women of European ancestry[32]. The subjects for the study were 2625 non-demented women who had cognitive testing at baseline and at 6-8 years of follow-up. The frequency of PvuII genotypes among the women was 549 (21%) with PP, 1217 (46%) with Pp and 859 (33%) with pp. The frequency of XbaI genotype was 315 (12%) with XX, 1232 (47%) with Xx and 1078 (41%) with xx. Women with at least one p allele had a greater decline in 6-8-year cognitive score, adjusted for age, education and baseline score (p for trend = 0.01), and there was a greater 6-8-year adjusted cognitive score decline in women with at least one x allele (p for trend = 0.02).

ERα allele frequencies differed among women who developed cognitive impairment compared with those who did not, with more women who developed cognitive impairment having a p allele (62% vs. 56%, $p = 0.03$; age- and education-adjusted odds ratio (OR) 1.35, 95% confidence interval (CI) 1.07-1.72). Similarly, more women who developed cognitive impairment had an x allele (70% vs. 64%, $p = 0.03$; OR 1.32, 95% CI 1.03-1.68). Adjusting for age and education did not change the magnitude or statistical significance of the results. Among the 62 women who said they had received a diagnosis of dementia or AD from their physician, the gene frequency for p was 65% ($p = 0.03$, compared with those without a diagnosis of dementia) and for x was 74% ($p = 0.02$).

ERα genotype frequencies also differed among women who did and did not develop cognitive impairment. Using the PP genotype as a reference, women who had a pp or Pp genotype had an increased likelihood of developing cognitive impairment (OR 1.65, 95% CI 1.03-2.63 for pp and OR 1.32, 95% CI 0.84-2.09 for Pp). Similarly, the adjusted odds of developing impairment were higher in women with the xx genotype, but not in those with the Xx genotype, compared with women with the XX genotype (age- and education-adjusted OR 1.73, 95% CI 0.99-3.02 for xx; adjusted OR 1.17, 95% CI 0.66-2.06 for Xx). Compared with women with PP or XX, the age- and education-adjusted odds of receiving a physician-diagnosis of dementia or AD were increased by almost three-fold among women with pp (adjusted OR 2.68, 95% CI 1.14-6.31) or with xx (adjusted OR 3.06, 95% CI 1.06-8.83).

While the polymorphisms may affect ERα gene enhancer activity[25] or gene regulation[24], *in vitro* evidence indicates that the ERα PvuII polymorphism produces a functional myb transcription factor binding site, suggesting that it produces a novel promoter or intronic enhancer of ERα expression (David Herrington, personal communication). How the ERα polymorphisms may influence cognitive function is not known. It may be, for example, that ER polymorphisms are associated with different estradiol serum concentrations that in turn may predict cognitive decline[33]. Recent studies have described an interaction between the ERα polymorhisms and ApoE e4 allele on risk of developing AD[30]. The observed interaction between ApoE e4 and oral estrogen therapy on risk of developing cognitive impairment also supports the hypothesis that estrogen, and possibly ERα polymorphisms, and ApoE may be mechanistically linked in their effect on cognitive decline[34]. Several lines of evidence from *in vitro* and animal studies, including estradiol-induced synaptic sprouting and expression of ApoE mRNA in rodents, support an estrogen–ApoE interaction[35,36]. It is also possible that the increased risk of cognitive impairment observed with the ERα polymorphisms is due to linkage disequilibrium with nearby genes that may, in turn, cause an increased risk of developing AD or other dementias.

STUDIES IN ELDERLY MEN SUGGEST A ROLE FOR EXOGENOUS TESTOSTERONE IN IMPROVING COGNITION

There is increasing interest in the role of sex hormones, particularly testosterone, and cognition in older men. Several small trials of testosterone in older men have reported improvement in some, but not in all, cognitive domains. Janowsky and colleagues reported benefits in visuospatial abilities in a trial of older men randomized to testosterone or to placebo for 3 months[37]. This group more recently reported that testosterone improved working memory in older men, and that this improvement was positively associated with serum free testosterone level[38]. In another small trial enrolling healthy men, serum levels of testosterone and estradiol increased among those receiving testosterone, and improvements were noted for spatial memory, verbal memory and visuospatial ability[39]. It was not clear whether these better scores were a result of increases in testosterone directly or because of conversion to estradiol. Another trial failed to observe an improvement of cognitive function with testosterone[40]. The conflicting results may be due to small sample sizes, differences in types of cognitive tests and infrequent measurement of the forms of sex hormones available to the brain (free or bioavailable).

ANDROGEN RECEPTOR POLYMORPHISMS MAY BE LINKED TO COGNITION IN MEN

The AR gene contains a CAG repeat polymorphism within exon 1 that encodes a polyglutamate sequence of variable length in the transcriptional activation domain of the receptor[41]. The polymorphism influences AR transcriptional activity, with longer repeat length conferring relative androgen resistance *in vitro*[42,43]. This polymorphism may also influence androgen sensitivity *in vivo*, since longer repeat length has been associated with a decreased risk of prostate cancer and hyperplasia[44,45] and increased risk of osteoporosis in men[46]. Data on the AR polymorphism and its effects on clinical outcomes in women are lacking, although in premenopausal women, those with fewer CAG repeats have higher serum levels of total testosterone[47].

We recently investigated the association between CAG repeat length on the AR gene and cognitive function in older community-dwelling non-demented men. Among the 301 men (mean age 73.0 ± 7.1 years), greater CAG repeat length was associated with lower scores in all three cognitive tests (Mini-Mental Status Exam, Trails B, Digit Symbol) ($p < 0.05$ for all). In addition, 12 participants had cognitive impairment in the low tertile of CAG repeat length, whereas 29 had cognitive impairment in the two higher tertiles (OR 1.8, 95% CI 0.9–3.7)[48]. This supports the hypothesis that longer CAG repeat length in the AR gene is associated with lower cognitive functioning.

Several mechanisms could explain the relationship between longer CAG repeat length in the AR gene and lower cognition. Increased number of CAG repeats may influence androgen sensitivity by decreasing the ability of the AR to *trans*-activate androgen target genes[49]. In keeping with this, CAG repeats may modulate serum levels of testosterone, and this could affect cognition either directly[39] or by conversion to estradiol via aromatase. Longer CAG repeat length may also decrease cognitive functioning by promoting neurodegeneration, since, in rodent models, androgen receptor polyglutamine expansion induces neuronal dysfunction[50]. Finally, it may be possible that the CAG repeat is in linkage disequilibrium with alleles in a nearby gene that influences cognition.

CONCLUSIONS

If sex hormones play a role in the prevention of AD and other cognitive decline, it is likely that genetic variations in sex hormone receptors and metabolic genes are linked to risk of AD and cognitive decline. Preliminary data support an association between several ERα polymorphisms and risk of AD and cognitive decline in older women. Moreover, the CAG repeat polymorphism on AR exon 1 is associated with cognitive performance in older men. Further research should determine the mechanism for these associations. An important broader consideration is whether there are genetic factors in sex hormone pathways that modulate cognitive decline and the response to endogenous steroids in cognition. Indeed, the recent report from the National Institutes of Health-sponsored Genetics, Response and Cognitive Enhancers: Implications for Alzheimer's Disease Expert Panel highlights the need for more research into the genetics of AD. In particular, the Panel emphasized the need to investigate the role of ethnicity and genetic markers of AD and other cognitive impairment. Very little is known about allele frequencies of sex hormone-related polymorphisms in non-white populations, and almost nothing is known about how these polymorphisms may impact upon cognitive decline in non-white elders. If sex hormone-related polymorphisms are associated with cognitive decline, especially via an alteration in sex hormone level, it would enable identification of individuals who might benefit preferentially from hormone replacement in aging or those who might be especially sensitive to side-effects of hormone replacement.

References

1. Evans DA. Estimated prevalence of Alzheimer's disease in the United States. *Milbank Q* 1990;68: 267–89
2. Brandi ML, Becherini L, Gennari L, *et al.* Association of the estrogen receptor α gene polymorphisms with sporadic Alzheimer's disease. *Biochem Biophys Res Commun* 1999;265:335–8
3. Shughrue PJ, Lane MV, Merchenthaler I. Comparative distribution of estrogen receptor-α and -β mRNA in the rat central nervous system. *J Comp Neurol* 1997;388:507–25
4. Stoffel-Wagner B. Neurosteroid metabolism in the human brain. *Eur J Endocrinol* 2001;145:669–79
5. Fugger HN, Foster TC, Gustafsson J, Rissman EF. Novel effects of estradiol and estrogen receptor α and β on cognitive function. *Brain Res* 2000; 883:258–64
6. Savaskan E, Olivieri G, Meier F, Ravid R, Muller-Spahn F. Hippocampal estrogen β-receptor immunoreactivity is increased in Alzheimer's disease. *Brain Res* 2001;908:113–19
7. Osterlund MK, Grandien K, Keller E, Hurd YL. The human brain has distinct regional expression patterns of estrogen receptor α mRNA isoforms derived from alternative promoters. *J Neurochem* 2000;75:1390–7
8. Simerly R, Chang C, Muramatsu M, Swanson L. Distribution of androgen and estrogen receptor mRNA-containing cells in the rat brain: an *in situ* hybridization study. *J Comp Neurol* 1990; 294:76–95
9. Wozniak A, Hutchison RE, Morris CM, Hutchison JB. Neuroblastoma and Alzheimer's disease brain cells contain aromatase activity. *Steroids* 1998;63: 263–7
10. Gibbs RB, Hashash A, Johnson DA. Effects of estrogen on potassium-stimulated acetylcholine release in the hippocampus and overlying cortex of adult rats. *Brain Res* 1997;749:143–6
11. Luine VN. Estradiol increases choline acetyltransferase activity in specific basal forebrain nuclei and projection areas of female rats. *Exp Neurol* 1985;89:484–90
12. Flood JF, Farr SA, Kaiser FE, La Regina M, Morley JE. Age-related decrease of plasma testosterone in SAMP8 mice: replacement improves age-related impairment of learning and memory. *Physiol Behav* 1995;57:669–73

13. McEwen BS. Clinical review 108: the molecular and neuroanatomical basis for estrogen effects in the central nervous system. *J Clin Endocrinol Metab* 1999;84:1790–7
14. Matsumoto A. Synaptogenic action of sex steroids in developing and adult neuroendocrine brain. *Psychoneuroendocrinology* 1991;16:25–40
15. Behl C, Skutella T, Lezoualc'h F, *et al.* Neuroprotection against oxidative stress by estrogens: structure-activity relationship. *Mol Pharmacol* 1997;51:535–41
16. Pike CJ. Testosterone attenuates β-amyloid toxicity in cultured hippocampal neurons. *Brain Res* 2001; 919:160–5
17. Xu H, Gouras GK, Greenfield JP, *et al.* Estrogen reduces neuronal generation of Alzheimer β-amyloid peptides. *Nat Med* 1998;4:447–51
18. Gouras GK, Xu H, Gross RS, *et al.* Testosterone reduces neuronal secretion of Alzheimer's β-amyloid peptides. *Proc Natl Acad Sci USA* 2000; 97:1202–5
19. Resnick SM, Metter EJ, Zonderman AB. Estrogen replacement therapy and longitudinal decline in visual memory. A possible protective effect? *Neurology* 1997;49:1491–7
20. Sherwin BB. Estrogen and/or androgen replacement therapy and cognitive functioning in surgically menopausal women. *Psychoneuroendocrinology* 1988;13:345–57
21. Tang MX, Jacobs D, Stern Y, *et al.* Effect of oestrogen during menopause on risk and age at onset of Alzheimer's disease. *Lancet* 1996;348:429–32
22. Kawas C, Resnick S, Morrison A, *et al.* A prospective study of estrogen replacement therapy and the risk of developing Alzheimer's disease: the Baltimore Longitudinal Study of Aging. *Neurology* 1997;48:1517–21
23. Farrer LA, Cupples LA, Haines JL, *et al.* Effects of age, sex, and ethnicity on the association between apolipoprotein E genotype and Alzheimer disease. A meta-analysis. APOE and Alzheimer Disease Meta Analysis Consortium. *J Am Med Assoc* 1997;278:1349–56
24. Albagha OM, McGuigan FE, Reid DM, Ralston SH. Estrogen receptor α gene polymorphisms and bone mineral density: haplotype analysis in women from the United Kingdom. *J Bone Miner Res* 2001;16:128–34
25. Maruyama H, Toji H, Harrington CR, *et al.* Lack of an association of estrogen receptor α gene polymorphisms and transcriptional activity with Alzheimer disease. *Arch Neurol* 2000;57:236–40
26. Anderson TI, Wooster R, Laake K, *et al.* Screening for ESR mutations in breast and ovarian cancer patients. *Hum Mutat* 1997;9:531–6
27. Deng HW, Li J, Li JL, Johnson M, Gong G, Recker RR. Association of VDR and estrogen receptor genotypes with bone mass in postmenopausal Caucasian women: different conclusions with different analyses and the implications. *Osteoporos Int* 1999;9:499–507
28. Georgiou I, Syrrou M, Bouba I, *et al.* Association of estrogen receptor gene polymorphisms with endometriosis. *Fertil Steril* 1999;72:164–6
29. Isoe-Wada K, Maeda M, Yong J, *et al.* Positive association between an estrogen receptor gene polymorphism and Parkinson's disease with dementia. *Eur J Neurol* 1999;6:431–5
30. Mattila KM, Axelman K, Rinne JO, *et al.* Interaction between estrogen receptor 1 and the ε4 allele of apolipoprotein E increases the risk of familial Alzheimer's disease in women. *Neurosci Lett* 2000; 282:45–8
31. Lambert JC, Harris JM, Mann D, *et al.* Are the estrogen receptors involved in Alzheimer's disease? *Neurosci Lett* 2001;306:193–7
32. Yaffe K, Lui L, Grady D, Stone K, Morin P. Estrogen receptor I polymorphisms and risk of cognitive impairment in older women. *Biol Psychiatry* 2002;51:677–82
33. Yaffe K, Lui L-Y, Grady D, Cauley J, Kramer J, Cummings S. Cognitive decline in women in relation to non-protein-bound oestradiol concentrations. *Lancet* 2000;356:708–12
34. Yaffe K, Haan M, Byers A, Tangen C, Kuller L. Estrogen use, APOE, and cognitive decline: evidence of gene-environment interaction. *Neurology* 2000;54:1949–54
35. Srivastava RA, Srivastava N, Averna M, *et al.* Estrogen up-regulates apolipoprotein E (ApoE) gene expression by increasing ApoE mRNA in the translating pool via the estrogen receptor α-mediated pathway. *J Biol Chem* 1997;272:33360–6
36. Stone DJ, Rozovsky I, Morgan TE, Anderson CP, Finch CE. Increased synaptic sprouting in response to estrogen via an apolipoprotein E-dependent mechanism: implications for Alzheimer's disease. *J Neurosci* 1998;18:3180–5
37. Janowsky JS, Oviatt SK, Orwoll ES. Testosterone influences spatial cognition in older men. *Behav Neurosci* 1994;108:325–32
38. Janowsky JS, Chavez B, Orwoll E. Sex steroids modify working memory. *J Cogn Neurosci* 2000; 12:407–14
39. Cherrier MM, Asthana S, Plymate S, *et al.* Testosterone supplementation improves spatial and verbal memory in healthy older men. *Neurology* 2001;57:80–8
40. Wolf OT, Preut R, Hellhammer DH, Kudielka BM, Schurmeyer TH, Kirschbaum C. Testosterone and cognition in elderly men: a single testosterone injection blocks the practice effect in verbal fluency, but has no effect on spatial or verbal memory. *Biol Psychiatry* 2000;47:650–4
41. La Spada AR, Wilson EM, Lubahn DB, Harding AE, Fischbeck KH. Androgen receptor gene mutations in X-linked spinal and bulbar muscular atrophy. *Nature (London)* 1991;352:77–9

42. Chamberlain NL, Driver ED, Miesfeld RL. The length and location of CAG trinucleotide repeats in the androgen receptor N-terminal domain affect *trans*activation function. *Nucleic Acids Res* 1994; 22:3181-6
43. Kazemi-Esfarjani P, Trifiro MA, Pinsky L. Evidence for a repressive function of the long polyglutamine tract in the human androgen receptor: possible pathogenetic relevance for the (CAG)n-expanded neuronopathies. *Hum Mol Genet* 1995;4:523-7
44. Giovannucci E, Stampfer MJ, Krithivas K, *et al.* The CAG repeat within the androgen receptor gene and its relationship to prostate cancer. *Proc Natl Acad Sci USA* 1997;94:3320-3
45. Giovannucci E, Platz EA, Stampfer MJ, *et al.* The CAG repeat within the androgen receptor gene and benign prostatic hyperplasia. *Urology* 1999;53: 121-5
46. Zmuda JM, Cauley JA, Kuller LH, *et al.* Androgen receptor CAG repeat polymorphism: a novel molecular marker of osteoporotic risk in men. *Osteoporos Int* 2000;11:S151(abstr)
47. Westberg L, Baghaei F, Rosmond R, *et al.* Polymorphisms of the androgen receptor gene and the estrogen receptor β gene are associated with androgen levels in women. *J Clin Endocrinol Metab* 2001;86:2562-8
48. Yaffe K, Edwards E, Lui L, Zmuda JM, Ferrell RE, Cauley JA. Androgen receptor CAG repeat polymorphism is associated with cognitive function in older men. *Biol Psychiatry* 2003;in press
49. Tut TG, Ghadessy FJ, Trifiro MA, Pinsky L, Yong EL. Long polyglutamine tracts in the androgen receptor are associated with reduced *trans*-activation, impaired sperm production, and male infertility. *J Clin Endocrinol Metab* 1997;82:3777-82
50. Adachi H, Kume A, Li M, *et al.* Transgenic mice with an expanded CAG repeat controlled by the human AR promoter show polyglutamine nuclear inclusions and neuronal dysfunction without neuronal cell death. *Hum Mol Genet* 2001;10: 1039-48

Menopause: risk factor for memory loss or Alzheimer's disease? 23

V. W. Henderson

INTRODUCTION

Menopause represents the permanent cessation of menstruation due to the loss of ovarian follicular function. The ovaries are the source of gonadal hormones, including estradiol and progesterone. Mean serum concentrations of estradiol begin to decline a year or so before the final menstrual period, and within 2 years levels have fallen to about 10% of values characteristic of the reproductive years[1,2]. Since natural menopause occurs at a mean age of about 51 years, endogenous estrogen production is quite low well before most women reach age 60. This change in the hormonal milieu affects a variety of reproductive and non-reproductive tissues, including the central nervous system.

In the brain, as in other target organ systems, estrogen interacts with specific intranuclear receptors to regulate transcription of target genes, and many neurons express receptors for estrogen, either estrogen receptor α or estrogen receptor β[3]. Some central nervous system effects of estrogen occur within a matter of seconds or minutes. These responses may be too rapid to implicate genomic activation, and may instead represent non-genomic effects mediated through estrogen receptors located within the cell membrane[4]. Estrogen also influences brain functions indirectly, through actions on non-neuronal tissues, including glial cells, the cerebral vasculature and the immune system[5].

Because estrogen has the potential to exert profound effects on the brain, estrogen loss after the menopause thus has the potential to affect a number of disorders, including memory deficits that occur during the course of aging and severe cognitive impairment characteristic of Alzheimer's disease. However, as described below, it is still controversial whether hormonal changes associated with the menopause, or the use of estrogen-containing hormone therapy after the menopause, have substantial, long-term effects on either memory or Alzheimer's disease.

MENOPAUSE, HORMONE THERAPY AND MEMORY LOSS

There are several neural systems for learning and memory. The most important of these is concerned with a kind of memory referred to as 'episodic' memory. Episodic memory represents the ability to learn new information presented during a discrete episode and then consciously recall this information after an interval of several minutes or more[6]. For many persons, mild decrements in episodic memory begin in midlife and become more apparent during old age. This age-associated decline is generally much smaller than obvious deficits found in persons with dementia, and memory changes that represent 'usual' accompaniments of aging are not usually viewed as pathological. For Alzheimer's disease, the most prevalent form of dementia, episodic memory impairment is usually severe, and substantial memory problems are often evident even in preclinical stages of the disorder. Indeed, episodic memory deficits are viewed as an early marker for Alzheimer's disease[7].

Animal studies, as well as data from human patients, indicate that episodic memory is critically dependent upon the integrity of the hippocampus and other structures in the medial temporal lobes of the cerebral hemispheres[6]. Estrogen affects the hippocampus in a manner that would be predicted to enhance episodic memory. These include actions on neurogenesis[8], synaptic plasticity[9], long-term potentiation[10], acetylcholine[11] and regional cerebral blood flow[12]. In several behavioral paradigms designed to assess learning and memory in ovariectomized rodents, memory performance is enhanced by estrogen administration[13-15].

Memory during the menopausal transition and early postmenopause

Memory complaints are common during the climacteric[16], but few studies have assessed memory objectively in women around the time of the menopause. Two small randomized controlled trials report beneficial effects of estrogen begun immediately after a surgical menopause[17,18]. When tested after intervals of up to 3 months in these trials, women randomized to estrogen therapy performed better on several tasks than those receiving placebo. For episodic memory, estrogen effects were more apparent when testing involved recall of verbal, as opposed to non-verbal, information[17,18].

In contrast to the abrupt loss of estrogen associated with an induced menopause, a natural menopause may not lead to substantial deficits in episodic memory, at least when assessed during the early postmenopausal period. Verbal memory was recently studied among participants in the Melbourne Women's Midlife Health Project[19]. For this population-derived cohort, eligible women were initially 45–55 years of age, menstruating and not taking hormone therapy. Memory was assessed 8 years after cohort inception. Women who had undergone a surgical menopause were excluded, but 326 other participants were administered a ten-item word-list memory task (three immediate recall trials and one delayed recall trial)[19]. Recall scores did not differ significantly among current, past and never-users of hormone therapy. However, *post hoc* analyses suggested that timing of hormone therapy might be important. Memory scores were better for women who began hormone therapy during the menopausal transition before their last menstrual period than for those who began hormone therapy after the menopause[19]. Mean immediate recall scores were 21.8 words in the early starters compared with 19.8 in the late starters ($p = 0.03$), and mean delayed recall scores were 8.0 words versus 7.3 ($p = 0.1$).

Memory during the late postmenopause

There are some hints from the clinical literature - but no strong evidence at present - that early use of hormone therapy could be relevant to cognitive performance in the late postmenopausal period. Some observational studies find no consistent benefit of hormone therapy in older women[20,21]. Among observational studies that do suggest a beneficial effect of hormone therapy on cognition, past use appears to be as effective as current use[22-24]. In Cache County, Utah, 2073 older women were tested on two occasions 3 years apart[24]. In this particular cohort, hormone therapy use was associated with less decline on a general cognitive measure. Current hormone therapy users performed equivalently to former hormone therapy users; recent use of hormone therapy was no more beneficial than more remote use; and longer use of hormone therapy was equivalent to shorter use[24]. In another prospective cohort study, 9651 older women were tested on two occasions 4-6 years apart[23]. At baseline, both current and past hormone therapy users performed better on a global cognitive measure than never-users. On follow-up, only past users showed milder declines than never-users. These findings, if valid, imply that past hormone therapy use might be equivalent to current use in terms of reducing age-associated cognitive decline, and also imply no additional cognitive benefit for long-term use. These findings must be interpreted cautiously, however, as observational studies are subject to unrecognized confounding and important biases.

Among older women, several studies of episodic memory have been conducted as randomized, double-blind, placebo-controlled trials, and here the evidence indicates no important effect of estrogen[25]. Among 52 women (mean age 81 years) who completed a 9-month study of unopposed estrogen versus placebo, there was no difference between treatment groups on a paired associate learning task[26]. Similarly, secondary analyses in a randomized controlled trial of 1063 women with coronary heart disease revealed no significant effect of estrogen plus progestin on word-list learning[27].

The Women's Health Initiative Memory Study (WHIMS) assessed the effects of estrogen plus progestin using a global cognitive measure[28]. Memory was not separately evaluated. In this randomized, placebo-controlled trial, 4532 women aged 65–79 were followed for approximately 4 years. During this time, cognitive scores tended to increase, presumably related to practice effects. However, the rate of increase was slightly but significantly diminished in the hormone therapy arm compared to the placebo group[28].

MENOPAUSE, HORMONE THERAPY AND ALZHEIMER'S DISEASE

Alzheimer's disease is rare before the age of menopause, but its prevalence increases exponentially over the ensuing four decades. Most studies do not show a relationship between age at menopause and the subsequent development of Alzheimer's disease. The prevalence of Alzheimer's disease for women is approximately twice that for men[29], in part because of sex differences in longevity. However, Alzheimer incidence also appears to be increased for women[30], especially among the very old[31,32].

Theoretically, neurotrophic and neuroprotective effects of estrogen might benefit Alzheimer's disease[5]. Drugs that increase cholinergic activity in the brain are therapeutically useful in Alzheimer's disease[33]; basal forebrain cholinergic neurons express estrogen receptors[34]; and estrogen helps to maintain the cholinergic neurotransmitter system after experimental lesions[11]. Protection against apoptosis[35] and oxidative stress[36] is also relevant to Alzheimer treatment and prevention. In animals, estrogen reduces accumulation of β-amyloid[37], an abnormal protein found in the Alzheimer brain.

Alzheimer's disease treatment

Observational studies imply that hormone therapy may be associated with milder cognitive deficits in women diagnosed with Alzheimer's disease[38,39]. However, this conclusion is not supported by results from randomized, placebo-controlled clinical trials. Decidedly negative findings were reported from clinical trials of estrogen involving 42 women treated for 4 months[40], 50 women treated for 3 months[41] and 120 women without a uterus treated for 12 months[42]. Positive findings for estrogen were reported from a 3-week study of 14 demented women[43] and mixed findings from an 8-week trial of 20 women with Alzheimer's disease[44]. One interesting difference between positive observational studies and the generally negative clinical trials is that, in the former, hormone therapy is likely to have been used for a number of years, presumably antedating Alzheimer symptoms in many instances. This difference is consistent with the argument that early hormone therapy use could lead to milder dementia symptoms later on, but in the absence of additional evidence, this supposition is tenuous.

Alzheimer's disease prevention

A number of observational studies indicate an association between women who have ever used hormone therapy and a reduced Alzheimer risk. In meta-analyses, estimates of overall Alzheimer risk reduction range from 34 to 44%[45,46]. Most of these studies have considered current hormone therapy users and past users as one combined group, but these two groups were analyzed separately in the Cache County cohort[32]. Here, 1889 women, whose mean age was 75 years, were without dementia at baseline. Eighty-eight cases of Alzheimer's disease were identified during a 3-year follow-up period, and ever-use of hormone therapy was associated with a significant overall risk reduction (relative risk estimate 0.41). However, this association was significant only for past users of hormone therapy (relative risk 0.33) and not for current users (relative risk 1.1)[32].

Two important negative studies of hormone therapy and Alzheimer's disease risk involved the use of computerized pharmacy databases. The first of these, conducted in a US health maintenance organization, identified 107 women with incident Alzheimer's disease and 120 matched controls (mean age approximately 77 years)[47]. The second study, which used a general practice research database from the UK, matched 59 women with recently diagnosed Alzheimer's disease to 221 controls (mean age approximately 66 years)[48]. Although both studies provided valid data on recent hormone therapy exposure, obviously neither database was able to assess hormone therapy use before the databases were established. Thus, estrogen exposure during the menopausal transition and early postmenopause could not be captured for older women.

If estrogen-containing hormone therapy protects against Alzheimer's disease, then the duration of hormone therapy treatment might be associated with a greater reduction in Alzheimer risk. In fact, several studies of estrogen exposure support this supposition. Significant associations between the duration of estrogen use and the degree of risk reduction were reported from a nested case-control study in a California retirement community[49], from cohorts in New York City[50] and Cache County, Utah[32], and from a case-control study conducted in Rochester, Minnesota[51]. In the Baltimore Longitudinal Study of Aging, however, there was no connection between duration of hormone therapy use and the magnitude of Alzheimer's disease risk reduction[52]. Because early hormone therapy use is associated with longer use[53], the relationship between duration of hormone therapy use and risk reduction also implies a relationship between earlier hormone therapy use and reduced Alzheimer risk.

The WHIMS trial represents the first randomized clinical trial to test whether postmenopausal hormone therapy actually can reduce dementia risk[54]. Contrary to earlier predictions, findings showed a two-fold increase in dementia risk among study participants who received continuous, combined estrogen plus progestin. Over a 4-year follow-up, 61 women were adjudicated as having dementia (hazard ratio of 2.05, 95% confidence interval of 1.21–3.48). Slightly over half of WHIMS cases were Alzheimer's disease (20 in the active treatment group and 12 in the placebo group). WHIMS did not include women younger than age 65 years, and outcomes have not yet been analyzed for women without a uterus using unopposed estrogen. For this reason, these important WHIMS findings are most directly applicable to older women using estrogen plus a progestin.

CONCLUSIONS AND SPECULATION

Data regarding effects of menopause on memory loss and Alzheimer's disease are incomplete[55]. As described above, limited clinical trial data indicate that estrogen-containing hormone therapy improves memory after abrupt cessation of ovarian function (induced menopause), but evidence is less secure after a natural menopause. In particular, clinical trial evidence shows that estrogen plus a progestin initiated in the late postmenopause does not benefit global cognition.

Limited data from randomized controlled trials in women with Alzheimer's disease do not support a role for hormone therapy begun after the onset of dementia symptoms. Although observational data imply that hormone therapy users face a reduced Alzeheimer risk, results from the WHIMS clinical trial show that estrogen plus progestin increases overall dementia risk when initiated in older postmenopausal women. Results from women treated with unopposed estrogen will not be available from the WHIMS trial for several years, and no current clinical trial addresses issues concerning timing of hormone therapy initiation.

Most women begin hormone therapy near the time of the menopause, and continue hormone therapy for only a relatively short period of time. In the third National Health and Nutrition Examination Survey conducted in the USA between 1988 and 1994, only 15% of women initiated hormone therapy more than 1 year after their final menstrual period[56]. Among women at least 10 years beyond the menopause, 24% of hormone therapy use was for less than 1 year and 34% was for 1–5 years; only 42% of women reported use of hormone therapy for more than 5 years[56].

This pattern of hormone therapy use raises questions about observational studies in older women that link ever-use of hormone therapy with putative cognitive benefit, and randomized trials that have failed to confirm benefit. For both memory and Alzheimer's disease, positive associations of course may be spurious, reflecting bias (e.g. the healthy-user bias) or confounding. Indeed, this is the most reasonable explanation for some of the discrepancies between observational and experimental results. However, these intriguing data also suggest the possibility that early hormone therapy use, perhaps initiated during a so-called critical window in the menopausal transition or early postmenopausal period[57], could benefit memory in later years or could have a favorable impact on Alzheimer's disease risk. At present, this perspective is purely speculative and should not be used as a basis for clinical decisions. Further research into the menopause and hormone therapy may clarify any relationship between timing or duration of hormone therapy exposure and age-associated memory loss or Alzheimer's disease.

ACKNOWLEDGEMENT

Studies from the Melbourne Women's Midlife Health Project were supported in part by Alzheimer's Association grant IIRG-01-2684.

References

1. Judd HL, Judd GE, Lucas WE, Yen SSC. Endocrine function of the postmenopausal ovary: concentration of androgens and estrogens in ovarian and peripheral vein blood. *J Clin Endocrinol Metab* 1974;39:1020–4
2. Trévoux R, De Brux J, Castanier M, Nahoul K, Soule J-P, Scholler R. Endometrium and plasma hormone profile in the perimenopause and postmenopause. *Maturitas* 1986;8:309–26
3. Shughrue PJ, Lane MV, Merchenthaler I. Comparative distribution of estrogen receptor-α and -β mRNA in the rat central nervous system. *J Comp Neurol* 1997;388:507–25
4. Wong M, Thompson TL, Moss RL. Nongenomic actions of estrogen in the brain: physiological significance and cellular mechanisms. *Crit Rev Neurobiol* 1996;10:189–203
5. Henderson VW. *Hormone Therapy and the Brain: A Clinical Perspective on the Role of Estrogen*. New York: Parthenon Publishing, 2000
6. Squire LT, Zola-Morgan S. The medial temporal lobe memory system. *Science* 1991;253:1380–6
7. Petersen RC, Doody R, Kurz A, *et al.* Current concepts in mild cognitive impairment. *Arch Neurol* 2001;58:1985–92
8. Tanapat P, Hastings NB, Reeves AJ, Gould E. Estrogen stimulates a transient increase in the number of new neurons in the dentate gyrus of the adult female rat. *J Neurosci* 1999;19:5792–801
9. Foy MR, Henderson VW, Berger TW, Thompson RF. Estrogen and neural plasticity. *Curr Direct Psychol Sci* 2000;9:148–52
10. Foy MR, Xu J, Xie X, Brinton RD, Thompson RF, Berger TW. 17β-Estradiol enhances NMDA receptor-mediated EPSPs and long-term potentiation. *J Neurophysiol* 1999;81:925–9
11. Luine V. Estradiol increases choline acetyltransferase activity in specific basal forebrain nuclei and projection areas of female rats. *Exp Neurol* 1985;89:484–90
12. Maki PM, Resnick SM. Longitudinal effects of estrogen replacement therapy on PET cerebral blood flow and cognition. *Neurobiol Aging* 2000; 21:373–83
13. Fader AJ, Hendricson AW, Dohanich GP. Estrogen improves performance of reinforced T-maze alternation and prevents the amnestic effects of scopolamine administered systemically or intrahippocampally. *Neurobiol Learn Mem* 1998;69: 225–40
14. Singh M, Meyer EM, Millard WJ, Simpkins JW. Ovarian steroid deprivation results in a reversible learning impairment and compromised cholinergic function in female Sprague–Dawley rats. *Brain Res* 1994;644:305–12
15. Gibbs RB. Long-term treatment with estrogen and progesterone enhances acquisition of a spatial memory task by ovariectomized aged rats. *Neurobiol Aging* 2000;21:107–16
16. Woods NF, Mitchell ES, Adams C. Memory functioning among midlife women: observations from the Seattle Midlife Women's Health Study. *Menopause* 2000;7:257–65
17. Sherwin BB. Estrogen and/or androgen replacement therapy and cognitive functioning in surgically menopausal women. *Psychoneuroendocrinology* 1988;13:345–57
18. Phillips SM, Sherwin BB. Effects of estrogen on memory function in surgically menopausal women. *Psychoneuroendocrinology* 1992;17:485–95
19. Henderson VW, Dudley EC, Guthrie JR, Burger HG, Dennerstein L. Estrogen exposures and

memory at midlife: a population-based study of women. *Neurology* 2003;60:1369–71

20. Barrett-Connor E, Kritz-Silverstein D. Estrogen replacement therapy and cognitive function in older women. *J Am Med Assoc* 1993;269:2637–41
21. Grodstein F, Chen J, Pollen DA, *et al.* Post-menopausal hormone therapy and cognitive function in healthy older women. *J Am Geriatr Soc* 2000;48:746–52
22. Jacobs DM, Tang MX, Stern Y, *et al.* Cognitive function in nondemented older women who took estrogen after menopause. *Neurology* 1998;50: 368–73
23. Matthews K, Cauley J, Yaffe K, Zmuda JM. Estrogen replacement therapy and cognitive decline in older community women. *J Am Geriatr Soc* 1999;47:518–23
24. Carlson MC, Zandi PP, Plassman BL, *et al.* Hormone replacement therapy and reduced cognitive decline in older women: the Cache County study. *Neurology* 2001;57:2210–16
25. Henderson VW. Randomized trials of estrogen for memory and dementia. In Lobo RA, Crosignani PG, Paoletti R, Bruschi F, eds. *Women's Health and Menopause: New Strategies - Improved Quality of Life.* Dordrecht, The Netherlands: Kluwer Academic Publishers, 2002:279–90
26. Binder EF, Schechtman KB, Birge SJ, Williams DB, Kohrt WM. Effects of hormone replacement therapy on cognitive performance in elderly women. *Maturitas* 2001;38:137–46
27. Grady D, Yaffe K, Kristof M, Lin F, Richards C, Barrett-Connor E. Effect of postmenopausal hormone therapy on cognitive function: the Heart and Estrogen/progestin Replacement Study. *Am J Med* 2002,113.543–8
28. Rapp SR, Espeland MA, Shumaker SA, *et al.* The effect of estrogen with progestin treatment on global cognitive function in postmenopausal women: results from the Women's Health Initiative Memory Study. *J Am Med Assoc* 2003;289:2663–72
29. Jorm AF, Korten AE, Henderson AS. The prevalence of dementia: a quantitative integration of the literature. *Acta Psychiatr Scand* 1987;76:465–79
30. Gao S, Hendrie HC, Hall KS, Hui S. The relationships between age, sex, and incidence of dementia and Alzheimer disease: a meta-analysis. *Arch Gen Psychiatry* 1998;55:809–15
31. Fratiglioni L, Viitanen M, von Strauss E, Tontodonati V, Herlitz A, Winblad B. Very old women at highest risk of dementia and Alzheimer's disease: incidence data from the Kungsholmen Project, Stockholm. *Neurology* 1997;48:132–8
32. Zandi PP, Carlson MC, Plassman BL, *et al.* Hormone replacement therapy and incidence of Alzheimer's disease in older women: the Cache County study. *J Am Med Assoc* 2002;288:2123–9
33. Feldman H, Gauthier S, Hecker J, Vellas B, Subbiah P, Whalen E. A 24-week, randomized, double-blind study of donepezil in moderate to severe Alzheimer's disease. *Neurology* 2001;57:613–20
34. Shughrue PJ, Scrimo PJ, Merchenthaler I. Estrogen binding and estrogen receptor characterization (ERα and ERβ) in the cholinergic neurons of the rat basal forebrain. *Neuroscience* 2000;96:41–9
35. Pike CJ. Estrogen modulates neuronal Bcl-x_L expression and β-amyloid-induced apoptosis: relevance to Alzheimer's disease. *J Neurochem* 1999; 72:1552–63
36. Behl C, Skutella T, Lezoualch F, *et al.* Neuroprotection against oxidative stress by estrogens: structure-activity relationship. *Mol Pharmacol* 1997;51:535–41
37. Petanceska SS, Nagy G, Frail D, Gandy S. Ovariectomy and 17β-estradiol modulate the levels of Alzheimer's amyloid β peptides in brain. *Neurology* 2000;54:2212–17
38. Henderson VW, Watt L, Buckwalter JG. Cognitive skills associated with estrogen replacement in women with Alzheimer's disease. *Psychoneuroendocrinology* 1996;21:421–30
39. Doraiswamy PM, Bieber F, Kaiser L, Krishnan KR, Reuning-Scherer J, Gulanski B. The Alzheimer's disease assessment scale: patterns and predictors of baseline cognitive performance in multicenter Alzheimer's disease trials. *Neurology* 1997;48: 1511–17
40. Henderson VW, Paganini-Hill A, Miller BL, *et al.* Estrogen for Alzheimer's disease in women: randomized, double-blind, placebo-controlled trial. *Neurology* 2000;54:295–301
41. Wang PN, Liao SQ, Liu RS, *et al.* Effects of estrogen on cognition, mood, and cerebral blood flow in AD: a controlled study. *Neurology* 2000;54:2061–6
42. Mulnard RA, Cotman CW, Kawas C, *et al.* Estrogen replacement therapy for treatment of mild to moderate Alzheimer disease: a randomized controlled trial. *J Am Med Assoc* 2000;283:1007–15
43. Honjo H, Ogino Y, Tanaka K, *et al.* An effect of conjugated estrogen to cognitive impairment in women with senile dementia - Alzheimer's type: a placebo-controlled double blind study. *J Jpn Menopause Soc* 1993;1:167–71
44. Asthana S, Baker LD, Craft S, *et al.* High-dose estradiol improves cognition for women with AD: results of a randomized study. *Neurology* 2001;57:605–12
45. LeBlanc ES, Janowsky J, Chan BKS, Nelson HD. Hormone replacement therapy and cognition: systemic review and meta-analysis. *J Am Med Assoc* 2001;285:1489–99
46. Hogervorst E, Williams J, Budge M, Riedel W, Jolles J. The nature of the effect of female gonadal hormone replacement therapy on cognitive function in postmenopausal women: a meta-analysis. *Neuroscience* 2000;101:485–512
47. Brenner DE, Kukull WA, Stergachis A, *et al.* Postmenopausal estrogen replacement therapy

and the risk of Alzheimer's disease: a population-based case-control study. *Am J Epidemiol* 1994; 140:262-7
48. Seshadri S, Zomberg GL, Derby LE, Myers MW, Jick H, Drachman DA. Postmenopausal estrogen replacement therapy and the risk of Alzheimer's disease. *Arch Neurol* 2001;58:435-40
49. Paganini-Hill A, Henderson VW. Estrogen replacement therapy and risk of Alzheimer's disease. *Arch Intern Med* 1996;156:2213-17
50. Tang M-X, Jacobs D, Stern Y, *et al.* Effect of oestrogen during menopause on risk and age at onset of Alzheimer's disease. *Lancet* 1996;348: 429-32
51. Waring SC, Rocca WA, Petersen RC, O'Brien PC, Tangalos EG, Kokmen E. Postmenopausal estrogen replacement therapy and risk of AD: a population-based study. *Neurology* 1999;52:965-70
52. Kawas C, Resnick S, Morrison A, *et al.* A prospective study of estrogen replacement therapy and the risk of developing Alzheimer's disease: the Baltimore Longitudinal Study of Aging. *Neurology* 1997;48:1517-21
53. Ettinger B, Pressman A, Silver P. Effect of age on reasons for initiation and discontinuation of hormone replacement therapy. *Menopause* 1999; 6:282-9
54. Shumaker SA, Legault C, Rapp SR, *et al.* Estrogen plus progestin and the incidence of dementia and mild cognitive impairment in postmenopausal women: the Women's Health Initiative Memory Study (WHIMS). *J Am Med Assoc* 2003;289:2651-62
55. Henderson VW, Klein BEK, Resnick SM. Menopause and disorders of neurologic function, mental health, and the eye. In Wenger NK, Paoletti R, Lenfant CJM, Pinn VW, eds. *International Position Paper on Women's Health and Menopause: A Comprehensive Approach*. Bethesda, MD: National Institutes of Health, 2002;02-3284:251-70
56. Brett KM, Chong Y. *Hormone Replacement Therapy: Knowledge and Use in the United States*. Hyattsville, MD: National Center for Health Statistics, 2001
57. Resnick SM, Henderson VW. Hormone therapy and risk of Alzheimer disease: a critical time. *J Am Med Assoc* 2002;288:2170-2

Depression, aging and the metabolic syndrome

24

P. W. Gold

INTRODUCTORY OVERVIEW

The stress system

Stress precipitates major depression and influences its incidence, severity and course[1,2]. The stress response and major depression share many features because of similar brain circuitries and mediators (reviewed in references 3-5). Each is associated with a diminution of cognitive and affective flexibility, alterations in arousal and perturbations in neuroendocrine and autonomic function (reviewed in reference 5). In addition, we now know that the biologies of the stress response and major depression resemble those of some of the neuroendocrine responses that occur with advancing age.

The stress system promotes survival during threatening situations. Anxiety, fear-related behaviors and heightened vigilance are essential. Cognitive processes shift from complex, sequence-dependent modes to relatively well-rehearsed programs consolidated during exposure to previous stressors. These emotional memories are held in abeyance until exposure to the next significantly stressful situation. Heart rate and blood pressure rise, while neurovegetative phenomena, whose execution would diminish the likelihood of survival during threatening circumstances, are inhibited. These include sleep, food intake, sexual activity and the endocrine programs for growth and reproduction. In some instances, there is an anticipatory activation of coagulation and inflammation.

Any delineation of specific structures in the brain that serves as a discrete stress system is, of course, an oversimplification. The following refers to four components whose effects and interactions have been best elucidated: the medial prefrontal cortex, the amygdala, the locus ceruleus-norepinephrine system (LC-NE) and the corticotropin-releasing hormone (CRH) system/hypothalamic-pituitary-adrenal (HPA) axis.

Components of the stress system

Medial prefrontal cortex and amygdala

Critical central nervous system (CNS) structures that mediate the stress response include the medial prefrontal cortex, the amygdala, the CRH system and brainstem noradrenergic nuclei, especially the locus ceruleus. The medial prefrontal cortex determines whether a situation is likely to result in reward or punishment. It shifts affect appropriately, based on internal or external cues. It is essential for complex cognitive processes such as sequencing and planning. The medial prefrontal cortex is the cortical structure that inhibits the amygdala fear system, the CRH system and the locus ceruleus. Ordinarily, the medial prefrontal cortex keeps amygdala generated in fear in check, and restrains the hypothalamic CRH systems and the locus ceruleus-norepinephrine system. Thus, the medial prefrontal cortex fundamentally restrains the key components of the stress system during ordinary times when the organism is not exposed to dangerous stimuli.

The amygdala plays a key role in activating structures that promote the stress response such as the CRH system and the locus ceruleus-norepinephrine (LC-NE), and inhibits components that restrain the stress system, especially the medial prefrontal cortex. While the amygdala stores only conditioned fear responses, it is crucial for the relay of aversive stimuli for consolidation and storage in higher centers in the brain. The amygdala is essential for the conscious experience of fear. It is restrained by the medial prefrontal cortex, but when activated, also inhibits the functions of the medial prefrontal cortex. Moreover, the amygdala also activates the CRH system and the LC-NE.

Locus ceruleus-norepinephrine system

The LC-NE system is the general alarm system of the brain. It also contributes significantly to selective attention by improving the signal/noise ratio in many key brain structures. The LC-NE system activates the CRH system and the amygdala while inhibiting the medial prefrontal cortex. Rather than playing a role in the higher cognitive and emotional components of the stress response and behavior in general, the LC-NE plays an important role in modulating its intensity. The LC-NE also plays an important role in regulating blood pressure and heart rate. While the LC-NE and the sympathetic nervous system are not synonymous, the LC-NE plays an important role in modulating sympathetic outflow.

Corticotropin-releasing hormone was first isolated as the hypothalamic releasing hormone for the HPA axis. Cortisol is essential for a successful response to stress, and its functions include breaking down tissue and mobilizing fuel for the brain, improving cardiac contractility and tissue responses to norepinephrine, inhibiting programs for growth and reproduction, and activating the amygdala. While the short-term effects of cortisol are of key positive value to survival during stressful situations, its sustained activation is almost always deleterious.

Many possible positive feedback loops are potentially emergent in the stress system, including bidirectional effects of each component on the other and the redundant effects of some structures upon others, such as the amygdala's capacity to activate the CRH and LC-NE systems while inhibiting the prefrontal cortex, essential in restraining the amygdala and the CRH and LC-NE systems.

The corticotropin-releasing hormone system

Corticotropin-releasing hormone was first isolated as the principal hypothalamic hormone that releases corticotropin (or adrenocorticotropic hormone, ACTH), which in turn activates adrenocorticosteroid secretion. Over the years, a series of painstaking studies in rodents has established roles for CRH in the stress response, other than that of HPA axis regulation. These include activation of the locus ceruleus, the sympathetic nervous system and the adrenal medulla, as well as inhibition of a variety of neurovegetative functions such as food intake, sexual activity and the endocrine programs for growth and reproduction (reviewed in references 3, 4 and 6). Extrahypothalamic CRH-containing neurons in the amygdala, although technically outside the core stress system, also play a key role in the stress response by activating fear-related behaviors while inhibiting exploration (reviewed in references 3, 4 and 6). Taken as a whole, CRH in the rat participates in virtually the entire cascade of the physiological and behavioral alterations occurring in response to stressors.

CRH-mediated glucocorticoid secretion has an abundance of adaptive and adverse effects. Acute glucocorticoid secretion during stress plays several roles, including enhancement of cardiovascular function and mobilization of fuel. Cortisol (along with CRH) also significantly contributes to the inhibition of programs for growth and reproduction via inhibition of the growth hormone and gonadal axes, as well as to feedback restraint upon an activated immune system. For the most part, the adaptive advantages conferred by cortisol secretion during stress are limited to its acute rather than chronic release.

MAJOR DEPRESSION

Major depression is a heritable disorder that affects approximately 8% of men and 15% of women[1]. For over 75% of patients, major depression is a recurrent, lifetime illness, characterized by repeated remissions and exacerbations[7]. Over 50% of patients who recover from a first depressive episode will have a second within 6 months unless they are given maintenance antidepressant treatment[2]. For those who never receive treatment, as many as 15% will succumb to suicide[8].

Depression not only causes great mental anguish, but also intrudes upon fundamental biological processes that regulate sleep, appetite, metabolic activity, autonomic function and neuroendocrine regulation (reviewed in references 3, 4 and 9). These disturbances are likely to contribute to premature coronary artery disease[10,11], premature osteoporosis[12] and the doubling of mortality in patients with major depression at any age, independent of suicide, smoking or significant physical illness[10,11].

Classification of major depression

The Diagnostic and Statistical Manual of Mental Disorders IV (DSM IV) lists two distinct clinical depressive syndromes that seem to be the antithesis of one another, melancholic and atypical depression. This distinction is based on the pattern of psychological and neurovegetative symptoms[13], is independent of the unipolar-bipolar distinction and provides direction for the appropriate choice of antidepressant medication[14].

Melancholic depression belies the term depression in that it is a state of pathological hyperarousal. Intense anxiety is often focused on the self, and takes the form of feelings of worthlessness and recollections of past transgressions, failures and helplessness. As a corollary, melancholics are beset by dread about future prospects for so deficient a self. It matters little that their self-assessments and emotional memories are discordant with the facts of their lives. Rather, their feelings of personal deficiency pervade thought and affect (reviewed in references 3, 4 and 6).

Patients with melancholic depression also manifest evidence of physiological hyperarousal such as hypercortisolism, suppression of the growth hormone and reproductive axes, insomnia (most often early-morning awakening) and loss of appetite. Another consistent feature of melancholia is a diurnal variation in the severity of depressed mood, which is greatest early in the morning (reviewed in references 5 and 15). Atypical depression seems to be the antithesis of melancholia, and is characterized by lethargy, fatigue, hyperphagia and hypersomnia. A discussion of atypical depression and its biology is beyond the scope of this chapter. While the findings in depression reported here might be somewhat more common in patients with melancholic depression, only one study refers specifically to data in melancholics.

BIOLOGICAL STUDIES IN MAJOR DEPRESSION

Prefrontal cortex and amygdala in major depression: neuroimaging studies

The principal finding of note in patients with major depression is a significant decrease in the size and metabolic activity of the subgenual prefrontal cortex. This region is particularly involved in estimating the likelihood of punishment or reward, shifting mood from one state to the other, promoting complex cognitive and behavioral sequences rather than relatively reflexive ones. The loss of volume is primarily due to the loss of glial cells. Thus, depression may be, in part, a neurotoxic state. We now know that antidepressant drugs such as depakote, lithium and imipramine are neurotropic, and, hence, may act to replenish some of the cells that have been lost.

Patients with major depression showed increased cerebral blood flow and metabolism in the amygdala[16]. Activation in the left amygdala persisted after recovery from depression. During depression, amygdala activation correlated positively with depression severity and baseline plasma cortisol levels[16]. The latter finding is of interest in light of the fact that the amygdala activates the CRH system. The loss of function in the medial prefrontal cortex disinhibits the amygdala. Increased amygdala function, on the other hand, would inhibit the medial prefrontal cortex. This sets the stage for a reverberatory positive feedback loop.

The locus ceruleus-norepinephrine system in major depression

For many years, the catecholamine hypothesis of major depression predominated, stating that major depression was associated with a pathologically reduced secretion of norepinephrine. These studies failed to take into account heterogeneity in clinical subtypes, the clinical state, the impact of various psychotropic agents and the acquisition of a single data point. Nevertheless, many studies reported decreased norepinephrine secretion. A recent elegant study explored the levels of norepinephrine spillover into carotid artery plasma, and found it to be reduced in a group of patients predominantly non-melancholic. In a group of severely depressed drug-free melancholic patients with prolonged depression, we found a significant increase in around-the-clock levels of cerebrospinal fluid (CSF) norepinephrine that was greatest at night, while patients slept (Figure 1). We subsequently found that these CSF norepinephrine levels fell significantly when patients were studied longitudinally. The increase in an arousal-producing compound in melancholic depression is consistent with a syndrome characterized by pathological hyperarousal.

The corticotropin-releasing hormone system in major depression

The hypercortisolism of depression is one of the most frequent findings in biological psychiatry, although many articles cite normal cortisol levels as well. It is generally accepted that hypothalamic

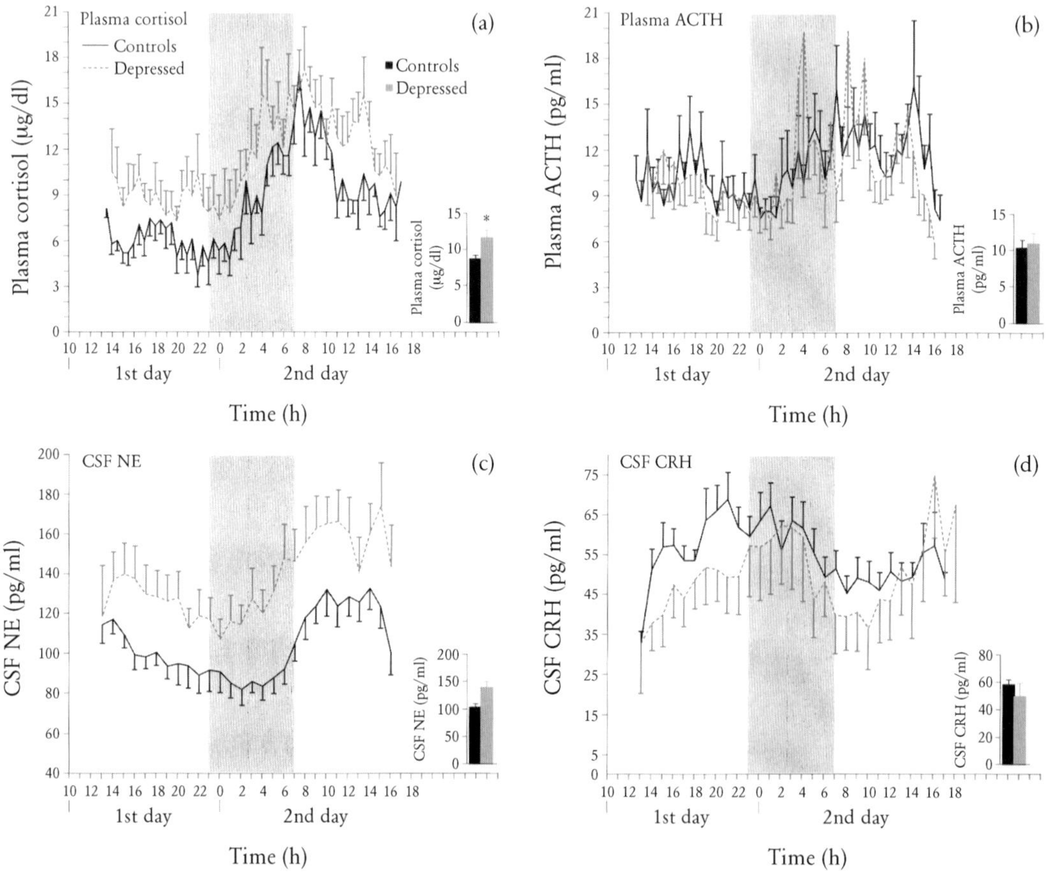

Figure 1 Thirty-hour patterns of cerebrospinal fluid (CSF) corticotropin-releasing hormone (CRH) and norepinephrine (NE) and plasma corticotropin (ACTH) and cortisol in patients with melancholic depression. Diurnal curves of (a) plasma cortisol, (b) plasma ACTH, (c) CSF NE and (d) CSF CRH levels (mean ± SE) in 14 healthy volunteers and ten patients with major depression, melancholic type. Curves are resultant from the averaged measurement per time point across a group of subjects using the cropped hormonal series. The shaded area represents lights off (23.00–07.00). In the right corner inserts under each pair of curves, bar graphs represent the average of the mean value for each series of hormonal measurements (mean ± SE); $^*p < 0.02$. Despite around-the-clock increases in plasma cortisol and CSF NE levels, CSF CRH and plasma ACTH are similar to those in controls, although inappropriately high for the degree of hypercortisolism. Note that the diurnal rhythms for plasma cortisol and CSF NE are virtually superimposable

CRH is elevated in depression. We first reported data consistent with pathological hypersecretion of CRH in patients with depression via stimulation studies with synthetic CRH. Surprisingly, although cortisol levels were elevated, plasma ACTH levels were normal. Holsboer and colleagues subsequently confirmed this finding[17]. Nemeroff and associates found that CSF CRH levels in depressed patients were elevated[18]. Nemeroff and co-workers found that CRH receptor numbers were reduced in the frontal cortex in post-mortem samples taken from patients who had died by suicide[19]. In our group, DeBellis found that fluoxetine significantly lowered CSF CRH levels when depression remitted[20]. In addition, we found that the chronic administration of imipramine to healthy volunteers produced effects compatible with a central down-regulation of the CRH system[21]. Finally, in experimental animals, we showed that the chronic, but not acute, administration of imipramine significantly reduced CRH mRNA levels while significantly increasing mRNA levels of the type I glucocorticoid receptor in the hippocampus, thought to be an important element in the feedback inhibition of the CRH system[9].

In a study of the 30-h pattern of CSF CRH levels in severely depressed in-patient melancholic subjects and normal controls, we found inappropriately 'normal' integrated 30-h CSF CRH concentrations, despite significant hypercortisolism and around-the-clock elevations of CSF norepinephrine[22] (Figure 1). Because the overall pool of CSF CRH and plasma ACTH levels are glucocorticoid-suppressible[15], we previously suggested that quantitatively 'normal' CSF CRH and plasma ACTH levels in the face of hypercortisolism are, nevertheless, inappropriate for the patients' degree of hypercortisolism[23], given significant hypertrophy and hyper-responsiveness of the adrenal to ACTH.

The predominant work on the behavioral and biological effects of CRH has been conducted in rodents. We recently found that the administration of the CRH-R1 receptor antagonist, anatalarmin, significantly reduced the effects of a social stressor in rhesus macaques on anxiety, HPA axis responses and adrenomedullary activation. Antalarmin also significantly decreased the levels of CSF CRH in response to the social stressor (Figure 2).

Interactions among the four components of the stress system and their implications

The confluence of long-term activation of the CRH and noradrenergic systems in depression, in association with glucocorticoid hypersecretion, is a highly pathological state that could readily produce the profound hyperarousal and anxiety that occur in melancholic depression. The capacity for components of the CRH and norepinephrine systems to activate one another and to lead to glucocorticoid excess, and for key components of each (for example, the amygdala CRH neurons) to respond positively to glucocorticoids, establishes the context for a pernicious cycle of stress-mediator activation that can be exceedingly difficult to break. Excessive secretion of norepinephrine and cortisol, regardless of the primary cause, could intensify this pathophysiological picture in several ways. By activating the amygdala and inhibiting the medial prefrontal cortex, norepinephrine would promote well-rehearsed rather than novel programs of behavior, and accentuate the activity of the amygdala. Glucocorticoid excess could set into motion several vicious cycles, including damage to hippocampal glucocorticoid-containing neurons that restrain the HPA axis, activation of the amygdala and extra-amygdala sites involved in conditioned fear and declarative emotionally laden memories (that would in turn lead to more hypercortisolism) and activation of descending hypothalamic CRH pathways to potentiate brainstem noradrenergic activity further.

LONG-TERM MEDICAL CONSEQUENCES OF MAJOR DEPRESSION

Patients with major depression show a doubling of the mortality rate at any age, independent of suicide[10,24]. Premature ischemic heart disease is likely to play an important role, and the relative risk for clinically significant coronary artery disease in patients with major depression is 2.0 or

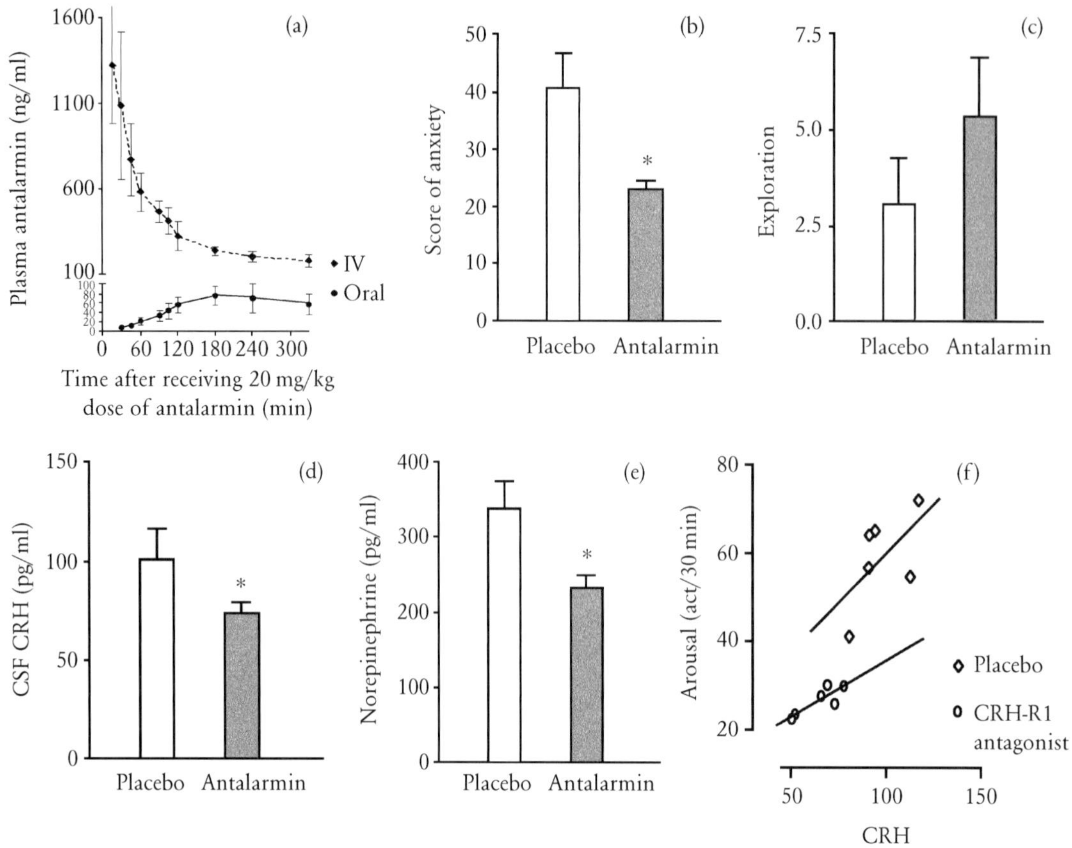

Figure 2 Effects of antalarmin, a non-peptide corticotropin-releasing hormone (CRH) antagonist, on behavioral and physiological responses to a severe social stressor in rhesus macaques (e.g. two unfamiliar male rhesus macaques placed on either side of a plexiglass barrier). Pharmacokinetics of antalarmin in rhesus macaques (a), and the effects of antalarmin to a social stressor on anxiety (b), exploration (c), cerebrospinal fluid (CSF) CRH (d) and plasma norepinephrine (e). Note that for a given level of CSF CRH, anxiety levels in rhesus macaques are significantly reduced (f)

more in studies that independently controlled for risk factors such as smoking and hypertension[10,24].

Potential mechanisms for premature ischemic heart disease in major depression include a vicious spiral between insulin resistance and increased visceral fat, potentially leading to hypertension, dyslipidemia, hypercoagulation and enhanced inflammation[25,26]. Increased sympathetic outflows seen in both our severely depressed in-patients and less severely depressed out-patients also further add to cardiac risk in several other ways. Norepinephrine is well known to promote insulin resistance, left ventricular hypertrophy[27] and increases in myocyte growth, arteriolar and ventricular remodelling[28,29], blood volume and blood viscosity[30]. In addition, norepinephrine also activates platelets and cytokine release and is arrhythmogenic[31].

In a study in which individual controls were matched to each patient based on body mass index, gender, age, race and other factors known to be independent risk factors for osteoporosis, we found that a cohort of over 30% of premenopausal women (average age 41) with severe affective disorder had bone density that was two standard deviations (or 20%) below their peak[12] (for biopsy sample in a 41-year-old woman, see Figure 3). We also showed that these premenopausal women had an almost 40% incidence of premature osteoporosis at either the hip or the spine, which usually occurred in the mid- to late 20s[12]. Ordinarily, bone mineral density does not fall 20% below peak density until women are in their 60s. This finding was associated with a significant increase in plasma cortisol secretion and a significant decrease in the secretion of osteocalcin. Three other studies have also found decreases in bone mineral density with depression. In addition, it was found that depressed patients lost bone faster than did controls, and that depressed men were particularly susceptible to losses in bone mineral density.

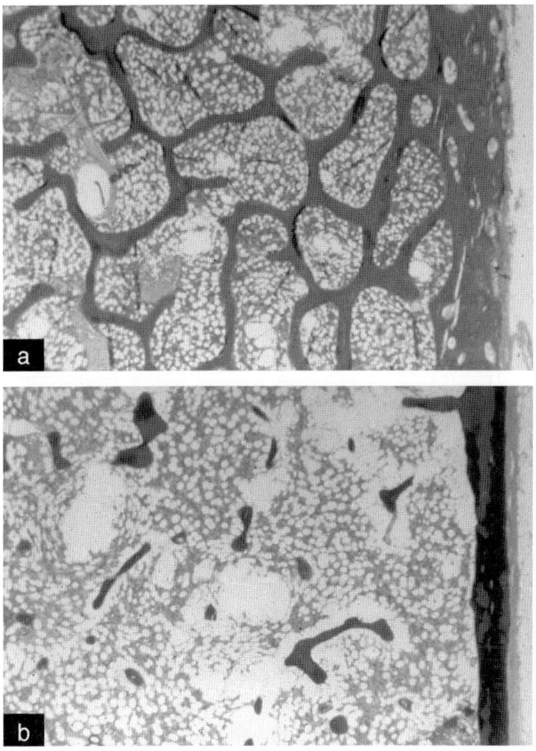

Figure 3 Pathological bone loss in depression. Bone biopsy of the anterior iliac crest of a 40-year-old female with major depression, currently in remission. There are two striking features. The trabeculations are markedly reduced in the depressed patient. These trabeculae are critical scaffolding for the bone and confer much of its strength. Note that the cortex is also thinner in the depressed patient. Ordinarily, glucocorticoids have much more effect on trabeculae *per se* than on the cortex. This suggests that factors other than glucocorticoids are operative in the bone loss of depression. Parenthetically, bone loss in depression is greater in the hip than in the spine. Glucocorticoid-mediated bone loss occurs predominantly in the spine

MAJOR DEPRESSION AND AGING

Aging consists of an age-related deterioration of physiological functions necessary for fertility and survival. There is an inability to compensate for stress or injury, and increased susceptibility to age-related illnesses such as coronary artery disease and osteoporosis. As individuals age, they show decreases in lean body mass, secretion of growth hormone and insulin sensitivity. Advanced age may also be associated with some loss in cognitive and affective flexibility. The extent to which many of these changes reflect loss of function of the prefrontal cortex remains to be determined.

Depression and aging share many features. As noted above, patients with major depression show suppression of the hypogonadal axis and increased mortality, at any age, independent of smoking and other risk factors for poor health. Patients with major depression also have decrements in gonadal function, reduced levels of plasma testosterone and hypothalamic amenorrhea. Such patients also show decreased lean body mass and insulin resistance (Gabry and Gold, unpublished observation). Finally, as noted above, patients with major depression have premature coronary artery disease and osteoporosis

The stress response also overlaps with both depression and aging. It is adaptive during stress to inhibit programs for growth and reproduction, to conserve crucial substrates in the struggle for survival. It is adaptive to be insulin resistant, to supply glucose to the brain and peripheral effectors of the stress response, especially muscle (including myocardium). Elderly individuals, patients with major depression and those under stress are in a catabolic state. The endocrine and autonomic changes in major depression lead gradually to coronary artery disease and osteoporosis. Finally, during stress, it is adaptive to call upon well-rehearsed, relatively stereotyped cognitive processes encoded during previous threatening situations, and to maintain a constant state rather than shifting affective states.

SUMMARY

This chapter presents an overview of data that suggest the possibility that major depression has many features in common not only with the stress response, but also with aging. In an elegant article, Seymour Benzer's group brought together the stress response and aging when they screened for gene mutations that extended life in drosophila. They found that the mutant line methuselah displayed an approximately 35% increase in average life span and enhanced resistance to various forms of stress including starvation, high temperature and free radical generation[32]. Preliminary analysis of the methuselah gene predicted a protein with homology to a well-known family of transmembrane receptors involved in neurotransmission, endocrine regulation and metabolism. In *Caenorhabditis elegans*, life span and stress are also closely associated, and organisms selected for postponed senescence also show increased tolerance to heat, starvation and oxidative damage[32]. Thus, there is likely to be a price for each activation of the stress response, and a higher price for patients with an illness that involves its long-term, more frequent activations.

References

1. Kessler RC, McGonagle KA, Zhao S, *et al.* Lifetime and 12-month prevalence of DSM-III-R psychiatric disorders in the United States. Results from the National Comorbidity Survey. *Arch Gen Psychiatry* 1994;51:8–19
2. Frank E KD, Perel JM, *et al.* Three year outcomes for maintenance in therapies in recurrent depression. *Arch Gen Psychiatry* 1990;47:1093–9
3. Gold PW, Goodwin FK, Chrousos GP. Clinical and biochemical manifestations of depression: relation to the neurobiology of stress (Part 1). *N Engl J Med* 1988;319:348–53
4. Gold PW, Goodwin FK, Chrousos GP. Clinical and biochemical manifestations of depression: relation to the neurobiology of stress (Part 2). *N Engl J Med* 1988;319:413–20
5. Gold P, Chrousos G. The endocrinology of melancholic and atypical depression: relation to neurocircuitry and somatic consequences. *Proc Assoc Am Phys* 1999;111:22–34
6. Chrousos GP, Gold PW. The concepts of stress and stress system disorders. Overview of physical and behavioral homeostasis [published erratum appears in *J Am Med Assoc* 1992;268:200]. *J Am Med Assoc* 1992;267:1244–52
7. Frank EaT, M. Natural history and preventive treatment of recurrent mood disorders. *Annu Rev Med* 1999;50:453–68
8. Guze S, Robins E. Suicide among primary affective disorders. *Br J Psychiatry* 1970;117:433–8
9. Brady LS, Whitfield HJ, Fox RJ, Gold PW, Herkenham M. Long-term antidepressant administration alters corticotropin-releasing hormone, tyrosine hydroxylase, and mineralocorticoid receptor gene expression in rat brain. Therapeutic implications. *J Clin Invest* 1991;87:831–7
10. Barefoot JC, Schroll M. Symptoms of depression, acute myocardial infarction, and total mortality in a community sample [see Comments]. *Circulation* 1996;93:1976–80
11. Penninx BW, Geerlings SW, Deeg DJ, van Eijk JT, van Tilburg W, Beekman AT. Minor and major depression and the risk of death in older persons. *Arch Gen Psychiatry* 1999;56:889–95
12. Michelson D, Stratakis C, Hill L, *et al.* Bone mineral density in women with depression. *N Engl J Med* 1996;335:1176–81
13. Levitan R, Lesage A, Parikh S, Goering P, Kennedy S. Reversed neurovegetative symptoms of depression: a community study. *Am J Psychiatry* 1997; 154:934–40
14. Quitkin FM SJ, McGrath PJ, *et al.* Columbia atypical depression. A subgroup of depressives with better responses to MAOI than to tricyclic antidepressants or placebo. *Br J Psychiatry* 1993; 163(Suppl 21):30–4
15. Gold PW, Licinio J, Wong ML, Chrousos GP. Corticotropin releasing hormone in the pathophysiology of melancholic and atypical depression and in the mechanism of action of antidepressant drugs. *Ann NY Acad Sci* 1995;771:716–29
16. Drevets W, Videen T, al JPe. A functional anatomical study of unipolar depression. *J Neurosci* 1992; 12:3628–41
17. Holsboer F, Girken A, Stalia GK, Muller OA. Blunted corticotropin and normal cortisol

response to human corticotropin-releasing factor in depression. 1984;311:1127
18. Nemeroff CB, Wilderlov E, Bisette G. Elevated concentrations of CSF corticotropin-releasing-factor-like immunoreactivity in depressed patients. 1984;226:1342–4
19. Nemeroff CB, Owens MJ, Bissette G, Andorn AC, Stanley M. Reduced corticotropin releasing factor binding sites in the frontal cortex of suicide victims. *Arch Gen Psychiatry* 1988;45:577–9
20. Kling MA, DeBellis MD, O'Rourke DK, *et al.* Diurnal variation of cerebrospinal fluid immunoreactive corticotropin-releasing hormone levels in healthy volunteers [Published erratum appears in *J Clin Endocrinol Metab* 1994;79:1762]. *J Clin Endocrinol Metab* 1994;79:233–9
21. Michelson D, Galliven E, Hill L, Demitrack M, Chrousos G, Gold P. Chronic imipramine is associated with diminished hypothalamic-pituitary-adrenal axis responsivity in healthy humans. *J Clin Endocrinol Metab* 1997;82:2601–6
22. Wong M-L, Kling MA, Munson PJ, *et al.* Pronounced and sustained central hypernoradrenergic function in major depression with melancholic features: relation to hypercortisolism and corticotropin-releasing hormone. *Proc Natl Acad Sci USA* 2000;97:325–30
23. Gold PW, Gwirtsman H, Avgerinos PC, *et al.* Abnormal hypothalamic-pituitary-adrenal function in anorexia nervosa. Pathophysiologic mechanisms in underweight and weight-corrected patients. *N Engl J Med* 1986;314:1335–42
24. Anda R, Williamson D, Jones D, *et al.* Depressed affect, hopelessness, and the risk of ischemic heart disease in a cohort of US adults [see Comments]. *Epidemiology* 1993;4:285–94
25. Chambers JC, Eda S, Bassett P, *et al.* C-reactive protein, insulin resistance, central obesity, and coronary heart disease risk in Indian Asians from the United Kingdom compared with European whites. *Circulation* 2001;104:145–50
26. Yudkin JS, Kumari M, Humphries SE, Mohamed-Ali V. Inflammation, obesity, stress and coronary heart disease: is interleukin-6 the link? *Atherosclerosis* 2000;148:209–14
27. Sen C, Teumpus R. Cardiac hypertrophy in spontaneously hypertensive rats. *Circ Res* 1974;35:775–81
28. Dzau VJ. Contributions of neuroendocrine and local autocrine-paracrine mechanisms to the pathophysiology and pharmacology of congestive heart failure. *Am J Cardiol* 1988;62:76E–81E
29. Colucci WS. The effects of norepinephrine on myocardial biology: implications for the therapy of heart failure. *Clin Cardiol* 1998;21:I20–4
30. Chababel A, Chien S. Blood viscosity in human hypertension. In Laragh J, Brenner F, eds. *Hypertension: Pathophysiology, Diagnosis, and Treatment.* New York: Raven Press, 1995:365–76
31. Podrid P, Fuchs T, Candinas R. Role of the sympathetic nervous system in the genesis of ventricular arrhythmia. *Circulation* 1990;82:103–13
32. Lin YJ, Seroude L, Benzer S. Extended life-span and stress resistance in the *Drosophila* mutant methuselah. *Science* 1998;282:943–6

Hormone replacement therapy and risk of Parkinson's disease

25

E. Martignoni, R. E. Nappi, D. Calandrella, R. Zagaglia, A. Sommacal, G. Riboldazzi, F. Polatti, C. Pacchetti and G. Nappi

INTRODUCTION

Parkinson's disease (PD) is a quite common degenerative disorder of the nervous system. The clinical picture is mainly due to progressive impairment of the control of movement, which becomes clumsy, slow and tremulous, but alterations of mood, behavior, cognition and autonomic function may also be symptoms of the disease.

The major pathological feature of PD is progressive loss of the dopamine-producing neurons of the substantia nigra, resulting in a reduction of the dopamine content in the target field of these neurons, the striatum. The cause of the death of dopamine-producing neurons is still unknown, and genetic and environmental factors may contribute to the pathogenesis and progression of the disease[1].

Parkinson's disease shows a larger prevalence in males compared with females[2-4], more severe motor impairment and behavioral problems in men[5] and more levodopa-induced dyskinesia and depression[6] and higher prescription rates of anxiolytics, hypnotics and sedatives among women[7]. All of these gender differences are marked when comparing men with age-matched premenopausal women, but are less apparent when comparisons are made with postmenopausal women not receiving hormone replacement therapy (HRT). That being so, a possible role of gonadal hormones in the gender difference and lower risk of PD in women could be proposed, also taking into account the role of estrogen in the nigrostriatal dopaminergic pathway[8,9].

Estrogen has a wide range of actions on the central nervous system, both genomic and non-genomic, not restricted to areas critical for reproduction, but also involving cognitive function, control of movement, pain and affective state, and its withdrawal after natural or surgical menopause can lead to a host of changes in brain function and behavior[10]. Some studies have suggested a possible protective role for menopausal estrogen therapy against cognitive decline in older women[11]. But HRT was also found to be protective against the development of dementia within the setting of Parkinson's disease, but did not affect the risk of PD[12]. On the other hand, estrogen influences the control of movement by influencing dopamine neurotransmission directly in nigrostriatal areas. It can stimulate dopamine synthesis by directly enhancing striatal tyrosine hydroxylase activity[13]. Estrogen can increase the density of presynaptic striatal dopamine intake sites, and the density and sensitivity of postsynaptic dopamine receptors[14]. Indirect estrogenic effects on the nigrostriatum via opioid, glutamatergic and γ-aminobutyric acid systems have also been proposed[10].

A number of animal studies indicate that estrogen protects dopamine neurons from injury, in animal models of PD using 1-methyl-4-phenyl-1,2,3,6-tetrahydropyridine (MPTP)[15] and 6-hydroxydopamine (6-OHDA)[16]. A recent study[17] suggests that lesions resulting from a submaximal dose of the neurotoxin 6-OHDA are exacerbated by gonadal factors in the male, whereas in the female the presence of physiological levels of circulating gonadal hormones, specifically estrogen, is neuroprotective. A neuroprotective role for estrogen is further supported by other evidence demonstrating that estrogen can attenuate neuronal damage in experimental models of central nervous system injury. For example, in cultured rat ventral mesencephalon, estradiol has been shown to attenuate significantly the formation of the toxin hydrogen peroxide and nitric oxide free radicals by glutamate[18]. Other studies suggest that estrogen may protect dopamine neurons via antioxidant effects, possibly independent of estrogen receptors but intrinsic to their phenolic structure[19]. Estrogen may also exert neuroprotective effects on dopamine neurons by regulating the expression of neurotrophic molecules as brain-derived neurotrophic factor (BDNF)[20]. Menstrual cycle-dependent changes have also been observed in striatal dopamine uptake, binding and metabolism. Menstrual cycle variations in dopamine uptake sites and release have been reported, and peak density of striatal dopamine uptake sites was shown to occur in the morning of proestrus when estrogen levels are highest[21] and to fluctuate during the estrous cycle[22].

ESTROGEN AND WOMEN WITH PARKINSON'S DISEASE

Cyclical fluctuations of hormone levels influence PD symptoms. In a study of premenopausal women with PD, 11 of these 12 women had subjective deterioration in their parkinsonism which began at a mean of 5 days before, and ended a mean of 2.2 days after, the onset of menses, corresponding to low estrogen levels[23]. The data were confirmed by another study of 352 women: 75% of PD women with natural menstrual cycles and 48% of those with exogenous hormone-mediated cycles noted worsening of PD symptoms before and during their menses[24].

The above observations were made only in PD women, so a recent study[25] was aimed towards describing reproductive milestones in 150 PD women in comparison with 300 healthy postmenopausal subjects (PM). Moreover, the premenopausal or postmenopausal onset of PD symptoms was evaluated, to verify whether estrogenic state may be relevant to clinical expression of the disease.

In respect of women comparable for age and geographical and cultural environment, PD women had a similar length of reproductive life, but complained about more premenstrual symptoms, had fewer children and fewer spontaneous and voluntary abortions and reported a lower use of contraception. The menopause occurred at the same age in PD and PM women. Even the characteristics of onset and type of menopause were similar between PD and PM women. Women with PD reported that they had had more hot flushes ($p = 0.001$), while depression, insomnia, urinary incontinence and dyspareunia were more frequently recalled by PM women ($p = 0.001$) and no difference was found in terms of irritability, anxiety and vaginal dryness. The percentage of women who assumed HRT was significantly lower among PD patients ($p = 0.001$).

The PD onset, before or after the menopause, was associated with dysmenorrhea, premenstrual syndrome and oral contraception, found significantly ($p = 0.001$) more frequently among subjects with disease onset during fertile life. A premenstrual worsening of parkinsonism and of response to treatments was found in 52.6% of PD women diagnosed before the menopause, while 43.3% (13 patients) of the 30 postmenopausal PD women reported a worsening of the disease when menses stopped, as this was related to an increase of drugs dose or reduced mobility with need of help. Disease length and severity were not significantly different in contraceptive users and non-users, but the contraceptive users were significantly younger ($p = 0.0001$), with significantly more years of education ($p = 0.036$) and a lower age at PD onset ($p = 0.001$) than the non-users.

A therapy for the menopause was taken by 23 of the 142 postmenopausal women, and these women were slightly younger, with longer education. Concerning symptoms of the menopause, women with PD onset before the menopause showed a significantly lesser degree of hot flushes ($p < 0.05$), but higher incidence of insomnia ($p < 0.01$), urinary incontinence ($p < 0.02$) and dyspareunia ($p < 0.01$) when compared with women with PD onset after the menopause. PD women had a lower use of HRT than healthy women (23 of 142 postmenopausal PD women were taking HRT), with no clinical difference in respect of untreated PD women. Among those patients taking HRT it was interesting to observe that, when treatment induced withdrawal bleeding (ten of 23), no clinical changes were recorded.

This study provided evidence that women with PD have a substantially normal fertile life, from the aspect of time-related events. The disease involves rather the qualitative aspects of the various stages of fertile life such as menstruation, pregnancy or menopause. PD worsened premenstrually in about 50% of cases, as other diseases do[26,27]. Menopause worsened PD in 40% of the women with disease onset during fertile life.

HORMONE REPLACEMENT THERAPY AND PARKINSON'S DISEASE

The role of estrogen replacement in symptom severity or in response to levodopa has been evaluated by various authors. Saunders-Pullman and colleagues[28] found a positive association between estrogen use and lower symptom severity in women with early PD not yet taking levodopa. They carried out a retrospective analysis of a database of patients, including only women who had symptoms of presumed PD for less than 5 years and who had not yet taken levodopa at their first clinic visit. The effects of estrogen on disease were measured by the Unified Parkinson's Disease Rating Scale (UPDRS) score. Age at onset and symptom duration were positively correlated with UPDRS score, while the use of estrogen was higher in women with less severe disease. The most common form of estrogen therapy was Premarin®, while Provera® was the most common progesterone derivative; the usual dose was 0.625 mg of estrogen and 2.5 mg of progestin. The results of the above analysis indicate that estrogen therapy should not be avoided and may be beneficial in early PD, at least prior to the initiation of levodopa. Tsang and associates[29] tested efficacy, tolerance and safety of low-dose oral estrogen in postmenopausal women with more advanced disease, as PD was associated with motor fluctuations. Patients were randomized to receive conjugated estrogen (oral Premarin 0.625 mg) or placebo over 8 weeks. Both treatment groups were similar in age, duration of disease and menopause, and PD medication. On and off times and motor score (UPDRS) improved with estrogen. Mean on time improved by 7% in estrogen-treated patients, while a deterioration of 0.5% was found in placebo-treated patients. Mean off time improved by 4% in estrogen-treated patients, but no change was detected in placebo-treated patients. These authors concluded that low-dose estrogen is a safe and effective adjunct therapy to existing antiparkinsonian treatment in reducing motor disability in postmenopausal women with PD associated with motor fluctuations. Blanchet and co-workers[30] examined the effect of transdermal 17β-estradiol on the severity of the signs of PD in eight postmenopausal women. Patients were randomized initially to either hormonal treatment or placebo for 2 weeks, followed by a 2-week wash-out period, and then another 2-week cross-over treatment period. All patients applied four skin patches of 17β-estradiol (and matching placebo), each of which contained 8 mg of 17β-estradiol designed to deliver 0.1 mg daily. 17β-Estradiol appeared to display a slight prodopaminergic (or antiparkinsonian) effect without consistently altering dyskinesias; standard postmenopausal replacement therapy with transdermal 17β-estradiol is likely to be well tolerated by many female parkinsonian patients. Moreover, a negative effect of the premenstrual phase on symptom severity and response to therapy was observed, even though parkinsonism and hormone levels measured premenstrually were not significantly related. Kompoliti and colleagues[31] studied women with PD and regular menstrual cycles and without taking estrogen or progesterone supplements. They found no significant correlation between objective or subjective measures of parkinsonism and estrogen and progesterone levels, although PD severity fluctuated during the study period.

In evaluating the above studies, a lack of consensus on the potential role of estrogen emerges. Indeed, some evidence[32] points towards PD improvement during the hypoestrogenic state. Conversely, conditions causing an early reduction in endogenous estrogens may promote the risk of PD, while in a short placebo-controlled, randomized, double-blind trial, no significant effect of estradiol could be demonstrated on PD symptoms in postmenopausal women. De Benedetti and colleagues[33] studied the association of PD with type of menopause (natural or surgical), age at menopause and postmenopausal estrogen replacement therapy using a case-control design. They found that PD women had undergone hysterectomy (with or without unilateral oophorectomy) significantly more often than controls, and had an early menopause (< 46 years) more commonly than controls. In addition, PD cases had used oral or parenteral estrogen for at least 6 months after the menopause less frequently than control subjects. These authors hypothesized that there is an increased risk of PD in conditions causing an early reduction in endogenous estrogen. Strijks and co-workers[34] examined the clinical effects of chronic administration of sex steroids on the symptoms of PD in postmenopausal women. They demonstrated that estradiol had no significant dopaminergic effect and progesterone seemed to have an anti-dopaminergic effect. Another interesting point concerns the possible relationship between estrogen replacement use and the risk of developing PD. A beneficial effect of estrogen could explain the lower risk of PD in women compared with men, and the decline of hormone levels has been suggested to increase the risk of PD among postmenopausal women. Studies concerning the association of risk of PD and hormone use or not have given inconsistent results, because they were small or relied on retrospective assessment of use of postmenopausal hormones. A recent study[35], performed during an 18-year follow-up of over 77 000 postmenopausal women, demonstrated that in the 154 cases with definite or probable PD, overall, neither use of postmenopausal hormones nor duration of use was associated with incidence of PD. The authors also examined the interaction of caffeine with use of hormones, which showed that caffeine alone reduces the risk of PD among women who do not use postmenopausal hormones, but increases the risk among hormone users. In particular, the use of HRT was associated with a lower risk of PD among women with a low caffeine intake, but with an increased risk among women with a high caffeine intake. The authors concluded that the inconsistency of the association between use of HRT and risk of PD in previous studies could be due to a caffeine-estrogen interaction.

In conclusion, women have a lower risk of PD than men, but it remains uncertain whether this difference is attributable to estrogens alone. The association between use of HRT and risk of PD should be evaluated also taking into account behaviors and use of substances whose metabolism could be influenced by hormones.

References

1. Blandini F, Nappi G, Tassorelli C, Martignoni E. Functional changes of the basal ganglia circuitry in PD. *Prog Neurobiol* 2000;62:63–88
2. Bharucha NE, Bharucha EP, Bharucha AE, *et al.* Prevalence of Parkinson's disease in the Parsi community of Bombay, India. *Arch Neurol* 1988; 45:1321–3
3. Bower JH, Maraganore DM, McDonnel SK, *et al.* Incidence and distribution of parkinsonism in Olmsted County, Minnesota, 1976–1990. *Neurology* 1999;52:1214–20
4. Baldereschi M, Di Carlo A, Rocca WA, *et al.* Parkinson's disease and parkinsonism in a longitudinal study: two-fold higher incidence in men. ILSA working group. Italian Longitudinal Study on Aging. *Neurology* 2000;55:1358–63
5. Fernandez HH, Lapane KL, Ott BR, Friedman JH. Gender differences in the frequency and treatment of behavior problems in Parkinson's disease. *Mov Disord* 2000;15:490–6
6. Lyons KE, Hubble JP, Troster AI, *et al.* Gender differences in Parkinson's disease. *Clin Neuropharmacol* 1998;21:118–21
7. Leoni O, Martignoni E, Cosentino M, *et al.* Drug prescribing patterns in Parkinson's disease. A pharmacoepidemiological survey in a cohort of ambulatory patients. *Pharmacoepidemiol Drug Saf* 2002;11:149–57
8. Shulman LM. Is there a connection between estrogen and Parkinson's disease? *Parkinsonism Relat Disord* 2002;8:289–95
9. Dluzen DE, McDermott JL. Gender differences in neuritoxicity of the nigrostriatal dopaminergic

system: implications for Parkinson's disease. *J Gend Specif Med* 2000;3:36–42
10. McEwen BS, Alves SE. Estrogen actions in the central nervous system. *Endocr Rev* 1999;20: 279–307
11. Robertson DMW, Amelsvoort T, Daly E, *et al.* Effects of estrogen replacement therapy on human brain aging: an *in vivo* ^{1}H MRS study. *Neurology* 2001;57:2114–17
12. Marder K, Tang MX, Alfaro B, *et al.* Postmenopausal estrogen use and Parkinson's disease with and without dementia. *Neurology* 1998;50:1141–3
13. Pasqualini C, Olivier V, Guibert B, Frain O, Leviel V. Acute stimulatory effect of estradiol on striatal dopamine synthesis. *J Neurochem* 1995;65:1651–7
14. Hruska RE, Nowak MW. Estrogen treatment increases the density of D1 dopamine receptors in the rat striatum. *Brain Res* 1988;442:349–50
15. Disshon KA, Dluzen DE. Estrogen as a neuromodulator of MPTP-induced neurotoxicity: effects upon striatal dopamine release. *Brain Res* 1997; 764:9–13
16. Dluzen D. Estrogen decreases corpus striatal neurotoxicity in response to 6-hydroxydopamine. *Brain Res* 1997;767:340–4
17. Murray HE, Pillai AV, McArthur SR, *et al.* Dose- and sex-dependent effects of the neurotoxin 6-hydroxydopamine on the nigrostriatal dopaminergic pathway of adult rats: differential actions of estrogen in males and females. *Neuroscience* 2003;116:213–22
18. Sawada H, Ibi M, Kihara T, *et al.* Estradiol protects mesencephalic dopaminergic neurons from oxidative stress-induced neuronal death. *J Neurosci Res* 1998;54:707–19
19. Behl C, Skutella T, Lezoualc F, *et al.* Neuroprotection against oxidative stress by estrogens: structure-activity relationship. *Mol Pharmacol* 1997;51:535–41
20. Ivanova T, Kuppers E, Engele J, Beyer C. Estrogen stimulates brain-derived neurotrophic factor expression in embryonic mouse midbrain neurons through a membrane-mediated and calcium dependent mechanism. *J Neurosci Res* 2001;97: 297–303
21. Dluzen D, Ramirez VD. *In vitro* dopamine from rat striatum: diurnal rhythm and its modification by the estrous cycle. *Neuroendocrinology* 1985;41: 97–100
22. Morrisette M, Di Paolo T. Effect of chronic estradiol and progesterone treatments of ovariectomized rats on brain dopamine uptake sites. *J Neurochem* 1993;60:1876–83
23. Quinn NP, Marsden CD. Menstrual-related fluctuations in Parkinson's disease. *Mov Disord* 1986; 1:85–7
24. Thulin PC, Carter JH, Nichols MD, *et al.* Menstrual cycle related changes in Parkinson's disease. *Neurology* 1996;46:A376
25. Martignoni E, Nappi RE, Citterio A, *et al.* Reproductive life milestones in women with Parkinson's disease. *Funct Neurol* 2003;18:in press
26. Tarsy D, Thulin PC, Herzog AG. Spasmodic torticollis and reproductive function in women. *Parkinsonism Relat Disord* 2001;7:323–7
27. Gwinn-Hardy KA, Adler CH, Weaver AL, Fish NM, Newman SJ. Effect of hormone variations and other factors on symptoms severity in women with dystonia. *Mayo Clin Proc* 2000;75:234–40
28. Saunders-Pullman R, Gordon-Elliot J, Parides M, *et al.* The effect of estrogen replacement on early Parkinson's disease. *Neurology* 1999;52:1417–21
29. Tsang KL, Jiang H, Ramsden DB, Ho SL. The use of estrogen in the treatment of Parkinson's disease. *Parkinsonism Relat Disord* 2001;8:133–7
30. Blanchet PJ, Fang J, Hyland K, *et al.* Short-term effect of high-dose 17β-estradiol in postmenopausal PD patients. *Neurology* 1999;53:91–5
31. Kompoliti K, Comella CL, Jaglin JA, *et al.* Menstrual-related changes in motoric function in women with Parkinson's disease. *Neurology* 2000; 55:1572–4
32. Session DR, Pearlstone MM, Jewelwicz R, *et al.* Estrogens and Parkinson's disease. *Med Hypoth* 1994;42:280–2
33. De Benedetti MD, Maraganore DM, Bower JH, *et al.* Hysterectomy, menopause, and estrogen use preceding Parkinson's disease: an exploratory case-control study. *Mov Disord* 2001;16:830–7
34. Strijks E, Kremer JAM, Horstink MWIM. Effects of female sex steroids on Parkinson's disease in postmenopausal women. *Clin Neuropharmacol* 1999;2: 93–7
35. Ascherio A, Chen H, Schwarzchild MA, *et al.* Caffeine, postmenopausal estrogen, and risk of PD. *Neurology* 2003;60:790–5

Hormone replacement therapy and Alzheimer's disease

26

H. Honjo, S. Fushiki, K. Fukui, K. Iwasa, T. Hosoda, J. Kitawaki, T. Okubo, H. Tatsumi, N. Oida, M. Mihara, Y. Hirasugi, H. Yamamoto, N. Kikuchi and M. Kawata

INTRODUCTION

On 7 July 2002, shocking and striking news spread throughout the world, following the Women's Health Initiative (WHI) Investigators' report[1] that hormone replacement therapy (HRT) using conjugated equine estrogens 0.625 mg/day plus medroxyprogesterone acetate 2.5 mg/day (continuous combined method) could not prevent primary coronary heart disease (CHD), and the clinical trial was stopped. More recently, on 8 January 2003, the US Food and Drug Administration (FDA)[2] limited indications for general use of HRT to climacteric syndrome only. However, the Cache County Study[3] recommended HRT use after the menopause to prevent Alzheimer's disease (AD). This chapter discusses HRT in relation to AD.

GENDER DIFFERENCES IN ALZHEIMER'S DISEASE

Significant gender differences in the incidence of AD after age 85 years in Europe were shown by the EURODEM studies[4], namely 81.7 per 1000 person-years in women and 24.0 in men at 90 years of age. The cumulative risk for 65-year-old women to develop AD at the age of 95 years was 0.22, compared with 0.09 for men. The Cache County Study[3] in Utah, USA also showed that AD was significantly more common in women than in men: 88 women (4.7%) and 35 men (2.6%) in that study, $p = 0.002$. The same tendency was seen in Japan[5], with an incidence rate of AD in women of 10.9/1000 person-years, compared with 5.1/1000 in men.

Estrogen secretion from the ovaries ceases at the menopause. In men, the testes continue (decreasing only slowly) to produce androgens[6], which are partly aromatized to estrogens. Serum levels of estrogens in elderly women after the menopause become lower than those in same-aged men[7]. Hendrie[8] found gender to be an inconsistent or interactive risk factor, but estrogen replacement therapy to be a somewhat consistent factor in AD.

Dehydroepiandrosterone (DHEA) and dehydroepiandrosterone sulfate (DHEAS) are produced in large amounts in both male and female adrenals. Levels decrease linearly with aging in both men and women. DHEAS levels in peripheral blood were found to be higher in men than in women in each age group[9]. In this study, there were many cases of lower levels of DHEA and DHEAS in patients with AD, especially in those under 70 years of age. There may be a possibility that DHEA and DHEAS prevent AD in men. However, symptoms of AD were not improved with intravenous injection of 200 mg DHEAS/day for 8 weeks, but symptoms of vascular dementia were improved[9]. Sex-specific rates for various diseases in patients requiring care were reported by the Japanese Ministry of Welfare[10] (2000). Brain vascular diseases were responsible in 51.6% of men and 25.2% of women, and dementia was responsible in 8.4% of men and 16.6% of women. Dementia-free life expectancy among elderly people was assessed using data of the health maintenance organization Kaizer Permanente[11]. The trends of health expectancies suggested an extension of the duration of life with dementia for men and a compression of dementia for women. The latter might be related to frequent HRT use by US women.

Thus, research into the prevention and treatment of AD with estrogens or non-feminizing estrogen is essentially important in women and also important in men.

PSYCHOPATHOLOGY OF CENTRAL NERVOUS SYSTEM

The clock drawing test (CDT) is a useful tool for screening cognitive impairment. Previous neuropsychological studies have revealed that CDT performance requires several cognitive functions, including semantic memory, visuospatial function and executive function. Twenty-six patients satisfying the National Institute of Neurological and Communicative Disease and Stroke-Alzheimer's Disease and Related Disorders Association criteria for probable AD underwent the CDT and the Mini-Mental State Examination (MMSE), together with *N*-isopropyl-*p*-[^{123}I] iodoamphetamine (IMP) single-photon emission computed tomography measurements of the resting regional cerebral blood flow (rCBF)[12]. The CDT score correlated significantly with the MMSE score ($r = 0.582$; $p < 0.05$). Stepwise multiple regression analysis revealed that the MMSE score and the left posterior temporal rCBF were major predictors of CDT score. The results indicated the following formula: CDT score = 0.321(MMSE score) + 13.855(left posterior temporal rCBF) – 10.920. These findings suggest that the CDT score may reflect the severity of dementia, and that it has a close relationship with the left posterior temporal function. The above findings provide the first functional neuroimaging evidence for the neural substrates involved in CDT performance.

Although cognitive abilities of healthy women and men are similar in general, women tend to perform better on certain verbal tasks and men tend to score better on some visuospatial and mathematical reasoning tasks[13]. These phenomena may be related to sexual differences in blood supply and metabolism in the central nervous system; these parameters are higher in women in the gyrus cinguli and thalamus, and higher in men in the temporal lobe (important region for memory), cerebrolimbic system, hippocampus and the cerebellum[14]. A preliminary report of single-photon emission computed tomography (SPECT) in AD patients found that men had a greater reduction of temporoparietal perfusion than women[15]. Unilateral temporoparietal defects are seen more commonly on SPECT in women than in men with AD. Estrogen increases cerebral and cerebellar blood flows[16], but the increased areas are not yet clarified completely in patients with AD.

Sexual differentiation occurs in the human sexually dimorphic nucleus of the preoptic area (SDN) owing to a decrease in cell number in the SDN of women, whereas the cell number in men remains approximately unchanged up to the age of 50. In men the reduction in cell number in senescence is less dramatic than in women. However, in one study, cell numbers in the SDN of AD patients were found to be within the normal range for age and sex[17].

A marked decrease was found in human suprachiasmatic nucleus (SCN) cell number in subjects 80–100 years of age, and the changes were even more dramatic in AD[18]. This might be the neural basis for the nightly restlessness observed in AD, whereas alterations in the visual system might contribute to these functional disturbances.

In a study of risk factors for depression in AD, family history of mood disorder was associated with an increased risk of major depression only for women, suggesting that genetic influences may be more important in women than in men for expression of the disease[19]. Ott[19] suggested that women were increasingly vulnerable to genetic influences in relation to AD, with accumulating evidence.

ESTROGEN AND NON-FEMINIZING ESTROGEN

Epidemiological data including the above recent report[3] and much basic research have suggested a preventive effect of estrogens on AD. The therapeutic effects of estrogens on AD are still under discussion[20,21]. Ameliorative effects of estrogens and non-feminizing estrogen (J 861: 14α, 15α-methylenestra-1,3,5(10),8-tetraene-3,17α-diol), which has little effect on sexual organs, were investigated.

Effects of 17β-estradiol and J 861 on intracellular calcium, peroxidation and apoptosis induced by amyloid-β

Rat pheochromacytoma PC12 cells were induced and differentiated to neurotype by incubation for 6 days in RPMI 1640 medium containing 100 ng/ml nerve growth factor (NGF). Differentiated PC12 cells were treated with or without various concentrations (10^{-12}, 10^{-10}, 10^{-8} mol/l) of 17β-estradiol (E_2) or J 861 for 3 days before exposure to amyloid-β (Aβ), which consists of a cytotoxic sequence between amino acid residues 25 and 35. To investigate interaction with the estrogen receptor (ER), each cell mixture was cultured with and without pure antiestrogen, ER antagonist ICI 182780, in parallel. After preincubation, the supernatant was renewed with medium containing 10 μmol/l Aβ. Intracellular calcium concentrations in each culture were measured by flow cytometry with 5 μmol/l of Fluo-3-AM. To determine the quantity of peroxidation, fluorescence intensity was measured with 100 μmol/l of DCF0-DA. Statistical analysis was performed by one-way analysis of variance (ANOVA) and *post hoc* multiple comparison by Fisher's test.

Flow cytometric analysis revealed that exposure to Aβ increased intracellular calcium concentration. Preincubation with E_2 or J 861 for 3 days prevented the increase of intracellular calcium concentration dose-dependently. The inhibitory effect of J 861 was stronger than that of E_2. These inhibitory effects were attenuated by the administration of ICI 182780.

Peroxidation increased after exposure to Aβ, but this increase was prevented in cultures preincubated with E_2 or J 861. The inhibitory effect of J 861 was stronger than that of E_2, and ICI 182780 significantly attenuated the effect of E_2 and J 861. Hence, E_2 and J 861 are suggested to protect from both intracellular calcium increase and peroxidation induced by Aβ directly and via an ER-mediated system. The mechanism of neurotoxicity by Aβ is considered to be: the formation of calcium pores on the cell membrane accelerates calcium inflow to the cell, and activated NO synthetase induces intracellular peroxidation[22]. Physiological levels of E_2 are considered to have sufficient antioxidant effect. The antioxidant effect of J 861 is probably stronger than that of E_2.

Effects of 17β-estradiol on relationship between advanced glycation of amyloid-β protein and receptor-mediated neuronal loss

Interaction between advanced glycation end products (AGEs) of amyloid-β protein (Aβ) and their receptor (RAGE) has been suggested to play an important role in the pathogenesis of AD.

We examined the effects of E_2 on the relationship between AGE-degraded Aβ (AGE-Aβ) and RAGE to elucidate the mechanism of the beneficial effects of estrogen replacement therapy (ERT) in AD. AGE-degradation of Aβ progressed with incubation in medium under physiological conditions, and the cytotoxicity of Aβ in PC12 cells was increased as AGE formation progressed; unfortunately, E_2 had no inhibitory effect on the AGE-degradation of Aβ. On the other hand, expression of RAGE was detected by reverse transcriptase-polymerase chain reaction (RT-PCR) and immunochemical assay in PC12 cells, and was accelerated by the stimulation of AGEs. E_2 was revealed to have an inhibitory effect on its expression. Therefore, E_2 affects the expression of RAGE but not the AGE-degradation of Aβ.

These results suggest that AGE-degradation of Aβ plays a pivotal role in the pathogenesis of AD. Estrogen may have beneficial effects by inhibiting AGE–RAGE interaction in AD.

Effects of 17β-estradiol and J 861 on cholinergic neurons in substantia innominata

Wistar female rats were divided into three groups: ovariectomized, E_2-treated and J 861-treated. After oophorectomy, rats of the E_2-treated group were given 5 μg/day of E_2 for 2 weeks by subcutaneous injection, and rats of the J 861-treated group were similarly given 5 μg/day of J 861. Cholinacetyltransferase (ChAT) was stained using the ABC (avitin-biotin complex) method. The number of positive ChAT-immunoreactive cells and morphological changes were compared among the three groups. The number of positive ChAT-immunoreactive cells in the ovariectomized group was fewer than that in the E_2 or J 861 group. The length of axon in the ovariectomized group was shorter than in the E_2 or J 861 group. The number of dendrites in the ovariectomized group was fewer than in the E_2 or J 861 group. J 861, like E_2, showed neuroprotective and neurotrophic effects.

Effects of 17β-estradiol and J 861 on morphological differentiation and survival ratio of rat glia cells

The effect of pretreatment with J 861 was investigated by incubation with H_2O_2. Glia cells showed more proliferation with 3.5×10^{-9} mol/l J 861 than the control. Despite the oxidation effect of H_2O_2, most cells survived and proliferated after pretreatment with the above amount of J 861.

Effects of 17β-estradiol and J 861 on adhesive factors

Human umbilical venous endothelial cells (HUVECs) were cultured on 96-well tissue plates, and 10^{-7} or 10^{-5} E_2, J 861 or α-tocopherol were added. HUVECs were incubated for 24 h with or without ICI 182780, and stimulated with 40 μg/ml of interleukin-1β (IL-1β) for 4 h. Cellular enzyme-linked immunosorbent assay was performed using the streptavidin-biotin method. By means of adsorption spectrophotometry, optical density was measured at 490 nm.

A level of 10^{-7} mol/l E_2 did not inhibit expression of E-selectin induced by IL-1α stimulation. J 861, like α-tocopherol, suppressed expression of E-selectin induced by IL-1β stimulation. Approximately a 20% decrease was recognized with the addition of 10^{-7} mol/l J 861 or α-tocopherol, and about a 30% decrease was recognized with the addition of 10^{-5} mol/l J 861 or α-tocopherol. Suppression by J 861 or α-tocopherol was stronger than that by E_2. ICI 182780 did not change suppression by α-tocopherol, but reduced suppression by J 861.

The level of 10^{-7} mol/l E_2 did not suppress expression of intercellular adhesion molecule-1 (ICAM-1) induced by IL-1β stimulation. J 861, like α-tocopherol, suppressed expression of ICAM-1 induced by IL-1β stimulation. About a 20% decrease was recognized with the addition of 10^{-7} mol/l of J 861 or α-tocopherol, and about a 40% decrease was recognized with the addition of 10^{-5}mol/l of J 861 or α-tocopherol. Suppression by J 861 or α-tocopherol was stronger than that by E_2. ICI 182780 did not change suppression by α-tocopherol, but reduced suppression by J 861.

E_2, J 861 or α-tocopherol may suppress the adhesion of monocytes by suppressing the expression of E-selectin and ICAM-1 on endothelium of vessels. Physiological serum levels of E_2 probably do not suppress the expression of E-selectin and ICAM-1. Physiological serum levels of α-tocopherol are considered to suppress the expression of E-selectin and ICAM-1. J 861 is considered to suppress the expression of these adhesive factors directly and partially with the help of ERα.

Effects of 17β-estradiol and J 861 on adhesion of monocytes to endothelium under physiological flow conditions

HUVECs were cultured on gelatin- and fibronectin-coated glass slides; 10^{-7} or 10^{-5} mol/l E_2, J 861 or α-tocopherol were added. HUVECs were incubated for 24 h, then stimulated with 40 μg/ml IL-1β for 4 h. U937 cells derived from human myeloma, in Hank's balanced salt solution (HBSS) (10^5 cells/ml), were passed through the flow chamber at 1.0 dyn/cm^2 of shear stress for 7 min. The number of adherent U937 cells was counted in 20 microscopic fields by analyzing recorded videotape. The number of adherent U937 cells under each condition was compared with that under the condition without any reagents, stimulated with IL-1β alone for 4 h. A level of 10^{-7} mol/l E_2 did not inhibit the adhesion of monocytes. About a 25% decrease was recognized with the addition of 10^{-5} mol/l E_2. J 861 and α-tocopherol suppressed the adhesion of monocytes dose-dependently. About a 40% decrease was recognized in 10^{-5} mol/l J 861 or α-tocopherol. A level of 40 μg/ml IL-1β is equivalent to the serum level under shock status, and 1.0 dyn/cm^2 of shear stress is equivalent to that applied to the venous wall in conditions of slowest blood flow, so this model was similar to physiological blood flow conditions. E_2 probably does not suppress the adhesion of monocytes at the physiological serum level. α-Tocopherol is considered to suppress the adhesion of monocytes sufficiently at the physiological serum level. J 861 suppressed the adhesion of monocytes as did α-tocopherol. The permitted dose of J 861 administered to humans is not yet known, but may be larger than that of E_2 because it has little effect on the sexual organs.

The above effects on adhesive factors in the vascular system should be considered in patients with vascular dementia and AD.

CONCLUSION

Gender differences in the psychopathology of AD should be clarified further. It is possible that dementia-free life expectancy among elderly persons could be prolonged with the use of HRT, non-feminizing estrogen and other compounds, subject to further investigation.

ACKNOWLEDGEMENTS

This study was supported in part by a Grant-in-Aid for General Scientific Research (No. 03454401, No. 07557366 and No. 10671564), Health Sciences Research Grants, Research on Health Services H13-Health-015, The Research Institute for Neurological Disease and Geriatrics, and Works of Scientific Research and Technical Development, Public Health Department of the Kyoto Prefectural Government. We would like to thank Dr M. Oettel and his colleagues at Jenapharm GmbH for the kind donation of J 861 and their co-operation.

References

1. Writing Group for the Women's Health Initiative Investigators. Risks and benefits of estrogen plus progestin in healthy postmenopausal women, principal results from the Women's Health Initiative randomized controlled trial. *J Am Med Assoc* 2002;288:321–33
2. Food and Drug Administration. *FDA approves new labels for estrogen and estrogen with progestin therapies for postmenopausal women.* Press release, FDA, Rockville, DC, 8 January, 2003
3. Zandi PP, Carlson MC, Plassman BL, *et al.* Hormone replacement therapy and incidence of Alzheimer's disease in older women, the Cache County Study. *J Am Med Assoc* 2002;28:2123–9
4. Andersen K, Launer LJ, Dewey ME, *et al.* Gender differences in the incidence of AD and vascular dementia, the EURODEM studies. *Neurology* 1999; 53:1992–7
5. Yoshitake T, Kiyohara Y, Kato I, *et al.* Incidence and risk factors of vascular dementia and Alzheimer's disease in a defined elderly Japanese population: the Hisayama study. *Neurology* 1995;45:1161–8
6. Seem MV. Psychopathology in women and men: focus on female hormones. *Am J Psychiatry* 1997; 154:1641–7
7. Riggs BL, Khosla S, Melton LJ. Primary osteoporosis in men: role of sex steroid deficiency. *Mayo Clin Proc* 2000;75(Suppl):S46–50
8. Hendrie HC. Epidemiology of dementia and Alzheimer's disease. *Am J Geriatr Psychiatry* 1998; 6:S3–18
9. Sugino S. Adult disease and sex difference. Hormone substitution therapy (HRT) and sex difference. Suprarenal androgen [in Japanese]. *Seisa Igaku* 1998;4:82–91
10. Japanese Ministry of Welfare. http://www.mhlw.go.jp/toukei/saikin/hw/kaigo/setaioo/kekka-2.html
11. Sauvaget C, Tsuji I, Haan NM, *et al.* Trends in dementia-free life expectancy among elderly members of a large health maintenance organization. *Int J Epidemiol* 1999;28:1110–18
12. Ueda H, Kitabayashi Y, Fukui K, *et al.* Relationship between clock drawing test performance and regional cerebral blood flow in Alzheimer's disease: a single photon emission computed tomography study. *Psychiatry Clin Neurosci* 2002;56:25–9
13. Birkhäuser MH, Strnad J, Kämpt C, *et al.* Oestrogen and Alzheimer's disease. *Int J Geriatr Psychiatry* 2000;15:600–9

14. Matsuoka H. Pick up - recent topics about cerebro-blood flows [in Japanese]. *SPECT* 2001; 13:81-3
15. Swartz RH, Black SE, Iziboviten FS, *et al.* Sex and mental status, but not apolipoprotein E, correlate with parietal and temporal hypoperfusion on SPECT in Alzheimer's disease. *Neurology* 1998;50(Suppl): A159 (abstr)
16. Ohkura T, Teshima Y, Isse K, *et al.* Estrogen increases cerebral and cerebellar blood flows in postmenopausal women. *Menopause* 1995;2:13-18
17. Swaab DF, Hofman MA. Sexual differentiation of the human, hypothalamus: ontogeny of the sexually dimorphic nucleus of the preoptic area. *Dev Brain Res* 1998;44:314-18
18. Swaab DF, Goudsmit E, Kremen HPH, *et al.* The human hypothalamus in development, sexual differentiation, aging and Alzheimer's disease. *Prog Brain Res* 1992;91:465-72
19. Ott BR. Cognition and behavior in patients with Alzheimer's disease. *J Gend Specif Med* 1999; 2:63-9
20. Honjo H, Tanaka K, Kashiwagi T, *et al.* Senile dementia: Alzheimer's type and estrogen. *Horm Metab Res* 1995;27:204-7
21. Yoon BK, Kim DK, Kang Y, *et al.* Hormone replacement therapy in postmenopausal women with Alzheimer's disease: a randomized, prospective study. *Fertil Steril* 2003;79:274-80
22. Le WD, Colom LV, Xie WJ, *et al.* Cell death induced by β-amyloid 1-40 in MES 23.5 hybrid clone: the role of nitric oxide and NMDA-gated-channel activation leading to apoptosis. *Brain Res* 1995; 686:49-60

Menopause: it's all in the brain 27

J. M. Alt

HOT FLUSHES AND MENOPAUSE

Vasomotor symptoms are among the most characteristic symptoms of the climacteric, and are one of the most common complaints for which perimenopausal and postmenopausal women seek medical treatment. It is estimated that as many as 75–80% of women suffer from hot flushes at or around the time of the menopause. For most women, hot flushes begin before the menopause, when menstrual cycles are still regular, or within 1 year of the menopause. Symptoms often last 1 year or less, but almost one-third of postmenopausal women report symptoms that last up to 5 years after a natural menopause, and hot flushes can persist for up to 15 years in 20% or more of women[1–4]. A recent evaluation of data from the Heart and Estrogen/progestin Replacement Study (HERS) showed that 16% of the study participants, whose average age was 67 years and who averaged 18 years since the menopause, still had hot flushes and other symptoms that are typically attributed to the menopause[5].

For the many women who experience hot flushes, these have a profound impact on quality of life. Hot flushes may be accompanied by sweating, palpitations, anxiety and even panic[6]. Sleep may be disrupted several times a night in women who report night sweats, resulting in fatigue and irritability during the daytime. It is estimated that 25% of women are severely affected, and that a further 50% are affected to a moderate degree. Between 10 and 20% of postmenopausal women with hot flushes find them nearly intolerable[4]. Dennerstein and colleagues used a validated well-being scale to examine the relationship between well-being and menopausal transition, and found that well-being was decreased in the first 2 years after cessation of menses. Negative affect was highest in the category of women who were 1–2 years postmenopausal. This menopausal category also contained the highest percentage (57%) of women with bothersome hot flushes. The presence of hot flushes during the last 2 weeks adversely affected negative moods in this model. Positive affect was also significantly lower in the first 2 years after the menopause, but this effect of menopausal status did not remain when hot flushes were included in the analysis[7]. The decrease in well-being appears, however, to be only temporary, as improvement was shown in women who were more than 2 years postmenopausal.

Despite the high prevalence and severity of the symptoms in many women, little is known about the pathophysiology of hot flushes. Hot flushes are likely to arise as a result of an alteration in the body's thermoregulatory set-point, which is located in the anterior portion of the hypothalamus in the brain, and which controls physiological responses that conserve or dissipate heat, such as vasoconstriction and vasodilatation[8]. It is not clear what triggers the alteration in the hypothalamic thermoregulatory set-point, but the temporal relationship between loss of ovarian estradiol secretion and time of first onset of hot flushes indicates that decreased estrogen concentrations may play a key role, although a direct relationship between absolute estrogen deficiency *per se* or between individual levels of estradiol and incidence and severity of hot flushes was not found[9,10]. A close temporal relationship between the occurrence of hot flushes, skin temperature elevations (of up to 4.9°C) and the pulsatile secretion of luteinizing hormone (LH) has been demonstrated[11,12]. As pituitary LH release is directly and functionally related to hypothalamic gonadotropin-releasing hormone (GnRH) secretion, these data also point to a key role of the hypothalamus in the pathogenesis of hot flushes[13,14]. In rats, a thermoregulatory skin vasomotor response can be elicited through direct infusion of GnRH in the septal area[15]. It has been postulated that estrogens modulate the hypothalamic thermoregulatory set-point indirectly through an interaction with the serotoninergic (5-HT) pathways in the brain. In this model, the set-point in the hypothalamus would be dependent on the balance of at least two (sub)types of the 5-HT receptor: 5-HT_{1A}/5-HT_{2A}. Any change in the balance could induce a vasomotor response to internal or external stimuli to dissipate or preserve heat[8].

PHARMACOLOGICAL TREATMENT OF HOT FLUSHES

Several hormonal and non-hormonal therapies have been reported to have a beneficial effect on the frequency and severity of hot flushes, of which estrogen replacement therapy is the most efficacious.

Hormonal treatment of hot flushes

Estrogen replacement therapy dose-dependently reduces the number of hot flushes by over 90%. Notelovitz and colleagues performed a dose-ranging study in which 333 menopausal women with moderate to severe hot flushes received 12 weeks of treatment with 0.25, 0.5, 1 or 2 mg oral micronized 17β-estradiol or placebo, and found that dosages of 1 and 2 mg rapidly and extensively alleviated the symptoms. The difference versus placebo was statistically significant from week 4 onwards. At this time, half the women on placebo had a reduction in moderate to severe hot flushes of at least 52%; the corresponding figures were 56%, 69%, 86% and 91% for 0.25, 0.5, 1 and 2 mg 17β-estradiol-treated women, respectively[10]. A large placebo effect is consistently reported from studies of hot flushes, necessitating placebo controls to obtain reliable efficacy data. The statistically significant superiority of estrogens is clearly demonstrated as shown by a recent Cochrane systematic review that involved a meta-analysis of 21 trials with 2511 patients and treatment durations between 3 months and 3 years. This meta-analysis demonstrated that hormone replacement therapy (either estrogen-only or combined estrogen–progestogen therapy) was statistically significantly better than placebo for treatment of hot flushes, in terms of both symptom frequency and severity of symptoms[16]. A reduction of hot flushes by more than 80% as achieved with estradiol 1 mg/day or more than 90% as achieved with estradiol 2 mg/day was also clinically significant.

Non-hormonal treatment of hot flushes

Selective serotonin reuptake inhibitors (SSRIs), such as venlafaxine[17,18] and fluoxetine[19], are also effective for reduction of hot flushes, although less so than estrogens. In addition, this class of drugs is associated with moderate gastrointestinal and central nervous system side-effects, often leading to the patient's premature discontinuation with therapy. Although SSRIs may thus not be the treatment of choice in the case of hot flushes, the positive results provide insight into the mechanism of the disorder. Treatment with SSRIs leads to increased availability of 5-HT at the synaptic cleft, through blockade of the 5-HT reuptake pump. With prolonged treatment, the sensitivity of the different (sub)types of 5-HT receptors at different locations in the brain is altered. Up-regulation or sensitization of 5-HT_{1A} receptors occurs in the forebrain, whereas the inhibitory somatodendritic 5-HT_{1A} receptors in the raphe nucleus are down-regulated or desensitized. Furthermore, functional binding to the 5-HT_{2A} receptor in the prefrontal cortex decreases with long-term SSRI treatment. In rats, the blockade of 5-HT_{2A} prevents hyperthermia, whereas 5-HT_{1A} stimulation inhibits hypothermia. A similar mechanism could possibly account for the positive effects of SSRI treatment on the reduction of hot flushes in (post)menopausal women[8].

The benefits of other, non-hormonal therapies for hot flushes such as vitamin E and soya are largely unproven, and in many studies these therapies do not seem to be better than placebo[20,21].

PLACEBO EFFECTS IN THE TREATMENT OF HOT FLUSHES

Placebo responses are a common phenomenon in various aspects of clinical practice. Probably the first documented demonstration of a placebo effect comes from Sutton, who, in 1865, treated 20 patients with rheumatic fever with mint water[22]. More than 100 years later, Gribbin argued that many patients could effectively be treated by placebos, especially if the doctor was persuasive as to their value[23]. Both the patient's attitude to the illness as well as the illness itself may improve by a feeling that something is being done about it. This argument applies in psychiatric illness, such as depression or social anxiety disorder, but also, albeit to a lesser extent, in more physical ailments[24]. The magnitude of the response itself may vary, but the incidence of the placebo response in such disorders is fairly constant, being observed in 20–40% of patients in almost all studies[25].

A recent meta-analysis demonstrated that the placebo effect might account for over 50% reduction of hot flushes in double-blind randomized trials[16]. A high placebo effect is to be expected in studies of hot flushes in view of the natural variability and the decline in symptoms over time, and possibly also from an increased understanding, resulting in relief of anxiety over symptoms, owing to counselling received during the course of the trial[16].

The high placebo response in studies of menopausal hot flushes is not unlike that found in other conditions employing subjective response measures[26]. Trials that use objective outcome measures have generally lower placebo response rates than trials with subjective outcome measures[26], and this also holds for studies in which hot flushes are objectively quantified by digital thermography. Haas and colleagues studied the effects of 6 weeks' treatment with 50 μg/day of transdermal estradiol patch or placebo in 17 healthy postmenopausal women. The subjective symptoms of hot flushes were measured throughout the study by means of diary cards, and objectively by 8-h continuous thermography immediately after application of the first patch and after 6 weeks. Women in the active treatment group reported adequate relief of symptoms (up to 85% decrease from baseline), in terms of both subjective and objective outcome measures. The maximum decline in the placebo group was smaller (i.e. 27%), and symptoms were not statistically different from baseline[27]. The striking fact is, however, that during objective measurement of hot flushes with digital thermography, objective and subjective hot flushes coincide, as demonstrated by Meldrum and co-workers[11,12].

It has been stressed that the effects of hormone replacement therapy prescribed for vasomotor symptoms should be assessed in a blinded manner against placebo, so that the magnitude of the active treatment effect can be assessed as accurately as possible[16]. However, with sequentially combined treatment regimens, the bleeding pattern would reveal to the patient whether she received placebo or active treatment. A double-blind, prospectively randomized, placebo-controlled study to assess the effect of a sequential treatment with estradiol 0.5, 1.0 or 2 mg daily and dydrogesterone 10 mg on days 15–28 of each cycle indicated that there was a direct relationship between the reduction of hot flushes and the number of bleeding days (Solvay, unpublished data). To reduce the well-known placebo effect, only those women who did *not* respond during a 4-week placebo run-in phase were randomized to enter the double-blind period of the study. Consequently, only 42% of the initial study population were eligible for randomization and entered the double-blind 12-week treatment period. Nevertheless, the women who continued with placebo had a reduction of 51% in hot flushes over the following 12 weeks, which is close to the decrease in women not selected for placebo response. The decrease of hot flushes in women receiving estradiol 2 mg daily was 87%, which is close to that observed in studies without placebo run-in.

When the results for women treated with estradiol or placebo were combined, it appeared that the reduction in hot flushes in women who did not bleed was only 19%, compared with a reduction of between 75 and 95% (depending on the number of bleeding days) in women who had bleeding episodes (Figure 1a). However, as shown in Figure 1b, this relatively small decrease in the frequency of hot flushes in women who do not bleed does not prove to be an 'unblinding' effect, as the reduction in hot flushes and the mean number of bleeding days are linked through a common denominator, namely estradiol levels.

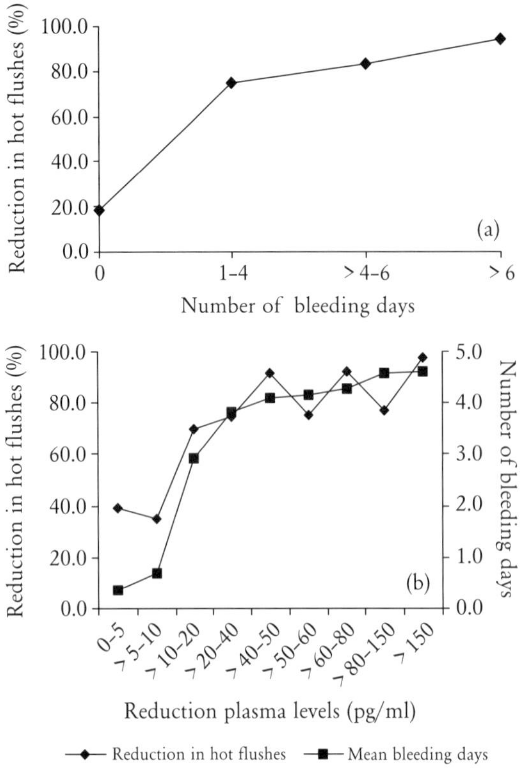

Figure 1 (a) Relationship between reduction of hot flushes and number of bleeding days in a double-blind placebo-controlled study in women with frequent hot flushes ($n = 93$ non-responders after 4-week placebo run-in, treatment duration 12 weeks, treatment 0.5, 1 or 2 mg estradiol daily and dydrogesterone 10 mg/day during days 15-28); (b) relationship between reduction of hot flushes, number of bleeding days and estradiol levels

An alternative hypothesis could therefore explain the considerable placebo effect: the 'frequent flushers' included in such trials are usually quite close to the menopause, and could be considered perimenopausal in spite of the low estradiol and high follicle stimulating hormone (FSH) levels required for inclusion. The mean age of the patients in this study was 51.1 years, the average duration of amenorrhea was 20.6 months and 74% of the patients were less than 2 years after the last natural menstruation. This could mean that there was still a certain fluctuation of estrogen levels obscuring the effect of the treatment.

A significant placebo effect of between 20 and 40% has also been reported in studies with other, non-hormonal - and often unconventional - treatment modalities, in which unblinding due to bleeding cannot play a role[8,20,21,28-32].

Another placebo-controlled study with patients who were *not* selected for frequent flushing showed a somewhat reduced placebo effect. The patients in this study were older, at 55.6 years on average, and 70.4 months on average after their last natural menstruation, and only 25% of the women were less than 2 years postmenopausal (Solvay, unpublished data). Although the end-point cannot be directly compared as it contained a quality-of-life element ('botheredness') instead of the number of hot flushes, the results show not only a greater difference between placebo and active treatment with estradiol 2 mg daily and dydrogesterone 10 mg/day from days 15 to 28 of each cycle, but also the persistence of the placebo effect which reached a maximum at the month-12 visit and persisted throughout the 2-year treatment period (Figure 2).

A more physiological explanation may serve as an alternative hypothesis for the mechanism underlying the observed placebo effect on hot flushes. It is known that variable, sometimes high, levels of endogenous estrogens are present in nearly all (peri)menopausal women[33,34]. The pulsatility of LH secretion is preserved until the postmenopausal years, although there is evidence that the amplitude of the pulse may change. And, although aging may impair the sensitivity of the hypothalamic–pituitary system to the negative feedback from gonadal steroids, there is evidence that this is not the case until after the early postmenopausal years[14,35]. It could thus be that fluctuating hormones affect the incidence and severity of hot flushes, especially in the perimenopausal years. Although LH pulses show no causal relationship with hot flushes, as they occur only later during such an event, they indicate the responsiveness of the pituitary in the context of residual ovarian activity. It is therefore highly plausible that not low estrogen levels *per se*, but rather rapidly fluctuating estrogen levels or estrogen withdrawal, is a causative factor underlying vasomotor instability[36]. This also fits in well with the observation of Simon and colleagues[9], who found that perimenopausal women show a higher placebo response than postmenopausal women.

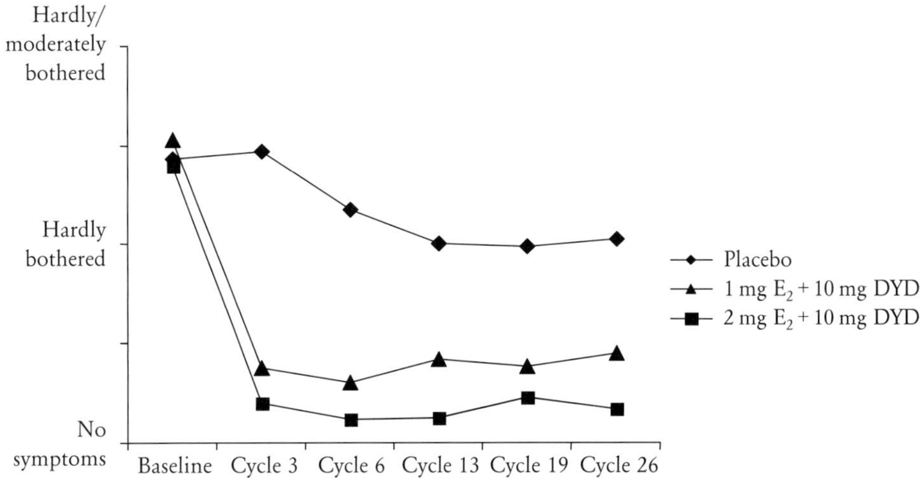

Figure 2 Improvement of 'botheredness' by hot flushes ($n = 344$ postmenopausal women unselected for vasomotor symptoms, placebo-controlled double-blind study). E_2, estradiol; DYD, dydroesterone

It remains to be determined in future studies whether placebo responders have higher estradiol levels, both at baseline and during treatment, or have a more responsive hypothalamic-pituitary system than placebo non-responders. Investigation of the etiology and pathophysiology of vasomotor symptoms, for example by examining the placebo effect, could help to develop effective non-hormonal treatment for women who do not tolerate estrogens or for whom estrogens are contraindicated. Because of the significant impact of hot flushes and night sweats on quality of life in climacteric women, such treatment would be highly welcome.

References

1. Oldenhave A, Jaszmann LJB, Haspels AA, *et al.* Impact of climacteric on well-being: a survey on 5213 women 39 to 60 years old. *Am J Obstet Gynecol* 1993;168:772–80
2. Haas S, Schiff I. Symptoms of oestrogen deficiency. In *The Menopause.* Oxford: Blackwell Scientific Publications, 1998;15:15–23
3. Maartens L, Leusink G, Knottnerus J, *et al.* Climacteric complaints in the community. *Fam Pract* 2001;18:189–94
4. Kronenberg F. Hot flashes: epidemiology and physiology. *Ann NY Acad Sci* 1990;592:52–86
5. Barnabei VM, Grady D, Stovall DW, *et al.* Menopausal symptoms in older women and the effects of treatment with hormone therapy. *Obstet Gynecol* 2002;100:1209–18
6. Kronenberg F. Hot flashes: phenomenology, quality of life and search for treatment options. *Exp Gerontol* 1994;29:319–36
7. Dennerstein L, Dudley E, Burger H. Well-being and the menopausal transition. *J Psychosom Obstet Gynecol* 1997;18:95–101
8. Stearns V, Ullmer L, Lopez JF. Hot flushes. *Lancet* 2002;360:1851–61
9. Simon JA, Stevens RE, Ayres SA, *et al.* Perimenopausal women in estrogen vasomotor trials: contribution to placebo effect and efficacy outcome. *Climacteric* 2001;4:19–27
10. Notelovitz M, Lenihan JP, McDermott M, *et al.* Initial 17β-estradiol dose for treating vasomotor symptoms. *Obstet Gynecol* 2000;95:726–31
11. Meldrum DR, Tataryn IV, Frumar AM, *et al.* Gonadotropins, estrogens, and adrenal steroids during the menopausal hot flash. *J Clin Endocrinol Metab* 1980;50:685–9
12. Meldrum DR, Shamonki IM, Frumar AM, *et al.* Elevations in skin temperature of the finger as an objective index of postmenopausal hot flashes:

standardization of the technique. *Am J Obstet Gynecol* 1979;135:713–17
13. Linsell CR, Lightman SL. Postmenopausal flashes: studies of chronological organisation. *Psychoneuroendocrinology* 1983;8:435–40
14. Rossmanith WG. Gonadotropin secretion during aging in women: review article. *Exp Gerontol* 1995; 30:369–81
15. Hosono T, Yanase-Fujiwara M, Zhang YH, *et al.* Effect of gonadotropin releasing hormone on thermoregulatory vasomotor activity in ovariectomized female rats. *Brain Res* 1997;754:88–94
16. MacLennan A, Lester S, Moore V. Oral oestrogen replacement therapy versus placebo for hot flushes (Cochrane Review). *The Cochrane Library*, 1. Oxford: Update Software, 2001
17. Loprinzi CL, Kugler JW, Sloan JA, *et al.* Venlafaxine in management of hot flashes in survivors of breast cancer: a randomised controlled trial. *Lancet* 2000;356:2059–63
18. Barton D, La Vasseur B, Loprinzi C, *et al.* Venlafaxine for the control of hot flashes: results of a longitudinal continuation study. *Oncol Nurse Forum* 2002;29:33–40
19. Loprinzi CL, Sloan JA, Perez EA, *et al.* Phase III evaluation of fluoxetine for treatment of hot flashes. *J Clin Oncol* 2002;20:1578–83
20. Barton DL, Loprinzi CL, Quella SK, *et al.* Prospective evaluation of vitamin E for hot flashes in breast cancer survivors. *J Clin Oncol* 1998;16:495–500
21. Quella SK, Loprinzi CL, Barton DL, *et al.* Evaluation of soy phytoestrogens for the treatment of hot flashes in breast cancer survivors: a North Central Cancer Treatment Group Trial. *J Clin Oncol* 2000;18:1068–74
22. Sutton HG. Cases of rheumatic fever treated for the most part by mint water. *Guy's Hosp Rep* 1865; 2:392
23. Gribbin M. Placebos: cheapest medicine in the world. *New Sci* 1981;89:64–5
24. Moyad MA. The placebo effect and randomized trials: analysis of conventional medicine. *Urol Clin North Am* 2002;29:125–33
25. Katzung BG, Berkowitz BA. Basic and clinical evaluation of new drugs. In Katzung BG, ed. *Basic and Clinical Pharmacology*. San Mateo: Appleton & Lange, 1989:51–8
26. Hrobjartsson A, Gotzsche PC. Is the placebo powerless? An analysis of clinical trials comparing placebo with no treatment. *N Engl J Med* 2001; 344:1594–602
27. Haas S, Walsh B, Evans S, *et al.* The effect of transdermal estradiol on hormone and metabolic dynamics over a six-week period. *Obstet Gynecol* 1988;71:671–6
28. Guttuso T, Kurlan R, McDermott MP, *et al.* Gabapentin's effects on hot flashes in postmenopausal women: a randomized controlled trial. *Obstet Gynecol* 2003;101:337–45
29. Davis SR, Briganti EM, Chen RQ, *et al.* The effects of Chinese medicinal herbs on postmenopausal vasomotor symptoms of Australian women. A randomised controlled trial. *Med J Aust* 2001; 174:68–71
30. Van Patten CL, Olivotto IA, Chambers GK, *et al.* Effect of soy phytoestrogens on hot flashes in postmenopausal women with breast cancer: a randomized, controlled clinical trial. *J Clin Oncol* 2002;20:1449–55
31. Upmalis DH, Lobo R, Bradley L, *et al.* Vasomotor symptom relief by soy isoflavone extract tablets in postmenopausal women: a multicenter, double-blind, randomized, placebo-controlled study. *Menopause* 2000;7:236–42
32. Nesheim BI, Saetre T. Reduction of menopausal hot flushes by methyldopa. A double blind crossover trial. *Eur J Clin Pharmacol* 1981; 20:413–16
33. Kuchel GA, Tannenbaum C, Greenspan SL, *et al.* Can variability in the hormonal status of elderly women assist in the decision to administer estrogens? *J Women's Health Gend Based Med* 2001;10:109–16
34. Johannes CB, Crawford SL. Menstrual bleeding, hormones, and the menopausal transition. *Semin Reprod Endocrinol* 1999;17:299–309
35. Rossmanith WG, Reichelt C, Scherbaum WA. Neuroendocrinology of aging in humans: attenuated sensitivity to sex steroid feedback in elderly postmenopausal women. *Neuroendocrinology* 1994;59:355–62
36. Prior JC. Perimenopause: the complex endocrinology of the menopausal transition. *Endocr Rev* 1998;19:397–428

Women, hormones and depression 28

J. Studd

INTRODUCTION

On Boxing Day 1851, Charles Dickens attended the patients' Christmas dance at St. Luke's Hospital for the Insane. On describing his visit in an article for *Household Words* he commented that the experience of the asylum proved that insanity was more prevalent among women than among men. Of the 18 759 inmates over the century, 11 162 had been women. He adds, 'it is well known that female servants are more frequently affected by lunacy than any other class of persons'.

Charles Dickens was as great an observer as any Nobel prize winner, and indeed this passage is one of the very few references in Victorian literature that makes a connection between gender and depression, but there are none, to the present author's knowledge, relating reproductive function to depression. Jane Eyre's red room and Bertha Mason's monthly madness in the same novel may be coded examples of this from Charlotte Brontë's pen. Modern epidemiology confirms that depression is more common in women than in men whether we look at hospital admissions, population studies, suicide attempts or the prescription of antidepressants[1]. The challenge remains to determine whether this increase in depression is environmental, reflecting women's perceived role in contemporary society, or whether it is due to hormonal changes.

It is clear that this excess of depression in women starts at puberty and is no longer present in the 6th and 7th decades. The peaks of depression occur at times of hormonal fluctuation in the premenstrual phase, the postpartum phase and the climacteric perimenopausal phase, particularly in the 1 or 2 years before menstruation ceases. This triad of hormone-responsive mood disorders often occurs in the same vulnerable women. Depression in these patients can usually be treated effectively by estrogens, preferably via the transdermal route and in a moderately high dose. Transdermal patches containing 200 μg estrogen have been used in our published placebo-controlled studies, but the 100-μg dose is frequently effective.

The 45-year-old depressed perimenopausal woman who is still menstruating will often give a history of previous postnatal depression as well as depression before menstrual periods. She will often be in very good mood during pregnancy and also have systemic manifestations of hormonal fluctuation in the form of menstrual headaches or menstrual migraine. Such a woman will often say that she last felt well during her last pregnancy. She then developed postnatal depression for several months. When her periods returned the depression became cyclical, and as she approached the menopause the depression became more constant. The problem with this clear clinical history of a woman who will probably respond to estrogens is that psychiatrists believe that such patients are ideal for the use of antidepressants. This is because they recognize that such women have a 'pre-morbid history of depression' and therefore they have chronic relapsing depressive illness, treated by psychiatrists. The fact that this depression is postnatal or premenstrual in timing usually escapes them. It is sad that both gynecologists and psychiatrists are products of their particular training, with too little overlap in knowledge. The patients thus become victims of this professional schism.

The clue to the use of estrogens came with the important and somewhat eccentric article of Klaiber and colleagues[2], who performed the first placebo-controlled study of very-high-dose estrogens in patients with chronic relapsing depression. The women had various diagnoses, and were both premenopausal and postmenopausal. They were initially given Premarin® 5 mg daily, with an

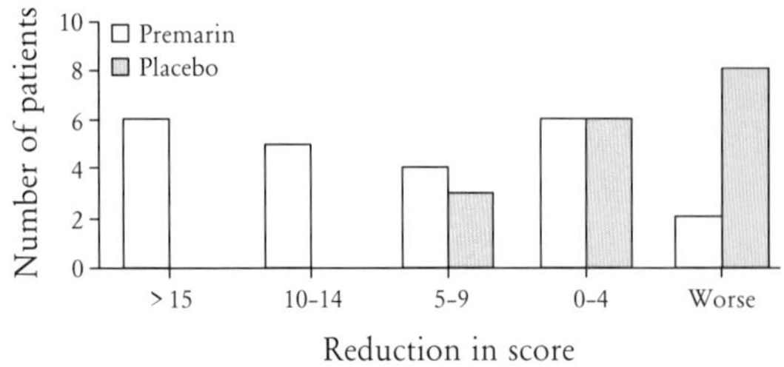

Figure 1 Placebo-controlled trial of women with chronic relapsing depression given large doses, up to 30 mg, of Premarin® per day showing a significant improvement in Hamilton depression score in women taking the active preparation

increase in dose of 5 mg each week until a maximum of 30 mg/day was used. There was a huge improvement in depression with these high doses (Figure 1), but this work has not been repeated because of anxiety over high-dose estrogens.

PREMENSTRUAL SYNDROME

This condition is mentioned in the fourth century BC by Hippocrates, but became a medical epidemic in the 19th century. Victorian physicians were aware of menstrual madness, hysteria, chlorosis and ovarian mania, as well as the more commonplace neurasthenia. In the 1870s Maudsley[3], the most distinguished psychiatrist of the time, wrote, '. . . the monthly activity of the ovaries which marks the advent of puberty in women has a notable effect upon the mind and body; wherefore it may become an important cause of mental and physical derangement . . .'. This and other female maladies were recognized, rightly or wrongly, to be due to the ovaries. As a consequence, bilateral oophorectomy – Battey's operation[4] – became fashionable, being performed in approximately 150 000 women in North America and Northern Europe in the 30 years from 1870. Longo[5], in his brilliant historical essay on the decline of Battey's operation, posed the question of whether it worked or not. Of course the physicians had no knowledge of osteoporosis and the devastation of long-term estrogen deficiency; therefore, on balance, the operation was not helpful as a long-term solution, but it probably did, as was claimed, cure the 'menstrual/ovarian madness', which would be a quaint Victorian way of labelling severe premenstrual syndrome (PMS). The essential logic of this operation was to remove cyclical ovarian function, but happily this can now effectively be achieved by simpler medical therapy.

Only in 1931 was the phrase 'premenstrual tension' introduced by Frank[6], who described 15 women with the typical symptoms of PMS as we know it. Greene and Dalton extended the definition to 'premenstrual syndrome' in 1953[7], recognizing the wider range of symptoms. Severe PMS is a poorly understood collection of cyclical symptoms, which cause considerable psychological and physical distress. The psychological symptoms of depression, loss of energy, irritability, loss of libido and abnormal behavior as well as the physical symptoms of headaches, breast discomfort and abdominal bloating may occur for up to 14 days each month. There may also be associated menstrual problems, pelvic pain and menstrual headaches, and the woman may enjoy only as few as 7 good days per month. It is obvious that the symptoms mentioned can have a significant impact on the day-to-day functioning of women.

It is estimated that up to 95% of women have some form of PMS, but about 5% of women of reproductive age will be affected severely, with disruption of their daily activities. Considering these figures, it is disturbing that many of the consultations at our specialist PMS clinics start with women saying that for many years they have been told that there are no treatments available, and that they should simply 'live with it'. In addition, many commonly used treatments of PMS, particularly progesterone or progestogens, have been shown by many placebo-controlled trials not only to be ineffective, but also to make the symptoms worse, as often women are progesterone- or progestogen-intolerant.

The exact cause of PMS is uncertain, but fundamentally it is due to the hormonal or biochemical changes (whatever they are) that occur with ovulation, and the resulting interaction between the ovarian steroids, the complex γ-aminobutyric acid (GABA) system in the brain, serotonin release and other neuroendocrine factors. These chemical fluctuations produce the varied symptoms in women who are somehow vulnerable to changes in their normal reproductive hormone levels.

These cyclical chemical changes, probably due to progesterone or one of its metabolites such as allopregnanalone, produce the cyclical symptoms of PMS.

ESTROGENS

Premenstrual syndrome does not occur if there is no ovarian function[8]. Obviously, it does not occur before puberty or after the menopause, or after oophorectomy. It also does not occur during pregnancy. However, it is important to realize that hysterectomy with conservation of the ovaries often does not cure PMS[9], as patients are left with the usual cyclical symptoms and cyclical headaches. This condition, best called 'the ovarian cycle syndrome'[10], is usually not recognized to be hormonal in etiology, as there is no reference point of menstruation. The failure to make this diagnosis is regrettable, because these monthly symptoms of depression, irritability, mood change, bloating and headaches, which might affect the woman for most days in the month with perhaps only a good week each month, can easily be treated with transdermal estrogens which suppress ovarian function and thus remove the symptoms.

A medical 'Battey's operation' can be achieved by the use of gonadotropin-releasing hormone (GnRH) analogs, and Leather and colleagues[11] have demonstrated that 3 months of Zoladex® therapy cures all of the symptom groups of PMS (Figure 2). The women do, of course, have hot flushes and sweats, but these are usually far preferable to the cyclical depression, irritability and headaches. The long-term risk of Zoladex therapy is bone demineralization, but the same group showed that add-back with a product containing 2 mg estradiol valerate and cyclical levonorgestrel (Nuvelle®; Schering Healthcare) maintain bone density at both the spine and the hip[12] (Figure 3). Most of the PMS symptoms remain improved with this 'add-back', but bloating, tension and irritability recur, probably due to the cyclical progestogen. Livial® may be a better add-back preparation.

In a Scandinavian study, Sundstrom and colleagues used low-dose GnRH analogs (100 μg buserelin) with good results for the symptoms of PMS, but the treatment still caused anovulation in as many as 56% of patients[13]. Danazol is another method used to treat PMS by inhibiting pituitary gonadotropins, but it has side-effects including androgenic and virilizing effects. When used in the luteal phase only[14], it relieved mastalgia but not the general symptoms of PMS, even though side-effects were minimal.

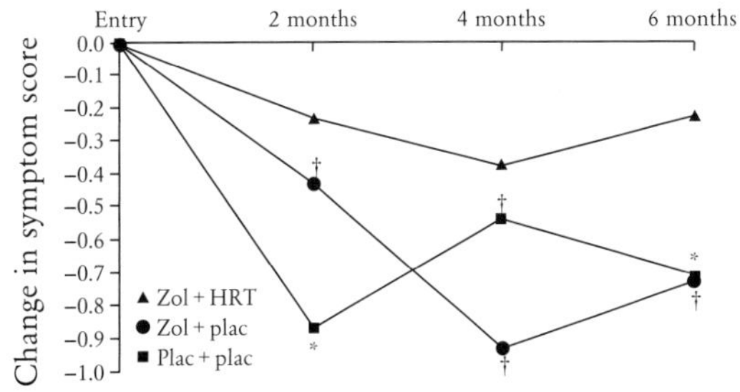

Figure 2 Improvement in depression in women with severe premenstrual syndrome, using Zoladex® (Zol) and Zoladex plus add-back estradiol-progestogen hormone replacement therapy (HRT). $^*p < 0.05$ vs. baseline and Plac + Plac; $^\dagger p < 0.05$ vs. baseline. Plac, placebo

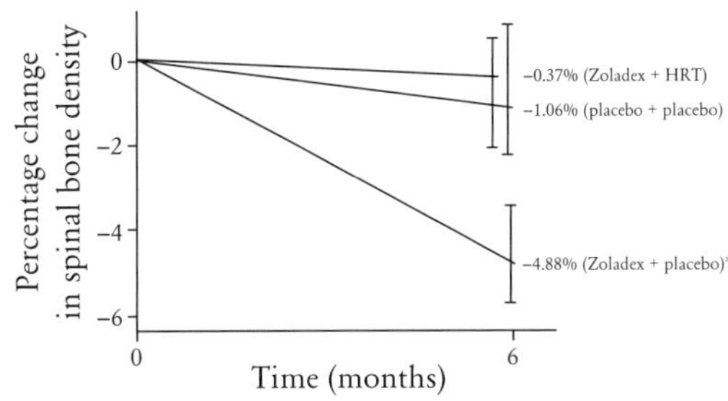

Figure 3 Loss of bone density at the lumbar spine after 6 months of Zoladex treatment being prevented by add-back with Nuvelle®: 2 mg estradiol plus norgestrel. $^*p < 0.005$ vs. placebo + placebo; $^\dagger p < 0.001$ vs. pretreatment. HRT, hormone replacement therapy

Greenblatt and colleagues showed the effects of an anovulatory dose of estrogen via an implant for contraception[15], and the first study of its use in PMS was carried out by Magos and associates[16] with 100-mg estradiol implants, the dose that had been shown to inhibit ovulation using ultrasound and day-21 progesterone measurements in earlier studies by the same group. This study demonstrated a huge 84% improvement with placebo implants, but improvement of every symptom cluster was greater in the active estradiol group. In addition, the placebo effect usually waned after a few months, compared with a continued response to estradiol. These patients, of course, were also given oral progestogen for 12 days each month to prevent endometrial hyperplasia and irregular bleeding[17]. It was clear that the addition of a progestogen attenuated the beneficial effect of the estrogen. Subsequently, a placebo-controlled trial of cyclical norethisterone in 'well-estrogenized' hysterectomized women reproduced the typical symptoms of PMS[18]. This study of cyclical oral progestogen in the estrogen-primed woman is the model for PMS. It is also significant that progestogen intolerance is one of the principal reasons why older, postmenopausal women stop taking hormone replacement therapy[19], particularly if they have a past history of PMS or progesterone intolerance. It is common for progestogens to cause PMS-like symptoms in these women in the same way as endogenous cyclical progesterone secretion is the probable fundamental cause of PMS.

Our group still uses estradiol implants in our PMS clinics, often with the addition of testosterone for loss of energy and loss of libido, but we have reduced the estradiol dose, never starting with 100 mg. We now insert pellets of estradiol 50 or 75 mg with 100 mg testosterone. These women must have endometrial protection by either oral progestogen or a Mirena® (Schering Healthcare) levonorgestrel-releasing intrauterine system (LNG IUS)[20]. As women with PMS respond well to estrogens but are often intolerant to progestogens, it is therefore commonplace for us to reduce the orthodox 13-day course of the progestogen to 10 or 7 days, starting, for convenience, on the first day of every calendar month. Thus, the menstrual cycle is reset, with the woman having the obvious additional advantage of 12 periods a year instead of 13. She can also easily plan her withdrawal bleeds to avoid holidays and other important functions.

The Mirena IUS also plays a vital part in preventing PMS-like symptoms, as it performs its role of protecting the endometrium without systemic absorption. A recent study has shown a 50% decrease in hysterectomies in our practice since the introduction of the Mirena IUS in 1995[17]. With its profound effect on menorrhagia and fewer progestogenic side-effects, Mirena appears to be a very promising component of PMS treatment in the future.

Hormone implants are not licensed in all countries, and are unsuitable for women who may wish to discontinue treatment easily to become pregnant. Estradiol patches are an alternative, and our original double-blind cross-over study used a 200-μg estradiol patch twice weekly[21]. This produced plasma estradiol levels of 800 pmol/l, and suppressed luteal-phase progesterone and ovulation. Once again this treatment was better than placebo in every symptom cluster of PMS. Figure 4 shows the responses to estradiol treatment and placebo in a 6-month cross-over study. This is now our treatment of choice in severe PMS.

Subsequently, a randomized but uncontrolled observational study from our PMS clinic indicated that PMS sufferers can have the same beneficial response to 100-μg patches as they do to the 200-μg dose. They also have fewer symptoms of breast

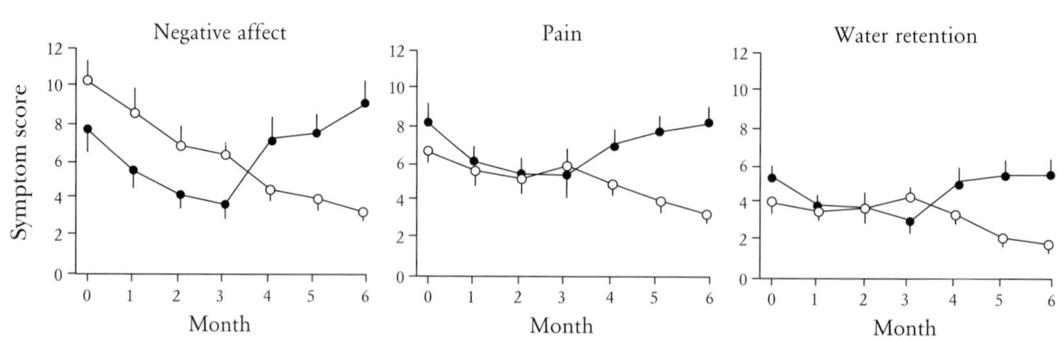

Figure 4 Results from a placebo-controlled cross-over trial of 200-μg estradiol patch (Estraderm®) effects on the symptoms of severe premenstrual syndrome. Open symbols, estradiol treatment; filled symbols, placebo treatment; MDQ, Mental Distress Questionnaire

discomfort and bloating, and there is less anxiety of the patient or general practitioner about high-dose estrogen therapy[22]. Day-21 progesterone assays in patients receiving 100 μg showed low anovulatory levels, prompting the intriguing question of whether even this moderate dose might reliably suppress ovulation and be contraceptive (Figure 5). Clearly, a great deal of work must be done before we can suggest that this treatment is an effective form of birth control, but it is of great importance, because many young women on this therapy for PMS would be pleased if it were also an effective contraceptive. This is a study which needs to be conducted.

The original studies outlined in this chapter are all scientifically valid placebo-controlled trials, showing a considerable improvement in PMS symptoms with estrogens. Although this treatment is used by most gynecologists in the UK, its value has not been exploited by psychiatrists anywhere in the world. We believe that the benefit of this therapy in severe PMS is due to the inhibition of ovulation, but there is probably also a central mental tonic effect. Klaiber and colleagues[2] in their study of high-dose Premarin demonstrated this, and our other psychoendocrine studies of climacteric depression[23] and postnatal depression[24] have shown the benefit of high-dose transdermal estrogens for these conditions, which is not related to or dependent upon suppression of ovulation.

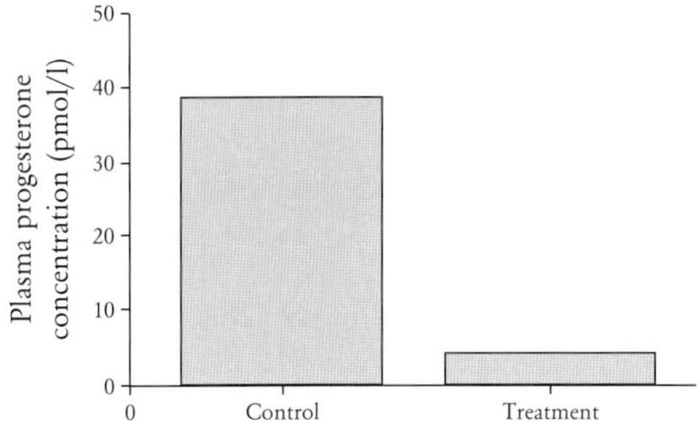

Figure 5 Day-21 plasma progesterone levels in women with premenstrual syndrome and those receiving 100-μg estradiol patches, indicating that such a dose suppresses ovulation in the majority of these women. However, it cannot be assumed that this treatment is contraceptive

Ultimately, there are some women who, after treatment with oestrogens and Mirena coils, will prefer to have a hysterectomy, to remove all cycles with a virtual guarantee of improvement of symptoms. This should not be seen as a failure or even the treatment of last resort, as it does carry many other advantages[25]. It is important that women who have had a hysterectomy and bilateral salpingo-oophorectomy have effective replacement therapy, ideally with replacement of the ovarian androgens. Implants of estradiol 50 mg and testosterone 100 mg are an ideal route and combination of hormones for this long-term therapy post-hysterectomy, with a continuation rate of 90% at 10 years[17]. We carried out a study of 47 such patients who had undergone a hysterectomy and bilateral salpingo-oophorectomy and subsequently had implants of estradiol and testosterone for severe PMS, who had experienced many years of treatment with transdermal estrogens and cyclical progestogens or a Mirena coil. The symptoms were removed in all patients, and all but one were 'very satisfied' with the outcome.

POSTNATAL DEPRESSION

Postnatal depression is another example of depression being caused by fluctuations of sex hormones and having the potential to be effectively treated by hormones. It is a common condition which affects 10–15% of women following childbirth, and may persist for over 1 year in 40% of those affected. There seems to be a lack of any overall influence of psychosocial background factors in determining vulnerability to this postpartum disorder, although it can be recurrent.

Although common, the disease is often not reported to the health-care professional, particularly the general practitioner or the visiting midwife, as the exhaustion and depression is regarded as normal. Indeed, the symptoms of postnatal depression may be confused with the normal sequelae of childbirth. The symptoms can consist of depressed mood with lack of pleasure with the baby or any interest in her surroundings. There may be sleep disturbance, either insomnia or hypersomnia. There may be loss of weight, loss of energy and certainly loss of libido, together with agitation, retardation and feelings of worthlessness or guilt. Frequent thoughts of death and suicide are common.

Postnatal depression is not more common after a long labor, difficult labor, Cesarean section or separation from the baby after birth, nor is it determined by education or socioeconomic group. The only environmental factor which seems to be important is the perceived amount of support given by the partner. There is no doubt that the first 6 months or more after delivery can be an exhausting time, full of anxiety and insecurity for mothers having the new responsibility of a baby. Even allowing for that, there does seem to be a clear hormonal aspect to this condition.

Postnatal depression is severe and more prolonged in women who are lactating, and lower estradiol levels are found in depressed women following delivery than in controls. It is probable that the low estradiol levels seen with breast-feeding and the higher incidence of depression are related in a causative way.

We studied the effect of high-dose transdermal estrogens on this condition, in an attempt to close the circle of studies investigating the triad of hormone-responsive mood disorders: premenstrual depression, climacteric depression and postnatal depression. This was a double-blind placebo-controlled trial of 60 women with major depression, which began within 3 months of childbirth and persisted for up to 18 months postnatally[24]. They had all been resistant to antidepressants, and the diagnosis of postnatal depression was made by two psychiatrists who are experts in the field. We excluded breast-feeding women from the study. Women were given either placebo patches or transdermal estradiol patches, 200 μg daily, for 3 months without any added progestogen. After 3 months, cyclical Duphaston® 10 μg daily was added for 12 days each month. The women were assessed monthly using a self-rating of depressive symptoms, the Edinburgh postnatal depression score (EPDS), and by clinical psychiatric interview. Both groups were severely depressed, with a mean EPDS score of 21.8 before treatment. During the first month of therapy, the women who received estrogen improved rapidly, and to a greater extent than controls. None of the other factors, age, psychiatric, obstetric or gynecological history, severity and duration of current episode of depression and concurrent antidepressant medication, influenced the response to treatment.

The study showed that the mean EPDS score was less in the active group at 1 month and then maintained for 8 months, and that the percentage with EPDS scores over 14 (diagnostic of postnatal depression) was reduced by 50% at 1 month and 90% at 5 months. This was much better than the placebo response (Figure 6).

Not only did this study show that transdermal estrogens were effective for the treatment of postnatal depression, but also a subsequent study by Lawrie and colleagues[26] showed that depot-progestogen was worse than placebo in causing a deterioration in the severity of postnatal depression. Thus, we have again the picture of the mood-elevating effect of estrogens and the depressing effect of a progestogen.

An uncontrolled study showed similar improvements using sublingual estradiol in 23 women with major postnatal depression[27]. These women had plasma levels of 79.0 pmol/l before treatment with sublingual estradiol. Estradiol levels were 342 pmol/l at 1 week and 480 pmol/l at 8 weeks. There was improvement in 12 of the 23 patients at 1 week, and after 2 weeks there was recovery in 19 of the 23 patients. The mean Montgomery Asberg depression rating scale (MADRS) was 40.7 before treatment, 11 at 1 week and 2 at 8 weeks. At the end of the second week of treatment, the MADRS scores were compatible

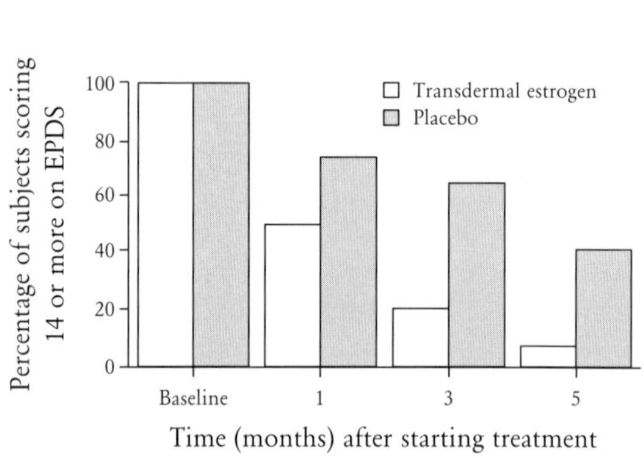

Figure 6 Improvement in Edinburgh postnatal depression score (EPDS) in women with postnatal depression using 200-μg estradiol patches compared with placebo

with clinical recovery in 19 of the 23 patients. This study stressed the rapidity of response to the estradiol therapy, and this was our observation also. However, it must be stressed that this was an uncontrolled study in women with a very low, almost postmenopausal level of estradiol. Another placebo-controlled study is required, together with information about bleeding patterns to support or refute our original article[24].

It would support the hormonal pathogenesis of this condition if we could mimic postnatal depression by hormonal manipulation. This was done in a study by Bloch and associates[28], who examined 16 women, eight with a history of postnatal depression. They induced hypogonadism with leuprolide acetate, and simulated pregnancy by 'add-back' supraphysiological doses of estradiol and progesterone for 8 weeks, then withdrawing both steroids. Five of the eight women (62.5%) with a history of postnatal depression and none of the women without a prior history developed significant mood symptoms during the withdrawal period.

This study supported the view that there is an involvement of the reproductive hormones, estradiol and progesterone, in the development of postpartum depression in a set group of women. Furthermore, the study showed that women with a history of postnatal depression are differentially sensitive to the mood-destabilizing effects of gonadal steroids.

CLIMACTERIC DEPRESSION

Like many aspects of depression in women, the diagnosis of climacteric depression and its treatment remain controversial. Whereas gynecologists who deal with the menopause have no difficulty in accepting the role of estrogens in the causation and treatment of this common disorder, psychiatrists seem to be implacably opposed to it. This may be because there is no real evidence of an excess of depression occurring *after* the menopause, nor any evidence that estrogens help *post*menopausal depression or what used to be called 'involutional melancholia'. This is quite true, and indeed many women with longstanding depression improve considerably when their periods stop. This is because the depression created by premenstrual syndrome, heavy painful periods, menstrual headaches and the exhaustion that attends excess blood loss disappears. Therefore, the longitudinal studies of depression carried out by many psychologists, particularly those as notable as Hunter[29], have shown no peak of depression in a large population of menopausal women. The depression that occurs in women around the time of the menopause is at its worst in the 2 or 3 years before menstruation ceases. This, of course, is perimenopausal depression, and is no doubt related to premenstrual depression as it becomes worse with age and with falling estrogen levels.

The earliest placebo-controlled study which defined the precise menopausal syndrome showed that estrogens helped hot flushes, night sweats and vaginal dryness. They also had a mood-elevating effect[30]. This work was further supported by the work of Campbell and Whitehead[31] who used Premarin, and by the study of Montgomery and colleagues[23] using higher-dose estradiol implants. This study of 90 peri- and postmenopausal women with depression showed considerable improvement in the treatment group compared with placebo, but only in the perimenopausal women (Figure 7). There was no improvement in depression in the postmenopausal women with this treatment, when compared with placebo. This effect is not transient, and we have shown that the improvement in depression is maintained even at 23 months. By this stage, the placebo patients had dropped out and there was no placebo group in the study. It was therefore decided not to publish this

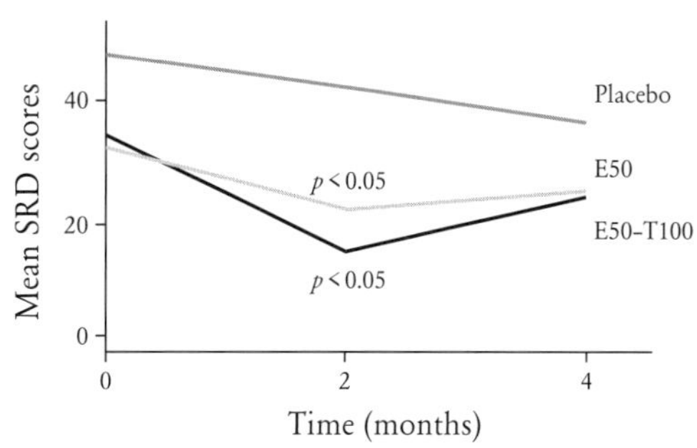

Figure 7 Improvement in depression and anxiety (self-rated depression, SRD30 score) at 2 months in women with perimenopausal depression treated with estradiol implants (E50) or estradiol-testosterone implants (E50–T100) compared with placebo

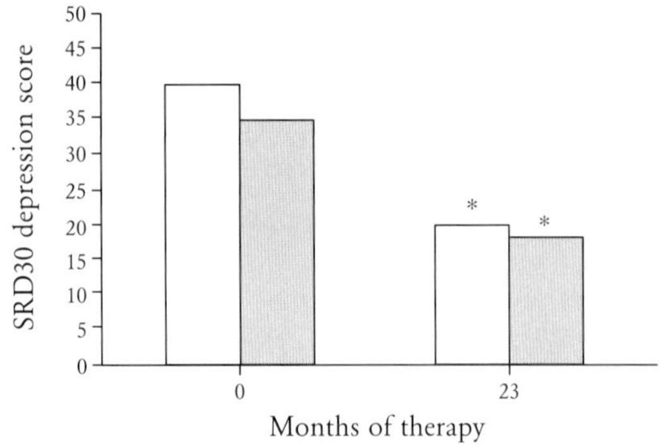

Figure 8 Sustained improvement in self-rated depression (SRD30) score after 23 months of treatment with estradiol implants (open bars) or estradiol plus testosterone implants (shaded bars)

uncontrolled observational study, but Figure 8 shows these data and the reader can draw whatever conclusion is necessary.

At last, after 15 years, psychiatrists particularly in the USA are coming round to the view that transdermal estrogens are effective in the treatment of depressed perimenopausal women. Soares and colleagues[32] in 2001 studied 50 such women, 26 with major depressive disorder, 11 with dysthymic depression and 30 with minor depressive illness. They treated them with 100-μg estradiol patches in a 12-week placebo-controlled study. There was a remission of depression in 17 out of 25 treatment patients (68%), and only five out of 25 placebo patients (20%). This improvement occurred regardless of the Diagnostic and Statistics Manual of Mental Disorders-IV (DSM-IV) diagnosis.

Rasgon and associates[33] studied 16 perimenopausal women with unipolar major depressive disorder in an 8-week open-protocol trial comparing low-dose 0.3 mg Premarin alone or plus fluoxetine daily. There was a greater response with estrogen alone. All but two of the total patients responded, but the response was greater in the estrogen-treated patients, and it was significant that the reduction of depression scores began rapidly after the first week of treatment.

More recently, Harlow and co-workers[34] studied a large number (976) of both perimenopausal women with a history of major depression and those without. Patients with a history of depression had higher follicle stimulating hormone levels and lower estradiol levels at enrolment to the study, and women with a history of antidepressant medication had three times the rate of early menopause, compared with women without depression. A similar excess rate was found in perimenopausal women who had a history of severe depression.

It is reassuring, for those 'menopausologists' who have been trying to persuade the world of psychiatry that estrogens have a place in the treatment of depressed women, and pleasing to read at last the view that, 'periods of intense hormonal fluctuations have been associated with the heightened prevalence and exacerbation of underlying psychiatric illness, particularly the occurrence of premenstrual dysphoria, puerperal depression and depressive treatment during the perimenopause. It is speculated that sex steroids such as oestrogens, progestogens [sic], testosterone and DHEA exert a significant modulation of brain functioning. There are preliminary, but promising, data on the use of estradiol (particularly transdermal) estradiol to alleviate depression during the menopause'[34].

At last we are getting through!

PROGESTOGEN INTOLERANCE

Those women having moderately high-dose estrogen therapy must of course take cyclical progestogen if they still have a uterus, to prevent irregular bleeding and endometrial hyperplasia. The problem is that women with hormone-responsive depression enjoy a mood-elevating effect with estrogens, but this is attenuated by the necessary progestogen[35]. This hormone can produce depression, tiredness, loss of libido, irritability, breast discomfort and, in fact, all of the symptoms of premenstrual syndrome, particularly in women with a history or previous history of PMS. A randomized trial of norethisterone against placebo in 'estrogenized' hysterectomized women, referred to above, clearly showed this, and indeed the article is subtitled 'a model for the premenstrual syndrome'[16].

If women become depressed with 10–12 days of progestogen, it may be necessary to halve the dose, decrease the duration or change the progestogen used[36]. It is our policy routinely to shorten the duration of progestogen in women with hormone-responsive depression, because adverse side-effects with any gestogen occur almost invariably. We would therefore use transdermal estrogens, either 100 or 200 μg in an estradiol patch, or a 50-mg estradiol implant, and then reset the menstrual bleeding by prescribing norethisterone 5 mg for the first 7 days of each calendar month. This will produce a regular bleed on about day 10 or 11 of each calendar month.

If heavy periods occur (and they usually do not), one should extend the duration of progestogen to the more orthodox 12 days each month. At this stage, many women would prefer to have a Mirena coil inserted, so that there will be no bleeding, no cycles nor any need to take oral progestogen with its side-effects. It is not unusual for women at this stage who understand the benefits of estrogens and the problems of their menstrual cycles to request hysterectomy and bilateral salpingo-oophorectomy with hormone replacement therapy with estradiol and testosterone[37]. This is a fact of medical life and patient choice, but it will be at least another 15 years before psychiatrists attempt to leap over that hurdle.

SUMMARY

(1) Estrogen therapy is effective for the treatment of postnatal depression, premenstrual depression and perimenopausal depression, the triad of hormone-responsive mood disorders.

(2) Transdermal estradiol in the form of 100- or 200-μg patches producing plasma levels of approximately 500 and 800 pmol/l, respectively, should be used.

(3) These patients often require plasma levels of more than 600 pmol/l for efficacy.

(4) Consider adding testosterone for improvement of depression, libido and energy.

(5) A cyclical progestogen or Mirena intrauterine system (IUS) is required if the patient still has a uterus.

(6) The most effective long-term medical therapy is use of estradiol patches or an implant of estradiol and testosterone with a Mirena IUS *in situ*.

(7) Ultimately, a hysterectomy plus bilateral salpingo-oophorectomy and an implant with estradiol and testosterone may be requested.

ACKNOWLEDGEMENT

This chapter has been reproduced, with permission, from *Management of the Menopause*, edited by J. Studd and published by Parthenon Publishing in July, 2003.

References

1. Paney N, Studd JWW. The psychotherapeutic effects of oestrogens. *Gynecol Endocrinol* 1998; 12:353–65
2. Klaiber EL, Broverman DM, Vogel W, Kobayashi Y. Estrogen therapy for severe persistent depressions in women. *Arch Gen Psychiatry* 1979;36:550–4
3. Maudsley H. Sex in mind and education. *Fortnightly Rev* 1874
4. Battey R. Battey's operation – its matured results. *Trans Georgia Med Assoc* 1873
5. Longo LD. The rise and fall of Battey's operation: a fashion in surgery. *Bull Hist Med* 1979;53:244–67
6. Frank RT. The hormonal basis of premenstrual tension. *Arch Neurol Psychiatry* 1931;26:1053–7
7. Greene R, Dalton K. The premenstrual syndrome. *Br Med J* 1953;1:1007–14
8. Studd JWW. Premenstrual tension syndrome. *Br Med J* 1979;1:410
9. Backstrom T, Boyle H, Baird DT. Persistence of symptoms of premenstrual tension in hysterectomized women. *Br J Obstet Gynaecol* 1981;88: 530–6
10. Studd JWW. Prophylactic oophorectomy at hysterectomy. *Br J Obstet Gynaecol* 1989;96:506–9

11. Leather AT, Studd JWW, Watson NR, Holland EFN. The treatment of severe premenstrual syndrome with goserelin with and without 'add-back' estrogen therapy: a placebo-controlled study. *Gynecol Endocrinol* 1999;13:48–55
12. Leather AT, Studd JWW, Watson NR, Holland EFN. The prevention of bone loss in young women treated with GnRH analogues with 'add back' oestrogen therapy. *Obstet Gynecol* 1993;81:104–7
13. Sundstrom I, Myberg S, Bixo M, Hammarback S, Backstrom T. Treatment of premenstrual syndrome with gonadotropin-releasing hormone agonist in a low dose regimen. *Acta Obstet Gynecol Scand* 1999;78:891–9
14. O'Brien PM, Abukhalil IE. Randomized controlled trial of the management of premenstrual syndrome and premenstrual mastalgia using luteal phase-only danazol. *Am J Obstet Gynecol* 1999;180:18–23
15. Greenblatt RB, Asch RH, Mahesh VB, Bryner JR. Implantation of pure crystalline pellets of estradiol for conception control. *Am J Obstet Gynecol* 1977; 127:520–7
16. Magos AL, Brincat M, Studd J. Treatment of the premenstrual syndrome by subcutaneous estradiol implants and cyclical oral norethisterone: placebo controlled study. *Br Med J* 1986;292:1629–33
17. Studd JWW, Domoney C, Khastgir G. The place of hysterectomy in the treatment of menstrual disorders. In *Disorders of the Menstrual Cycle*. London: RCOG Press, 2000;29:313–232
18. Magos AL, Brewster E, Singh R, O'Dowd T, Brincat M, Studd JWW. The effects of norethisterone in postmenopausal women on oestrogen replacement therapy: a model for the premenstrual syndrome. *Br J Obstet Gynaecol* 1986;93:1290–6
19. Bjorn I, Backstrom T. Drug related negative side-effects is a common reason for poor compliance in hormone replacement therapy. *Maturitas* 1999;32: 77–86
20. Panay N, Studd JWW. Progestogen intolerance and compliance with hormone replacement therapy in menopausal women. *Hum Reprod Update* 1997; 3:159–71
21. Watson NR, Studd JWW, Savvas M, Garnett T, Baber RJ. Treatment of severe premenstrual syndrome with oestradiol patches and cyclical oral norethisterone. *Lancet* 1989;23:730–2
22. Smith RNH, Studd JWW, Zambleera D, Holland EFN. A randomised comparison over 8 months of 100 μg and 200 μg twice weekly doses in the treatment of severe premenstrual syndrome. *Br J Obstet Gynaecol* 1995;102:475–84
23. Montgomery JC, Brincat M, Tapp A, *et al.* Effect of oestrogen and testosterone implants on psychological disorders in the climacteric. *Lancet* 1987;1: 297–9
24. Gregoire AJP, Kumar R, Everitt B, Henderson A, Studd JWW. Transdermal oestrogen for treatment of severe postnatal depression. *Lancet* 1996;3347: 930–3
25. Khastgir G, Studd JWW. Patients' outlook, experience and satisfaction with hysterectomy, bilateral oophorectomy and subsequent continuation of hormone replacement therapy. *Am J Obstet Gynecol* 2000;183:1427–33
26. Lawrie TA, Hofmeyr GJ, De Jager M, *et al.* A double blind randomised placebo controlled study of postnatal norethisterone enanthate: the effect on postnatal depression and hormones. *Br J Obstet Gynaecol* 1998;105:1082–90
27. Ahokas A, Kaukoranta J, Wahlbeck K, Aitom M. Oestrogen deficiency in severe postpartum depression. Successful treatment with sublingual physiologic 17β-oestradiol: a preliminary study. *J Clin Psychiatry* 2001;62:332–6
28. Bloch M, Schmidt PJ, Danaceau M, Murphy J, Nieman L, Rubinow DR. Effects of denerbal steroids in women with a history of postpartum depression. *Am J Psychiatry* 2000;57:924–30
29. Hunter MS. Depression and the menopause. *Br Med J* 1996;313:1217–18
30. Utian WH. The true clinical features of post-menopause and oophorectomy and their response to oestrogen therapy. *South Afr Med J* 1972;46:732–7
31. Campbell S, Whitehead M. Oestrogen therapy and the menopausal syndrome. *Clin Obstet Gynecol* 1977;4:31–47
32. Soares CN, al Maida OP, Joffe E, Cohen LS. Efficacy of oestradiol for the treatment of depressive disorders in perimenopausal women: a double blind randomised placebo controlled trial. *Arch Gen Psychiatry* 2001;58:529–34
33. Rasgon NL, Altshuler LL, Fairbanks LA, *et al.* Estrogen replacement therapy in the treatment of major depressive disorder in perimenopausal women. *J Clin Psychiatry* 2002;63(Suppl 7):545–8
34. Harlow BL, Wise LA, Otto MW, Soares CN, Cohen LS. Depression and its influence on reproductive endocrine and menstrual cycle markers associated with perimenopause: the Harvard Study of Moods and Cycles. *Arch Gen Psychiatry* 2003;60:29–36
35. Smith RN, Holland ES, Studd JWW. The symptomatology of progestogen intolerance. *Maturitas* 1994;18:87–91
36. Panay N, Studd JWW. Progestogen intolerance and compliance with hormone replacement therapy in menopausal women. *Hum Reprod Update* 1997;3:159–71
37. Watson NR, Studd JWW, Savvas M, Bayber R. The long-term effects of oestrogen implant therapy for the treatment of premenstrual syndrome. *Gynecol Endocrinol* 1990;4:99–107

Methodological pitfalls in the study of estrogen effects on cognition and brain function

29

P. M. Maki

INTRODUCTION

Meta-analyses of observational data consistently show a lower risk of Alzheimer's disease among women who have received hormone replacement therapy (HRT)[1-3], although a recent study suggests that only early use confers this protection[4]. By contrast, the evidence on HRT and normal cognitive aging is inconsistent. Some of the variation in results may reflect true differences in hormone effects and the possibility that HRT confers cognitive benefits to some but not all women. Individual differences such as age, time since menopause, menopausal symptoms and surgical versus natural menopause may modulate the effects of estrogen on cognition. The effects might also vary with different regimens, treatment durations and doses. Additionally, some of the variation in results may reflect varying degrees of sensitivity of the measures and/or procedures selected to study cognitive function. This chapter focuses on specific issues in the collection and interpretation of neuropsychological data in studies of cognition and HRT.

WANTING TOO MANY DATA POINTS FROM YOUR SUBJECTS: THE PITFALLS OF PRACTICE

An inherent limitation in the study of cognitive interventions is that performance on cognitive tests can improve with practice, to the point where the individual reaches the maximum test score or her maximum performance. Thus, the effect of the cognitive intervention must not only be greater than the effect of no treatment or a placebo treatment, but also be evident within the limited range of improvement in a cognitive test. Two estimates of the maximum level of performance in a test can be distinguished (Figure 1). The psychometric ceiling is the maximum score obtainable in a test; in a test with 30 items, the ceiling is 30. The psychometric ceiling is equal across individuals and is easily reached in mental status tests and other tests with limited sensitivity. Although it can be quantified, it can be masked in group data wherein many but not all participants reach the ceiling. The individual ceiling, by contrast, is the highest score possible for a particular individual. This concept recognizes individual variation in cognitive skills. For example, the maximum score on a test of verbal memory may be 60, but the maximum score for one individual might be one standard deviation above the mean, and for another, two standard deviations above the mean. This ceiling effect is especially problematic because it is unrecognized, and is difficult to detect or quantify except by looking at individual trajectories of change over time. Frequent test sessions

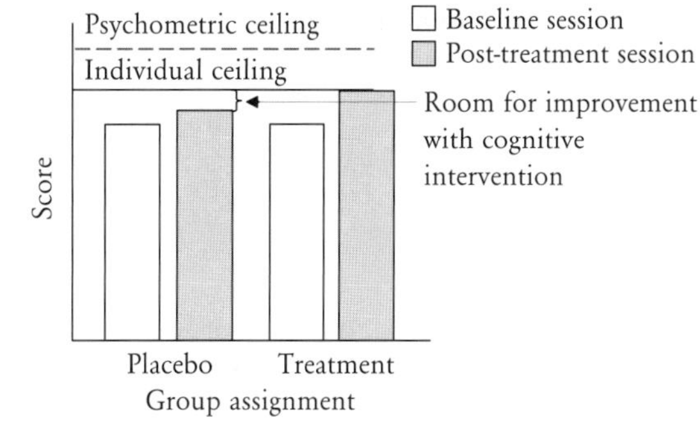

Figure 1 Ceiling effects in hypothetical randomized clinical trial

over a short interval increase the likelihood that an individual will reach her maximum performance.

There are two general approaches to minimizing these ceiling effects. One option is to conduct assessments at one time only and assume equal baselines, a methodological approach used in the recent ancillary study to the Heart and Estrogen/progestin Replacement Study[5]. This approach is more appropriate in large samples of women where equal baselines are more likely. The alternative is to conduct a repeated-measures analysis, but limit the number of longitudinal assessments and space test sessions to minimize practice effects. Practice effects in standardized cognitive tests are evident over intervals longer than a year even in older individuals[6]. Short-term intervention trials are especially vulnerable to practice effects, because practical considerations frequently limit the duration of the interval between test sessions. In contrast, it is often easier to space test sessions in observational studies. Because they typically involve longer intervals, observational studies may be more sensitive to the effects of HRT over time. In studies involving intervals of over a year between longitudinal assessments, beneficial effects of hormones were shown in tests of figural memory[7] and verbal memory[8].

EXTRAPOLATION OF MENTAL STATUS TO THE WHOLE OF COGNITION

A number of longitudinal studies have examined changes in mental status as a function of hormone use, because such measures are often used in epidemiological studies as a proxy for cognitive function. In studies involving large samples of older women, mental status instruments have been very useful in pointing to factors that might modulate cognitive aging, including apolipoprotein genotype[9], estrogen polymorphisms[10] and reproductive factors[11]. Mental status instruments, however, are non-specific, and insufficiently sensitive to normal, age-related changes in cognitive function. For instance, in a recent study, as many as 52% of women failed to make a single error in a test of mental status[12], and no effects of HRT were observed in the study. Despite the marked ceiling effect in performance in the mental status measure, the conclusion drawn from the study was that HRT 'is not protective for cognitive decline related to aging'[12]. It is important to be cautious in extrapolating mental status to cognitive aging and, in particular, to avoid interpreting the absence of changes in mental status to absence of changes in specific domains of cognitive function. Mental status measures are especially vulnerable to ceiling effects, lack sufficient sensitivity to age effects and do not measure specific domains of cognitive function that may be especially sensitive to hormone effects.

EXPECTING HRT TO AFFECT MORE COGNITIVE DOMAINS THAN IT DOES

Cognitive function is not unitary. Few factors, including age, affect all areas of cognitive function equally. In a recent review, we found that the most consistent finding from randomized clinical trials is of a beneficial effect of estradiol on verbal memory in recently surgically menopausal women[13]. The effects of HRT on verbal memory in older women are unclear. An observational study of women enrolled in the Baltimore Longitudinal Study of Aging suggested a significant beneficial effect of HRT on verbal memory and a trend towards better attention[14]. Similarly, a large randomized clinical trial of raloxifene found a lower risk of impairment in tests of verbal memory and attention among women on active treatment[15]. In contrast, the largest randomized clinical trial to date found worse performance in a test of verbal memory in older women with cardiovascular disease treated with conjugated equine estrogen and medroxyprogesterone acetate[5]. These studies suggest that tests of verbal memory may be especially sensitive to the effects of HRT. This is notable, given the female advantage over males in tests of verbal memory[16] and predictive validity of verbal memory tests in studies of preclinical dementia[17]. Hormone effects are also seen in tests of figural memory. A longitudinal study of women enrolled in the Baltimore Longitudinal Study of Aging demonstrated benefits of HRT for memory for designs in both cross-sectional and longitudinal analyses[7]. Notably, this measure also predicts dementia many years in advance of disease onset[18].

Evidence that the brain areas subserving memory performance, in particular the hippocampal formation, respond to estrogen in both humans and animals further supports the view that estrogen therapy may preferentially affect memory. Early animal studies demonstrated that exogenous and endogenous estradiol increased dendritic spine density in the CA1 region of the hippocampus[19,20]. In an early study, we found differential patterns of brain activation in those brain areas in HRT users and non-users as they performed verbal and figural memory tasks[21]. Specifically, activity during performance of a delayed verbal recognition memory task was compared with rest, and group differences were evident in the right parahippocampal gyrus, right precuneus, right dorsal frontal gyrus, right inferior frontal cortex and left hypothalamus. Areas showing alterations during performance of the figural memory task compared with rest included right inferior parietal lobe, right parahippocampal gyrus, left visual association cortex and left anterior thalamus. Importantly, the HRT users performed better in standardized measures of verbal memory and figural memory. In a longitudinal follow-up study, we found increased activation in the hippocampal formation in HRT users compared with non-users, suggesting HRT-related enhancements in neural activity in that brain region over time. Notably, the opposite pattern of activation is observed in individuals at increased risk for Alzheimer's disease[22]. Animal and human studies point to the hippocampus, and hippocampally mediated cognitive abilities, as particular targets of estrogen therapy. This underscores the biological plausibility of differential effects of estrogen in memory tests, compared with other cognitive functions (Figure 2).

FAILURE TO DISTINGUISH BETWEEN INDIRECT AND DIRECT EFFECTS OF HORMONES

Many reviews of HRT and cognitive function raise the criticism that studies do not control for menopausal symptoms, and that the cognitive effects of estrogens might be attributable to treatment-related improvements in sleep, mood, hot flushes and other menopausal symptoms. The argument is that the effects of hormones on cognitive function are indirect, and HRT has little direct effect on cognitive function. Although this argument has high face validity, there is ample evidence of direct effects of hormones on cognitive function and the brain areas underlying those functions as described above. It may be that the relative impact of direct and indirect influences varies across reproductive phases, with greater indirect effects during the perimenopause compared with the pre- and postmenopause.

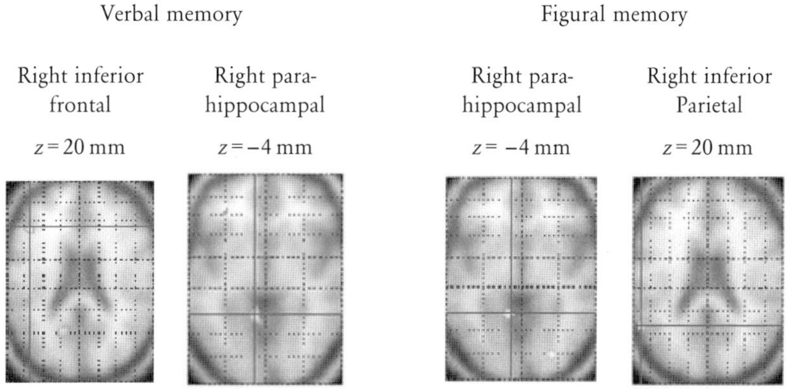

Figure 2 Hormone replacement therapy (HRT) is associated with improved memory and modulations in activity in brain areas subserving memory performance: voxel highlighted by cross-hair indicates region of altered activation for women on HRT. Reproduced from reference 21, with permission

In premenopausal women, ovarian hormones appear to exert direct effects on sexually dimorphic cognitive abilities. For example, in a recent study, young women completed a battery of neuropsychological tests at the early-follicular and mid-luteal phases of two successive menstrual cycles, with phase at first testing counterbalanced across participants. The pattern of results indicated a double dissociation, with enhancement of tests of fine motor skills, conceptual implicit memory and verbal fluency - tests that favor women over men - during the mid-luteal phase, and enhancement of a test of mental rotations during the early follicular phase (Figure 3)[23]. The finding of enhanced performance in tests of mental rotations when ovarian steroid hormone levels are lowest, and arguably most detrimental to cognitive function, contradict the theory that menstrual-cycle effects reflect hormone-related improvements in mood.

Fluctuations in circulating ovarian steroids appear to influence cognition indirectly in the perimenopause, through effects on mood and sleep. In a study of women followed across the menopausal transition in the Baltimore Longitudinal Study of Aging, no differences in performance in a standardized neuropsychological test battery were evident between pre- and perimenopausal women, suggesting no overall loss of cognitive function during the perimenopause. However, correlations between menopausal symptoms and cognitive test performance indicated an indirect effect of hormones on cognition. Mood and sleep disturbances correlated significantly with performance in effortful tests, such as tests of figural memory and mental rotations, but not in sexually dimorphic tests[24]. Notably, hot flush severity and frequency were unrelated to cognitive test performance, a finding reported in a sample of over 7478 women studied in the Multiple Outcomes of Raloxifene Evaluation (MORE)[15]. This suggests that perimenopausal hormone changes affect cognitive function indirectly through effects on sleep and mood, but not hot flushes.

A number of factors suggest that HRT-related improvements in memory in older women cannot be attributed primarily to improved menopausal symptoms or mood. First is the low frequency of menopausal symptoms in older women. Indeed, older women initiating HRT experience an increase of symptoms such as breakthrough bleeding and breast tenderness. Second, HRT-related improvements in cognition and brain function are seen in samples of HRT users and non-users who report similar, low levels of depressive symptoms[14,21,25]. Third, factors that are associated with increased endogenous estrogen but have little impact on menopausal symptoms are associated with enhancements of cognitive test performance in older postmenopausal women. These include estrogen receptor polymorphisms[10], bone mineral density[26] and circulating hormone levels[27] in older asymptomatic women. Moreover, reproductive factors associated with greater lifelong exposure

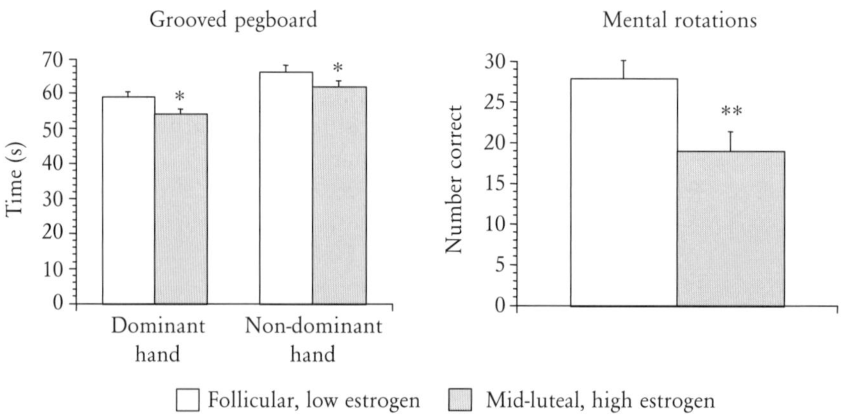

Figure 3 Performance in sexually dimorphic tests varies across the menstrual cycle, with mid-luteal enhancements in 'female' tasks such as fine motor performance (grooved pegboard) and decreases in 'male' tasks such as mental rotations ($n = 16$). $^*p < 0.01$, $^{**}p < 0.001$, significant difference compared with follicular phase

to estrogen, such as nulliparity and later age at menopause, are associated with better cognitive performance in older women[11]. Finally, HRT-related improvements in sleep are evident in younger symptomatic women, but not older asymptomatic women[28]. These converging lines of evidence contradict the argument that estrogen-related improvements in cognitive function in older women can be attributed to improvements in menopausal symptoms. Finally, improvements in mood and sleep would benefit cognition broadly, but HRT effects are frequently specific. Evidence of widespread benefit of HRT in samples of older women might suggest the influence of confounding factors such as education or health status, which tend to affect a broader range of cognitive abilities.

SUBOPTIMAL SELECTION OF CONTROL GROUPS

One of the primary limitations of observational cognitive studies is the need of control for differences between HRT users and non-users in education and health status, because, in most populations, HRT users are better educated and healthier than non-users[29]. There are two general approaches to controlling for the so-called healthy-user bias in observational studies: experimental control (matched samples) and *post hoc* statistical control. The conclusion drawn from observational studies varies, depending on which of these two approaches is used[13]. Of studies using direct experimental control, 92% showed a benefit of HRT on some aspect of cognitive function (11/12). Of studies using indirect statistical control, only 60% showed a benefit (9/15). Statistical adjustment increases scores of more poorly educated non-users and decreases scores of better-educated users, thereby lowering the difference between groups.

By definition, a control group differs from the experimental group in the factor of interest (e.g. HRT), and is similar to the experimental group in other factors. Insights into important clinical issues have been limited by suboptimal selection of control groups. For example, a recent study addressed the effects of HRT on cognition in women with a natural menopause, hysterectomy or hysterectomy plus oophorectomy[30]. The conclusion of the study was that 'Estrogen use did not improve the performance of hysterectomized women. In fact, among current estrogen users, women with a hysterectomy and bilateral oophorectomy performed significantly *worse* [emphasis theirs] than women without a hysterectomy . . . '. The inference appears to be that HRT in women with a hysterectomy and bilateral oophorectomy might be harmful. Note, however, that the appropriate analysis of this issue involves a comparison between hysterectomized and oophorectomized women receiving HRT and similar women not receiving HRT (not naturally menopausal women receiving HRT). When the appropriate control group is studied, no significant harmful effects are evident. Indeed, verbal memory performance was higher in HRT users in each group, and, although the effects were apparently non-significant, the data do not support the conclusion that estrogen therapy is harmful in women with a hysterectomy and oophorectomy.

EXCLUSIVE RELIANCE ON RANDOMIZED CLINICAL TRIAL DATA TO PROVIDE TRUTHFUL INSIGHTS

The randomized clinical trial is regarded as the gold standard in evidence-based medicine. In a randomized trial, we assemble study groups, intervene, follow them over time and quantify risk of disease. This design is in contrast with the prospective (observational) study in which we assemble the study group, follow them over time, identify those with exposure and those without exposure and quantify the risk of disease. The limitations of the prospective cohort design are well recognized, and include differential or biased exposure across groups, difficulty assessing the effects of initial exposure and imprecision in characterizing exposure. The limitations of randomized clinical trials are less well recognized, but have been brought to light in the area of HRT in recent critiques, particularly with regard to external validity[31].

There are clear limitations in prospective studies of HRT and cognitive function.

Differential exposure across study groups is seen in the healthy-user bias[29]. Individuals with high educational attainment are at decreased risk for Alzheimer's disease[32,33], and it might be the higher educational attainment rather than HRT that confers protection against Alzheimer's disease in studies of HRT. Current understanding of the effects of HRT on cognition is limited by another characteristic of observational trials, namely, difficulty in assessing the effects of initial exposure to HRT. This limitation may lead to an underestimation of the possible negative or beneficial effects on cognitive function. For example, subjects in the Women's Health Initiative (WHI) who were randomized to receive combined conjugated equine estrogen and medroxyprogesterone acetate showed an increased risk of stroke, and the yearly rates for venothrombolic events were highest in the initial year and decreased over the subsequent 5 years ($z = 2.45$, $p < 0.05$)[34]. That time effect, coupled with the rarity of the events (i.e. attributable risk of 8/10 000 women/year), may limit the sensitivity of prospective studies to detect cognitive impairment following stroke or transient ischemic attacks. Conversely, initial benefits of HRT on cognitive function owing to improvements in sleep and mood in younger menopausal women may not be evident in prospective studies of older women.

Randomized clinical trials address concerns about differential exposure across study groups and difficulty assessing initial exposure. However, other characteristics of randomized clinical trials can also mask truth. In her noted critique, the late Trudy Bush wrote: 'The truth is found only when there are sufficient numbers of appropriate studies, and no one study has a monopoly . . . the clinical trial is a very good study design, but not *necessarily* the ultimate study design'[35]. Some of the factors that can limit the validity of conclusions drawn from randomized clinical trials include intention-to-treat, external generalizability, volunteer bias, overall benefit of being in a trial, use of person-time for real time, placebo effect, effects that vary depending on length of trial and differential blindedness.

An examination of the literature on HRT and cognitive function raises some questions about the reliability and validity of clinical trial data in this area. Randomized clinical trials are not necessarily reliable; similar studies sometimes lead to different conclusions. For example, of three trials investigating reasoning, an executive function, two showed significant improvements following HRT treatment[36,37] while one did not[38]. Randomized clinical trials are not necessarily randomized. A recent review of studies published in the obstetrics and gynecology literature found evidence of non-random manipulation of study groups across studies, and inadequate allocation of treatment and concealment of treatment in the majority of studies[39]. Perhaps most important in the pursuit of evidence-based medicine is that randomized clinical trials are not always feasible; some issues cannot be addressed owing to cost and ethical considerations. One such issue is the effect of early versus late initiation of therapy. Evidence from a recently published prospective study indicates that estrogen might be most effective in lowering the risk of Alzheimer's disease when used earlier in life, and may have a detrimental effect when initiated later in life[4,40]. To investigate the possibility of a critical period of HRT use, a clinical trial would require randomization of large groups of women in their early 50s and ascertainment of Alzheimer's risk beginning 15 years later, when participants would reach an age associated with late-onset Alzheimer's disease. Such a study is cost-prohibitive.

Most observational data on HRT and Alzheimer's disease come from women who initiated HRT for the treatment of menopausal symptoms, because such women constitute the large majority of HRT users. In contrast, the only large-scale randomized clinical trial study of standard HRT and cognitive function is a study of combined conjugated equine estrogen plus medroxyprogesterone acetate in 1063 older women with cardiovascular disease[5]. Results indicated a statistically but not clinically significant detrimental effect of HRT on delayed verbal recall and a trend towards poorer verbal fluency. Older women with cardiovascular disease might not benefit from HRT, because they are more likely to have a genetic risk factor that has been shown to modulate the effects of HRT on cognitive function[41,42]. Can one then extrapolate from a randomized clinical trial in women with cardiovascular disease to women without cardiovascular disease? The WHI ancillary studies of dementia (WHI Memory Study or WHIMS) and cognitive aging (WHI Study of Cognitive Aging or WHISCA) will address this issue. These important studies will not, however, address another critical issue, namely, timing of initiation of HRT. Other issues concern the generalizability of these findings to estrogen alone, to regimens other than continuous combined and to other routes of administration.

The greater weight given to randomized clinical trials can lead to errors of extrapolation if the samples studied in randomized clinical trials and observational trials differ systematically. Samples studied in randomized clinical trials and observational studies differ in age at initiation of therapy and health status. High internal validity does not guarantee high external validity, and key questions will remain after the WHI. It is important to recognize the strengths and weaknesses of both observational and randomized clinical trials. Study findings from both approaches might be distributed around truth.

CONCLUSIONS

The ultimate determination of the efficacy of estrogen as a neuroprotective agent will come from clinical studies. That determination is a top priority in women's health, not only because Alzheimer's disease affects more women than men, but also because the base rate of the disease is high[30]. In perimenopausal women, the maintenance of cognitive skills is important in quality of life and career success. In all phases of a woman's life, consideration about possible benefits to cognitive function must be balanced against known health risks. Conclusions about the effects of HRT on cognitive function must be drawn from the best evidence available, and care must be taken in assessing external generalizability in important clinical questions. The expertise of epidemiologists, neuroscientists, cognitive neuropsychologists, obstetricians, gynecologists, endocrinologists and others must be brought together to develop the best research studies and best interpretation of available data. To this end, the field of cognitive neuropsychology offers insights into specific issues in cognitive assessment. Consideration of important methodological issues, including test sensitivity, specificity of HRT effects to particular cognitive domains during particular reproductive phases, practice effects, selection of appropriate control groups and caution in attributing direct effects of hormones to indirect effects will help us to determine the answer to this important question.

References

1. Yaffe K, Sawaya G, Lieberburg I, Grady D. Estrogen therapy in postmenopausal women: effects on cognitive function and dementia. *J Am Med Assoc* 1998;279:688–95
2. LeBlanc ES, Janowsky J, Chan BK, Nelson HD. Hormone replacement therapy and cognition: systematic review and meta-analysis. *J Am Med Assoc* 2001;285:1489–99
3. Hogervorst E, Williams J, Budge M, Riedel W, Jolles J. The nature of the effect of female gonadal hormone replacement therapy on cognitive function in post-menopausal women: a meta-analysis. *Neuroscience* 2000;101:485–512
4. Zandi PP, Carlson MC, Plassman BL, *et al.* Hormone replacement therapy and incidence of Alzheimer's disease in older women: The Cache County Study. *J Am Med Assoc* 2002;288:2123–9
5. Grady D, Yaffe K, Kristof M, Lin F, Richards C, Barrett-Connor E. Effect of postmenopausal hormone therapy on cognitive function: the Heart and Estrogen/progestin Replacement Study [Comment]. *Am J Med* 2002;113:543–8
6. Lamar M, Resnick SM, Zonderman AB. Longitudinal changes in verbal memory in older adults: distinguishing the effects of age from repeat testing. *Neurology* 2003;60:82–6

7. Resnick SM, Metter EJ, Zonderman AB. Estrogen replacement therapy and longitudinal decline in visual memory: a possible protective effect? *Neurology* 1997;49:1491–7
8. Jacobs DM, Tang MX, Stern Y, *et al.* Cognitive function in nondemented older women who took estrogen after menopause. *Neurology* 1998;50: 368–73
9. Yaffe K, Haan M, Byers A, Tangen C, Kuller L. Estrogen use, APOE, and cognitive decline: evidence of gene-environment interaction. *Neurology* 2000;54:1949–54
10. Yaffe K, Lui LY, Grady D, Stone K, Morin P. Estrogen receptor 1 polymorphisms and risk of cognitive impairment in older women. *Biol Psychiatry* 2002;51:677–82
11. McLay RN, Maki PM, Lyketsos CG. Effects of nulliparity and age at menopause on cognitive decline. *J Neuropsychiatry Clin Neurosci* 2003;in press
12. Fillenbaum G, Hanlon J, Landerman L, Schmader K. Impact of estrogen use on decline in cognitive function in a representative sample of older community-resident women. *Am J Epidemiol* 2001; 153:137–44
13. Maki PM, Hogervorst E. HRT and cognitive decline. *Best Pract Res Clin Endocrinol Metab* 2003;17:105–22
14. Maki P, Zonderman A, Resnick S. Enhanced verbal memory in nondemented elderly women receiving hormone-replacement therapy. *Am J Psychiatry* 2001;158:227–33
15. Yaffe K, Krueger K, Sarkar S, *et al.* Cognitive function in postmenopausal women treated with raloxifene. *N Engl J Med* 2001;344:1207–13
16. Kramer J, Delis D, Daniel M. Sex differences in verbal learning. *J Clin Psychol* 1988;44:907–15
17. Chodosh J, Reuben DB, Albert MS, Seeman TE. Predicting cognitive impairment in high-functioning community-dwelling older persons: MacArthur Studies of Successful Aging. *J Am Geriatr Soc* 2002;50:1051–60
18. Giambra LM, Arenberg D, Zonderman AB, Kawas C, Costa PT Jr. Adult life span changes in immediate visual memory and verbal intelligence. *Psychol. Aging* 1995;10:123–39
19. Woolley CS, Gould E, Frankfurt M, McEwen BS. Naturally occurring fluctuation in dendritic spine density on adult hippocampal pyramidal neurons. *J Neurosci* 1990;10:4035–9
20. Woolley CS, McEwen BS. Estradiol mediates fluctuation in hippocampal synapse density during estrous cycle in the adult rat. *J Neurosci* 1992; 12:2549–54
21. Resnick SM, Maki PM, Golski S, Kraut MA, Zonderman AB. Estrogen effects on PET cerebral blood flow and neuropsychological performance. *Horm Behav* 1998;34:171–84
22. Johnson KA, Jones K, Holman BL, *et al.* Preclinical prediction of Alzheimer's disease using SPECT. *Neurology* 1998;50:1563–71
23. Maki PM, Rich JB, Rosenbaum SR. Implicit memory varies across the menstrual cycle: estrogen effects in young women. *Neuropsychologia* 2002;40: 518–29
24. Mordecai K, Bellantoni M, Maki P. Cognition in pre- versus perimenopausal women: effects of menopausal symptoms. *J Int Neuropsychol Soc* 2002;8:312(abstr)
25. Maki PM, Resnick SM. Longitudinal effects of estrogen replacement therapy on PET cerebral blood flow and cognition. *Neurobiol Aging* 2000; 21:373–83
26. Zhang Y, Seshadri S, Ellison RC, Heeren T, Felson DT. Bone mineral density and verbal memory impairment: Third National Health and Nutrition Examination Survey. *Am J Epidemiol* 2001;154: 795–802
27. Yaffe K, Lui L, Grady D, Cauley J, Kramer J, Cummings S. Cognitive decline in women in relation to non-protein-bound oestradiol concentrations. *Lancet* 2000;356:708–12
28. Hays J, Ockene J, Brunner R, *et al.* Effects of estrogen plus progestin on health-related quality of life. *N Engl J Med* 2003;348:in press
29. Matthews KA, Kuller LH, Wing RR, Meilahn EN, Plantinga P. Prior to use of estrogen replacement therapy, are users healthier than nonusers? *Am J Epidemiol* 1996;143:971–8
30. Kritz-Silverstein D, Barrett-Connor E. Hysterectomy, oophorectomy, and cognitive function in older women. *J Am Geriatr Soc* 2002;50:55–61
31. Grimes DA, Lobo RA. Perspectives on the Women's Health Initiative trial of hormone replacement therapy. *Obstet Gynecol* 2002;100: 1344–53
32. Matthews K, Cauley J, Yaffe K, Zmuda JM. Estrogen replacement therapy and cognitive decline in older community women. *J Am Geriatr Soc* 1999;47:518–23
33. Launer LJ, Andersen K, Dewey ME, *et al.* Rates and risk factors for dementia and Alzheimer's disease: results from EURODEM pooled analyses. EURODEM Incidence Research Group and Work Groups. European Studies of Dementia. *Neurology* 1999;52:78–84
34. Writing Group for the Women's Health Initiative Investigators. Risks and benefits of estrogen plus progestin in healthy postmenopausal women: principal results from the Women's Health Initiative randomized controlled trial. *J Am Med Assoc* 2002;288:321–33
35. Bush T. Beyond HERS: some (not so) random thoughts on randomized clinical trials. *Int J Fertil Women's Med* 2001;46:55–9

36. Fedor-Freybergh P. The influence of oestrogens on the wellbeing and mental performance in climacteric and postmenopausal women. *Acta Obstet Gynecol Scand* 1977;64:1–91
37. Sherwin BB. Estrogen and/or androgen replacement therapy and cognitive functioning in surgically menopausal women. *Psychoneuroendocrinology* 1988;13:345–57
38. Rauramo L, Lagerspetz K, Engblom P, Punnonen R. The effect of castration and peroral estrogen therapy on some psychological functions. *Frontiers in Hormone Research*. 1975:94–104
39. Schulz KF. Assessing the quality of randomization from reports of controlled trials published in obstetrics and gynecology journals [Comment]. *J Am Med Assoc* 1994;272:125–8
40. Resnick SM, Henderson VW. Hormone therapy and risk of Alzheimer disease: a critical time. *J Am Med Assoc* 2002;288
41. Sano M, Bell K, Jacobs D. Cognitive effects of estrogens in women with cardiovascular disease: what we do not know. *Am J Med* 2002; 113:612–13
42. Saunders AM, Strittmatter WJ, Schmechel D, *et al.* Association of apolipoprotien E allele 4 with late-onset familial and sporadic Alzheimer's disease. *Neurology* 1993;43:1467–72

Safety and tolerability of transdermal testosterone therapy versus placebo in surgically menopausal women receiving oral or transdermal estrogen

30

J. A. Simon, S. R. Davis, N. B. Watts, V. P. Eymer, J. D. Lucas and G. D. Braunstein

The study was designed to evaluate the safety and tolerability of three doses of transdermal testosterone versus placebo in surgically menopausal women with hypoactive sexual desire disorder receiving oral or transdermal concomitant estrogen replacement therapy (ERT).

Two phase II clinical studies were performed. A total of 447 women receiving oral ERT, and varying by age, weight and time since surgical menopause, were enrolled in a 6-month, double-blind, multicenter trial. They were randomly assigned to receive placebo or testosterone 150, 300 or 450 μg/day by transdermal patch. A 6-month safety extension was added to this trial and 155 women consented to participate, continuing to receive the same dose. In the second trial, 77 women receiving transdermal ERT, and likewise diverse in baseline characteristics, were enrolled in a double-blind, 6-month multicenter trial in which they were randomized to receive placebo or a 300 μg/day transdermal testosterone patch.

Safety assessments, including liver function, hematology, carbohydrate metabolism, lipid profiles, clotting parameters, acne (assessed by the scale of Palatsi and colleagues[1]) and hirsutism (assessed by the Lorenzo pictorial rating scale[2]), were essentially unchanged from baseline in both studies at 6 months. Pooled adverse events for the two studies, including those of special interest discussed below, were comparable among all treatment groups (placebo and three testosterone doses), with no evidence of a dose-dependent effect at 6 months. Acne was reported as an adverse event in 14% of all patients and the reports were comparable among the four treatment groups. Breast pain was reported by 11% overall and the reports were also comparable among all groups. The occurrences of hot flushes (4%, overall), hirsutism (3%, overall) and alopecia (< 1%, overall) were not different among the four treatment groups. Fifty-four (10%) patients withdrew due to adverse events by 6 months. These were similarly distributed among the four treatment groups. In the 12-month extension, all safety assessments were again essentially unchanged from baseline. The adverse events of special interest remained low in frequency and comparable among the four treatment groups, except for an increase in hirsutism seen only in the 450-μg/day dose group. All adverse events involving hirsutism were assessed as mild or moderate in severity by the investigators. The patch showed good skin tolerability, with the majority of reactions at application sites assessed as mild. No deaths or drug-related, serious adverse events were reported in either study.

Overall, transdermal testosterone was well tolerated in a widely varied population of surgically menopausal patients. No clinically serious safety concerns were detected in patients treated with doses up to 450 μg/day of transdermal testosterone.

References

1. Palatsi R, Hirvensalo E, Liukko P, *et al.* Serum total and unbound testosterone and sex hormone binding globulin (SHBG) in female acne patients treated with two different oral contraceptives. *Acta Derm Venereol (Stockh)* 1984;64:517–23
2. Lorenzo EM. Familial study of hirsutism. *J Clin Endocrinol* 1970;31:556–64

Selective estrogen receptor modulators: effects in the brain

31

H. U. Bryant, V. Krishnan and D. Agnusdei

The broad systemic effects of estrogen influence a wide spectrum of physiological functions throughout a woman's life. During the earliest phases of life, estrogen controls the development of primary and secondary sex organs, influences the growth of long bones and imprints various behavioral circuits in the brain. Throughout the reproductive years, estrogen is a key player in the regulation of reproductive cycles, continues to maintain a regulatory role in bone turnover and also influences the cardiovascular, immune and integumentary systems. Following the cessation of cyclic exposure to estrogen with the menopause, a variety of pathological states emerge with the relative absence of this important regulatory hormone. Most acutely apparent among the effects of estrogen withdrawal are the discontinuation of reproductive cycles and menses. However, the importance of other beneficial effects of estrogen emerges as well with time, most important being the rapid loss of bone mass, which occurs when bone turnover dramatically rises with estrogen deficiency and which leads to the development of osteoporosis. The incidence of mortality and morbidity due to heart disease also rapidly increases in women following the menopause. The important role of estrogen within the central nervous system (CNS) also becomes apparent when estrogen levels drop, with the incidence of vasomotor symptoms (hot flushes), depression, alterations in mood and cognitive decline.

Replacement of estrogen in postmenopausal women has dramatic effects, which include an improvement in bone density[1], reduction of vasomotor symptoms[2] and beneficial effects on mood and behavior[3]. However, these benefits are tempered by the occurrence of a number of undesired actions. The effects of estrogen on the cardiovascular system have been a topic of intense recent interest, given the reported adverse impact of estrogen-progestin replacement on cardiovascular mortality[4]. Compounding this concern are the well-documented effects of estrogen on the uterus (resumption of menses and increased incidence of endometrial cancer[4]) and the growing body of evidence suggesting an increase in the risk for breast cancer[4], which together markedly reduce initial use of, or continued compliance with, estrogen replacement strategies. The introduction of selective estrogen receptor modulators (SERMs) offers one potential alternative for many of the desired effects of estrogen replacement, without the most serious undesired effects. For example, in postmenopausal women, raloxifene (a SERM used for the treatment and prevention of osteoporosis) increases bone mineral density[5], reduces fracture incidence[6] and improves markers of cardiovascular health[7], without stimulating the uterus[8] or breast[5]. In fact, an added benefit of the SERM approach to postmenopausal health care is a marked reduction of the incidence of breast cancer[9].

Of particular interest is the effect of SERMs on the brain, given the clear benefit of estrogen for menopausal symptoms such as hot flushes, and the likely beneficial effects of estrogen on behavior and cognition[10]. Early reports of the increased incidence of vasomotor symptoms in women receiving raloxifene[5] led to erroneous concerns and speculation that the compound might generically antagonize estrogen effects across the brain, and lead to cognitive deficits, or impairment of neuromuscular function with an increased risk of fracture due to falls[11]. As reviewed in this chapter, there is now clear evidence that these early concerns are invalid, based on both preclinical as well as clinical observations. Following a brief review of the currently available SERMs, estrogen receptors (ERs) in the brain and the penetration of SERMs into the brain, and specific actions of various SERMs, are discussed on the basis of their neuroendocrine effects, as well as their cognition-relevant effects on synaptogenesis and mediation of neurotransmission, and effects on cognition and other properties that have been connected with the beneficial effects of estrogen on the brain. One key theme that emerges is that the estrogen-agonistic or -antagonistic properties of SERMs cannot be generalized across the multitude of actions that estrogen produces in the brain. Furthermore, also it is not possible to generalize effects of various SERMs for a given action in the brain, as in many instances different SERMs produce different effects (both qualitative and quantitative) on the same brain function or parameter.

SELECTIVE ESTROGEN RECEPTOR MODULATORS

Three SERMs are currently approved for use in humans, although for different indications. These molecules are depicted in Figure 1. As stated above, raloxifene is approved for the treatment and prevention of osteoporosis in postmenopausal women. Raloxifene is a benzothiophene SERM, as is arzoxifene (a SERM currently in clinical trials[12]) and LY117018 (Figure 1). Tamoxifen is a SERM indicated for use in humans for the treatment and prevention of breast cancer[13]. A third SERM currently used in humans is clomiphene, based on its ability to stimulate ovulation[14]. Tamoxifen and clomiphene are both in the triphenylethylene chemical class. Other chemical structures have served as a nucleus for the synthesis of molecules with a SERM activity profile; these include: tetrahydronaphthylenes (e.g. lasofoxifene[15]), benzopyrans (e.g. levormeloxifene[16]), naphthylenes (e.g. nafoxidene[17]) and indoles (e.g. bazedoxifene[18]), among others. As the bulk of the brain activity-related data for SERMs has been generated with the compounds depicted in Figure 1, this chapter limits its scope to those agents.

ESTROGEN RECEPTORS IN THE BRAIN

Estrogen exerts most of its effects via the estrogen receptor (ER), which acts as an intracellular transcription factor to activate estrogen response gene transcription. Recent work suggests the presence of a membrane receptor for estrogen linked to rapid cellular activation via signal transduction pathways (i.e. mitogen-activated protein (MAP) kinase)[19]. Two known subtypes of ER exist, ERα and ERβ, with distinct tissue distribution profiles that exhibit some overlap within the brain[20,21], as well as the potential to interact with each other. *In vivo* ER binding with

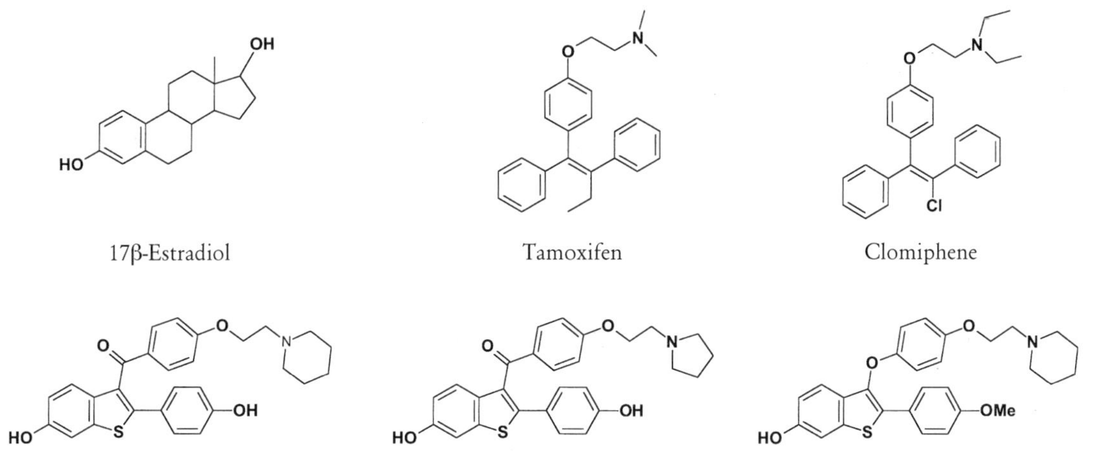

Figure 1 Structures of estradiol and various selective estrogen receptor modulators (SERMs)

^{125}I-estradiol shows nuclear binding sites in neurons associated with learning and memory, such as pyramidal cells throughout the CA1 and CA3 regions of the hippocampus and cortex[20], as well as in the midbrain regions traditionally associated with the regulation of temperature, feeding and neuroendocrine hormone production. Differential activity of SERMs such as raloxifene and tamoxifen, however, cannot be explained on the basis of differential ability to interact with either ERα or ERβ, either in the periphery or in the brain. Raloxifene, for example, shows very comparable affinity for, and ability to transactivate, either ER subtype[22].

BRAIN PENETRATION OF SERMS

Obviously, a central pharmacological tenet is that, for agents to exert their effect on a receptor, they must be available to the receptor. While physical-chemical properties of a molecule are generally the primary determinants of its overall bioavailability, exposure to the CNS is further complicated by the presence of the blood-brain barrier. Certainly, functional studies of the various SERMs argue strongly that there is sufficient exposure to exert an effect; however, critical factors such as dose, duration and agonist/antagonist potential may be severely or subtly affected by the ability of the molecule to penetrate the brain. In the case of tamoxifen, and its active metabolite 4-hydroxy-tamoxifen, ER binding studies suggested reduced (but not eliminated) penetration into the hypothalamus, compared with the pituitary or uterus[23]. Distributional studies of ^{3}H-raloxifene in ovariectomized rats demonstrated low-level penetration of raloxifene into blood-brain barrier-protected regions (i.e. cortex, hypothalamus, hippocampus[24]). As summarized in Table 1, the amount of radioactivity that was detected in the various brain structures was only 1–2% of the amount detected in the pituitary, a non-blood-brain barrier-protected structure. Thus, while the blood-brain barrier does appear to diminish the quantity of at least these two SERMs able to enter the brain, there still is appreciable uptake, which, based on the functional data reviewed below, is clearly capable of producing pharmacological effects in the brain.

Table 1 Distribution of 3H-raloxifene in ovariectomized rats

	1 h Post-injection	
Tissue	*Radioactivity* (dpm/g tissue)*	*Percentage of pituitary activity*
Liver	1 143 164 ± 96 422	481.7
Uterus	95 387 ± 10 570	40.2
Femur	130 930 ± 7650	55.2
Pituitary	237 300 ± 17 520	100
Brain		
cortex	2665 ± 250	1.1
hippocampus	3238 ± 707	1.4
striatum	2775 ± 702	1.2
thalamus	3388 ± 488	1.4
hypothalamus	1972 ± 524	0.8
brainstem	2781 ± 377	1.2
cerebellum	5139 ± 575	2.2

*Values represent mean ± SEM for five animals given 35 μCi of 3H-raloxifene (31.2 Ci/mmol)

NEUROENDOCRINE EFFECTS

Since tamoxifen and raloxifene were initially developed as anti-breast cancer agents, based on their ability to antagonize estrogen receptors in mammary tumor cells, initial attention regarding the CNS effects of these agents focused on their actions on neuroendocrine relationships, particularly with respect to the hypothalamic-gonadal axis. In cell culture studies, at the level of the hypothalamus and pituitary, raloxifene antagonized estrogen inhibition of luteinizing hormone (LH) secretion[25]. In estrogen-supplemented rats, raloxifene elevated the suppressed LH levels and blocked the elevation of prolactin induced by estrogen[26], and tamoxifen displayed estrogen-antagonist properties on LH release in other studies[27]. However, in the former study, a clear time of day dependency was noted[26]. In studies focusing on the pulsatile release of LH in ovariectomized rats without estrogen stimulation of the gonadal axis, raloxifene suppressed LH levels and elevated prolactin, indicating an estrogen-agonist profile[28], an observation that was consistent with the findings of Genazzani and colleagues[29]. Taken together, these studies suggest a classical partial agonist profile for raloxifene on the gonadal-ovarian axis. A similar partial agonist profile was also described for tamoxifen[27]. Interestingly, clomiphene is a SERM used explicitly to elevate LH and follicle stimulating hormone levels in order to induce ovulation, an effect probably due to increased sensitivity of the pituitary to gonadotropin-releasing hormone and prevention of the negative feedback effects of estrogen[30]. Of note, tamoxifen possessed a similar ability to that of clomiphene to induce ovulation in women[31].

With respect to higher neural circuitry regulating the gonadotropin axis, raloxifene and tamoxifen have estrogen-like effects on differentiation of hypothalamic circuitries controlling this function, when administered to neonates[28]. In other work, LY117018 produced estrogen-like effects on allopregnenolone levels in the hypothalamus, hippocampus and pituitary[29], and had an estrogen-like effect on β-endorphin levels in the hypothalamus and pituitary[32]. With respect to other neuroendocrine effects, raloxifene blocked estrogen-induced growth hormone release from somatotrophs in culture[33].

EFFECTS ON SYNAPTOGENESIS

Neuronal survival and synaptogenesis are key components of all higher neural functions, and beneficial effects of estrogen at this most basic level of neural function may form the foundation for the putative positive effects of estrogen on brain function. For example, dendritic spine density, a potential marker for synaptic interactions, is increased in the hippocampus when estrogen levels are high[34]. Cell culture systems have been quite useful for tracking the effects of estrogen on neurite outgrowth[35]. In PC12 cells, raloxifene at 10^{-7} mol/l produced an increase in neurite outgrowth that was comparable to that produced by nmol/l concentrations of 17β-estradiol, as determined by neurite length[36]. Raloxifene did not block the estrogen effect on neurite outgrowth in PC12 cells; in fact, the combination produced a slight additive effect[36]. In similar studies conducted in nerve growth factor (NGF)-treated SH-SY-5Y cells, 17β-estradiol-induced neurite outgrowth was antagonized by the pure estrogen antagonist, ICI-182-780, as well as by 4-hydroxy-tamoxifen[37]. Demonstrating a key difference between SERMs, raloxifene failed to block estradiol-induced neurite outgrowth in this neural cell line[37]. Thus, while there may be some differences between various SERMs, it is certain that at least some SERM molecules can mimic the synaptogenic effect of estrogen.

EFFECTS ON NEUROTRANSMISSION

Numerous connections have been made with respect to the beneficial effect of estrogen on various brain functions. Depression is associated with low levels of estrogen, and estrogen replacement improves or prevents depression[38]. Estrogen has also been associated with the symptoms of schizophrenia[39]. As already discussed, several links exist between estrogen and cognition. Each of these functions of the brain has been studied extensively with respect to the specific neurotransmitter systems that are affected. In most cases, multiple neurotransmitter systems are involved as various pharmacological approaches, or even agents with mixed pharmacology, provide symptomatic relief. A growing body of evidence is demonstrating a clear role for estrogen, as well as the SERMs, in regulating these neurotransmitter systems. Specific attention has been paid to: acetylcholine, serotonin, dopamine and the excitatory amino acids, each of which is discussed separately below.

Acetylcholine

Acetylcholine levels are depressed in the brains of patients with Alzheimer's disease[40], and treatments that increase cholinergic activity improve performance in learning and memory tasks[41]. Estrogen deficiency is associated with a reduction in hippocampal levels of choline acetyltransferase (ChAT), the rate-limiting enzyme in the synthesis of acetylcholine, and exposure to estrogen increases hippocampal ChAT levels[42]. The SERMs raloxifene and tamoxifen also increase ChAT levels in the hippocampus of ovariectomized rats[43]. Importantly, this effect of raloxifene is limited to ChAT activity in the hippocampus, as no effect of raloxifene was observed on ChAT activity in other brain regions such as the hypothalamus or cortex (regions which also failed to show dependency on estrogen for maintenance of ChAT activity)[43]. Consistent with likely reduced penetration of the blood-brain barrier, in ovariectomized rats the dose-response curve for hippocampal ChAT induction by raloxifene was shifted to the right, compared with efficacy in the maintenance of bone mineral density (i.e. effective dose - 50% (ED_{50}) of approximately 2.4 mg/kg for increase in ChAT activity with raloxifene vs. approximately 0.3 mg/kg for the bone protective effect ED_{50} in ovariectomized rats)[43]. In combination studies in animals, where raloxifene completely antagonized the uterine-stimulating activity of estrogen, no reduction in ChAT induction was observed, demonstrating simultaneously in two separate tissues estrogen antagonism by raloxifene (in the uterus) and complete estrogen agonism (for the hippocampal ChAT response)[43]. Thus, in the case of acetylcholine, raloxifene behaves as a complete estrogen agonist in the hippocampus.

Serotonin

The serotonin system plays an important role in the regulation of mood and anxiety and contributes to aspects of cognition, learning and memory. A clear connection between estrogen and regulation of serotoninergic outputs has been established, which may partially explain the beneficial effects of estrogen in the CNS[38,39]. In ovariectomized rats, site-specific alterations in various regulators of serotoninergic neurotransmission can be observed, such as the reduction of 5-hydroxytryptamine-2A ($5\text{-}HT_{2A}$) receptor mRNA in the cortex and midbrain[44]. Estrogen administration to ovariectomized rats[44], or in a genetic animal model of depression[45], was associated with an increase in $5\text{-}HT_{2A}$ receptor mRNA, as well as in serotonin transporter (SERT) mRNA in the forebrain. Studies with tamoxifen in ovariectomized rats showed no estrogen-like increases in forebrain or dorsal raphe $5\text{-}HT_{2A}$ receptor or SERT mRNA[46], but rather an antagonistic effect on the stimulatory effect of estrogen on $5\text{-}HT_{2A}$ receptor message induction, indicating an antagonist profile for tamoxifen. Alternatively, an estrogen-like increase in striatal levels of $5\text{-}HT_{2A}$ mRNA was detected in rats treated with tamoxifen[44]. Raloxifene, however, produces a much more estrogen-like overall profile in terms of $5\text{-}HT_{2A}$ receptor message in the forebrain and midbrain regions of ovariectomized rats[44]. While one report demonstrates minimal effects of raloxifene on SERT mRNA in the midbrain of ovariectomized rats[47], a 30-day study in ovariectomized macaques showed an estrogen-like effect on SERT mRNA in the midbrain. Notably in this study, raloxifene produced an estrogen-like elevation of tryptophan hydroxylase (TPH, a critical enzyme involved in neural serotonin production) activity in the midbrain of ovariectomized macaques[48]. TPH message was reduced by estrogen and raloxifene in the dorsal raphe of macaques[49]. In the ovariectomized monkey model, the SERM arzoxifene increased midbrain expression of TPH and reduced SERT, much like estrogen and raloxifene[48]. In summary, both raloxifene and tamoxifen mimicked some of the effects of estrogen on expression of key mediators of serotoninergic neurotransmission; however, raloxifene more closely paralleled the effects of estrogen than did tamoxifen. Furthermore, there was no indication of estrogen-antagonist effects with raloxifene, while in some instances a significant antagonist profile was observed with tamoxifen.

Dopamine

Yet another neurotransmitter associated with various psychoses, as well as neurodegenerative disorders of motor systems (i.e. Parkinson's disease), is dopamine. Several lines of evidence indicate an important role for estrogen in the modulation of striatal dopamine neurotransmission[50]. In ovariectomized rats, a reduction in specific binding to dopamine D_2 receptors was observed within 2 weeks[51]. 17β-Estradiol or raloxifene treatment for the 2-week period elevated D_2 binding in the lateral striatum, but tamoxifen at equivalent doses to raloxifene did not[51]. The effects of ovariectomy, 17β-estradiol and raloxifene were restricted to the striatum, as concomitant changes did not occur in other brain regions[51]. The pattern of changes in binding to the D_3 receptor were also similar for estrogen and raloxifene, but dissimilar for tamoxifen[51]. In a rat model of Parkinson's disease (1-methyl-4-phenyl-1,2,3,6-tetrahydropyridine (MPTP)-lesion model), a marked reduction of striatal content of dopamine and dopamine metabolites (i.e. 3,4-dihydroxyphenylacetic acid, homovanillic acid) was used as a marker of the extent of dopamine denervation[52]. 17β-Estradiol or raloxifene offered protection from the loss of dopamine and its metabolites in the striatum of MPTP-treated rats[52], an observation of potential importance given the reported beneficial effects of estrogen in Parkinson's disease[53].

Excitatory amino acids

Glutamate receptors represent one final area wherein important interactions with estrogen may explain some of the beneficial effects of estrogen on cognition and regulation of neuromuscular tone. *N*-methyl-D-aspartate (NMDA) and α-amino-3-hydroxy-5-methyl-4-isoxazoleproprionic acid (AMPA) receptors are subtypes of ionotropic glutamate receptors that have been implicated in memory[54] and excitotoxicity associated with Parkinson's disease[55]. Regional-specific effects of estrogen have been observed on NMDA receptor binding. For example, in the striatum, 17β-estradiol, raloxifene or tamoxifen reduced NMDA receptor binding[56], suggesting potential beneficial effects in Parkinson's as an excitatory amino acid antagonist. In other regions, such as the hippocampus, 17β-estradiol, raloxifene or tamoxifen increased NMDA receptor binding[56], consistent with a potential positive effect on learning and memory function. Cortical binding for both NMDA and AMPA receptors was reduced by 17β-estradiol, raloxifene or tamoxifen[57]. Thus, in contrast to the effects on serotoninergic and dopaminergic neurotransmission, tamoxifen and raloxifene produce a similar pattern of estrogen-agonist effects on glutamate receptors.

A summary of the effects of estrogen, raloxifene and tamoxifen on the various brain neurotransmitters is provided in Table 2. From this review, two important features emerge. First, the effects of the two SERM molecules do not perfectly parallel each other, particularly with respect to serotonin and dopamine effects. Second, the profile for raloxifene largely suggests that of a relatively complete estrogen agonist across these brain neurotransmitter effects. It is also important to note that some of the SERMs have been evaluated as well for effects on other important chemical messenger systems within the brain, which have been associated with beneficial effects on functions such as cognition. For example, in the cortical projections of basal forebrain neurons in ovariectomized rats, raloxifene produced an estrogen-like elevation of brain-derived neurotrophic factor (a neurotrophin associated with memory)[58]. LY117018 also produced an increase in hippocampal and cortical expression of TrkA (a component of the nerve growth factor receptor)[24].

EFFECTS ON COGNITION

Although there remains some controversy as to the beneficial effects of estrogen on cognition, there is a growing body of evidence demonstrating

Table 2 Effects of estrogen, raloxifene and tamoxifen on brain neurotransmission in ovariectomized rats and macaques: arrows indicate direction of response relative to ovariectomized controls[43–49,51,52,56,57]

	Acetylcholine	*Serotonin*					*Dopamine*	*Excitatory amino acid*		
		Cortex		*Striatum/hindbrain*						
	Hippocampal ChAT	*5-HT$_{2A}$-R*	*SERT*	*5-HT$_{2A}$-R*	*SERT*	*TPH*	*Striatum D$_2$-R*	*Striatum NMDA-R*	*Hippocampus NMDA-R*	*Cortex AMPA-R*
Estrogen	↑	↑	↑	↑	↓	↑	↑	↓	↑	↓
Raloxifene	↑	↑	no Δ	↑	↓	↑	↑	↓	↑	↓
Tamoxifen	↑	no Δ	no Δ	↑	no Δ	↓	no Δ	↓	↑	↓

ChAT, choline acetyltransferase; 5-HT$_{2A}$-R, serotonin 2A receptor; SERT, serotonin transporter; TPH, tryptophan hydroxylase; D$_2$-R, dopamine-2 receptor; NMDA-R, *N*-methyl-D-aspartate receptor; AMPA-R, α-amino-3-hydroxy-5-methyl-4-isoxazoleproprionic acid receptor; no Δ, no change enhanced cognitive performance in postmenopausal women who use estrogen[59]. However, concomitant use of progestin, to protect the uterus in most forms of hormone replacement therapy, complicates matters in the light of reported negative progestinal effects on cognition[60]. One disadvantage with respect to clinical studies of the effects of estrogens on cognition is that very few prospective, placebo-controlled, randomized trials have been conducted in a population of women at high risk for cognitive decline. This problem applies to the clinical evaluation of SERMs for cognitive effects as well, since the available cognition data for tamoxifen and raloxifene are the results of studies targeted at breast cancer and osteoporosis, respectively.

In women who used tamoxifen for 5 years for breast cancer, there was little difference in performance in a series of cognitive tests relative to women who had never used tamoxifen[61], although in women who had used tamoxifen there was an increase in physician visits for memory problems[61]. The confounding variable of the ongoing disease state in these women, however, must be factored into consideration, as more recent studies found no statistically significant differences in modified mental status examination, or in psychomotor speed[62].

Extensive evaluation of a raloxifene osteoporosis trial has been conducted in terms of effects of the agent on cognition. Driven primarily from an assessment of safety, the first report of 1-year data in approximately 140 women showed no negative effects on tests of cognitive performance[63]. The only difference observed in the study was a slight increase in performance of verbal memory in the raloxifene-treated women, at the 1-month time point[63]. Interestingly, this trend was consistent, at least, with the expected effect of estrogen typically associated with verbal memory[10]. A follow-up study in this population, following over 7700 women with an average 3-year exposure to raloxifene, showed similar results. While the ultimate conclusion of the study was that long-term exposure to raloxifene does not affect overall cognitive scores[64], two important additional results were clear. First, there was no evidence for untoward effects of raloxifene on memory function[64], and second, there continued to be a trend for lower risk of cognitive decline in raloxifene users in verbal memory tests, as well as in an attention test[64]. Despite earlier concerns with respect to potential adverse effects on cognition associated with hot flushes[11], this long-term study in osteoporosis patients showed no influence of hot flush incidence on cognitive performance across all treatment groups[64]. Subsequent study of the lowest decile from this study population (in terms of cognitive performance) suggested that the 120-mg dose of raloxifene (which is twice the normal 60-mg dose used for treatment of osteoporosis) reduced the risk of cognitive impairment in non-demented women, and tended to reduce the risk of Alzheimer's disease[65]. Given the limited uptake of raloxifene by the brain, this study suggests that higher doses of raloxifene, or perhaps SERMs with better brain penetration, might better be able to demonstrate positive effects in human cognition trials. Brain activation, as determined by whole brain functional magnetic resonance imaging, shows specific patterns during visual encoding with estrogen. In a study with raloxifene, shifts in activation were observed in the parahippocampal gyrus (decrease), lingual gyrus (decrease) and frontal gyrus (increase)[66], with an activity pattern similar to that observed with estrogen[67]. While raloxifene clearly affected brain activation patterns upon visual encoding, the impact of these changes is uncertain, as these changes were not accompanied by any changes in performance levels[66]. With respect to the central effects, chronic treatment of postmenopausal women with raloxifene also produced no untoward effects on mood, sexual behavior or sleep[68].

Relatively little animal work has been done with respect to SERM effects on cognition. In one trial, a small group of long-term post-ovariectomy monkeys were given raloxifene or ethinylestradiol. While estrogen improved spatial working memory in this aged animal model, no significant effects were observed for raloxifene, although some parameters demonstrated a trend in a favorable direction for the SERM[69].

OTHER SERM EFFECTS OF RELEVANCE TO THE BRAIN

There are numerous additional beneficial effects of estrogen and SERMs in the brain that exist outside the above categories. Perhaps most notable of these are the protective effects in experimental models of stroke, where estrogen is neuroprotective[70]. Tamoxifen, for example, was neuroprotective in rats following middle cerebral artery occlusion[71]. Various mechanisms may contribute to this activity, including inhibitory effects on excitatory amino acid release, and putative antioxidant properties, as well as inhibition of production of reactive oxynitrite species[72]. A beneficial effect on blood flow, via activation of endothelial-derived nitric oxide synthase[73], as has been described with raloxifene, might also contribute to neuroprotection against ischemic damage in the brain following stroke injury. Arzoxifene is one other SERM for which a neuroprotection from focal cerebral ischemia following middle cerebral artery occlusion was observed[74]. Interestingly, the beneficial effect of arzoxifene against stroke damage was dissociated from effects on cerebral blood flow[74].

The observation that raloxifene produces a slight but significant increase in the incidence of hot flushes in postmenopausal women was initially the focus of some concern, with respect to broader examples of estrogen antagonism in the brain[5,11]. Work in an animal model of vasomotor symptoms, however, suggests that in this case raloxifene may be demonstrating a partial agonist profile. In a morphine withdrawal model, tail skin temperature fluctuations are controllable by administration of exogenous estrogen, and raloxifene has been shown to block this effect of estrogen[75]. In work conducted in our laboratory with this model, pushing the dose of raloxifene high enough can lead to partial suppression of the increase in tail skin temperature (Figure 2), consistent with the profile of a partial agonist.

An effect very characteristic of estrogenic agents in the rat is a marked reduction of body weight, in large part due to a reduction in feeding behavior. Raloxifene and LY117018 both produce similar estrogen-like anorectic effects in ovariectomized rats[24]. Finally, one important potential mechanism for estrogen action in the brain, particularly the neuroprotective action, may be linked to antioxidative properties that are associated with the phenolic A ring of certain estrogens. These antioxidant effects have been linked with neuroprotection versus oxidative stress and activation of novel signalling pathways, or perhaps induction of antiapoptotic proteins[76]. In this regard, an antioxidant effect has been observed with raloxifene in rat brain[77].

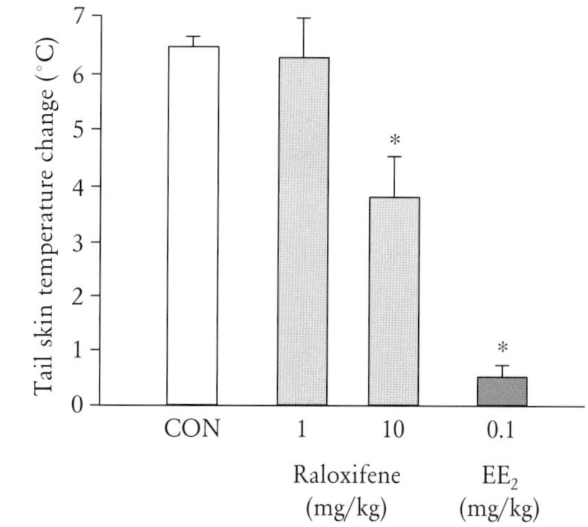

Figure 2 Effect of raloxifene and ethinylestradiol (EE_2) on tail skin temperature in the morphine withdrawal hot flush model. Bars represent the mean tail skin temperature change for six rats + SEM. *$p < 0.05$ vs. control (CON)

SUMMARY

Interest in the effects of estrogen on the brain is growing at a rapid rate. However, today, most of the available clinical information on estrogen effects on brain function is actually related to hormone replacement therapy, that is, combinations of estrogen and a progestin, to reduce the incidence of uterine endometrial cancer. Although not reviewed here, concerns have been raised elsewhere that progestins can in some cases inhibit estrogen effects in the brain, and progestins have been associated with increased depression scores. Since SERMs such as raloxifene do not have estrogen-like stimulatory effects on the uterus, they can be administered without concomitant use of a progestin, which creates the possibility of exploring the effects of ER modulation alone on brain

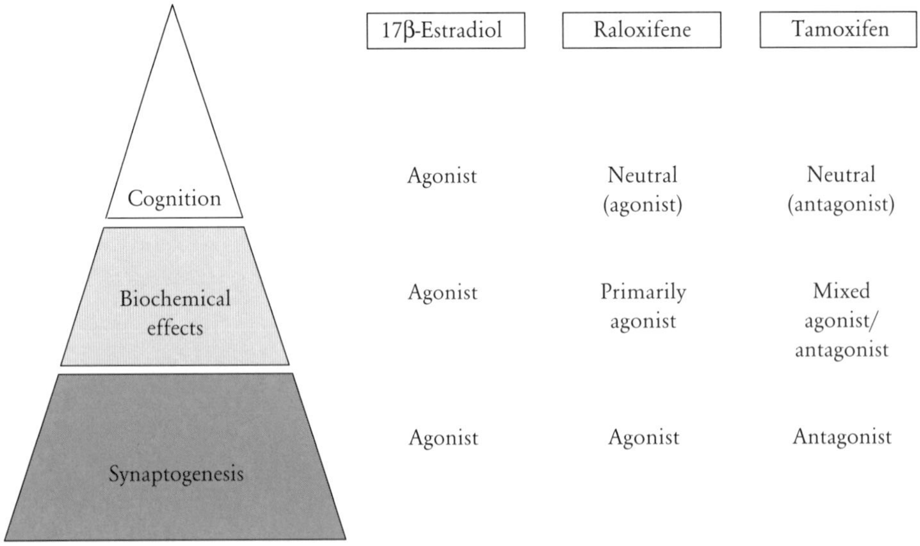

Figure 3 Summary of estradiol and selective estrogen receptor modulator (SERM) effects on central nervous system (CNS)

function. As depicted in Figure 3, the beneficial effects of estrogen on brain function can be considered as building upon each other, with neuronal viability and synaptogenesis underlying important effects of estrogen on key neurotransmitters and growth factors, which in turn combine to produce the beneficial effects that have been observed with functions such as cognition. In many cases, the effects of SERMs parallel those of natural estrogens. Several key points should be emphasized, however, when evaluating SERM action in the brain. These important points include:

(1) SERMs such as raloxifene and tamoxifen penetrate the blood-brain barrier, albeit to a lesser degree of exposure than found in peripheral organs. This does not mean necessarily, though, that all SERMs will have limited exposure to the brain.

(2) Antagonism of estrogen action with respect to one brain function by a SERM (i.e. hot flushes) does not indicate that a generic estrogen-antagonist profile will be detected throughout the brain. In fact, for a SERM like raloxifene, both estrogen-agonist and -antagonist effects can be observed in a site- and function-dependent manner. Furthermore, in most cases where an estrogen-antagonist character has been ascribed to SERMs like raloxifene in the brain, in actuality, a partial agonist profile is more likely to be the case (i.e. induction of hot flushes or neuroendocrine effects on LH release).

(3) Individual SERMs differ in their profile of activity in the CNS, as certainly is the case for tamoxifen and raloxifene. As CNS characteristics of other SERMs are determined, it may be possible to predict some activity profiles, but at present, each individual SERM molecule needs to be evaluated separately for effects in the brain. Generically associating class effects in this case should be avoided.

(4) The potential exists for either current or future SERMs to produce beneficial effects on brain functions ranging from cognition to mood to regulation of motor tone. Unfortunately, most clinical trials to date with SERM effects in the CNS have focused on other disease populations (i.e. breast cancer- or osteoporosis-patient studies), and to get a better understanding of potential beneficial effects in diseases such as Alzheimer's, studies focused on the disease population of interest are necessary. Preliminary evidence, such as that recently generated with raloxifene, is very encouraging.

References

1. Lindsay R, Aitken JM, Anderson JB. Long-term prevention of postmenopausal osteoporosis by estrogen. *Lancet* 1976;I:1038–41
2. Bachmann GA. Vasomotor flushes in menopausal women. *Am J Obstet Gynecol* 1999;180:S312–16
3. Finke G, Sumner BE, McQueen JK, *et al.* Sex steroid control of mood, mental state and memory. *Clin Exp Pharmacol Physiol* 1998;25:764–75
4. Rossouw JE, Anderson GL, Prentice RL, *et al.* Risks and benefits of estrogen plus progestin in healthy postmenopausal women: principal results from the Women's Health Initiative randomized controlled trial. *J Am Med Assoc* 2002;288:321–33
5. Delmas PD, Bjarnason NH, Mitlak BH, *et al.* Effects of raloxifene on bone mineral density, bone turnover, and serum cholesterol concentrations and uterine endometrium in postmenopausal women. *N Engl J Med* 1997;337:1641–7
6. Ettinger B, Black DM, Mitlak BH, *et al.* Reduction of vertebral fracture risk in postmenopausal women with osteoporosis treated with raloxifene. *J Am Med Assoc* 1999:282:637–45
7. Barrett-Connor E, Grady D, Sashegyi A, *et al.* Raloxifene and cardiovascular events in osteoporotic postmenopausal women: Four-year results from the MORE randomized trial. *J Am Med Assoc* 2002:287:847–57
8. Fugure P, Scheele WH, Shah A, *et al.* Uterine effects of raloxifene in comparison with continuous-combined hormone replacement therapy in postmenopausal women. *Am J Obstet Gynecol* 2000; 182:568–74
9. Cauley JA, Norton L, Lippman ME, *et al.* Continued breast cancer risk reduction in postmenopausal women treated with raloxifene: 4-year results from MORE trial. Multiple Outcomes of Raloxifene trial. *Breast Cancer Res Treat* 2001;65: 125–34
10. Sherwin BB. Cognitive assessment for postmenopausal women and general assessment of their mental health. *Psychpharmacol Bull* 1998;34: 323–6
11. Birge SJ. Can falls and hip fracture be prevented in frail older adults [Editorial]? *J Am Geriatr Soc* 1999;47:1265–6
12. Munster PH, Buzdar A, Dhingra K, *et al.* Phase I study of a third generation selective estrogen receptor modulator, LY353381.HCl, in metastatic breast cancer. *J Clin Oncol* 2001;19:2002–9
13. O'Reagan RM, Jordan VC. The evolution of tamoxifen therapy in breast cancer: selective oestrogen receptor modulators and down regulators. *Lancet Oncol* 2002;3:207–14
14. Tavaniotou A, Albano C, Smitz J, *et al.* Effect of clomiphene citrate on follicular and luteal phase luteinizing hormone concentrations in *in vitro* fertilization cycles stimulated with gonadotropins and gonadotropin-releasing hormone antagonist. *Fertil Steril* 2002;77:733–7
15. Ke HZ, Qi H, Crawford DT, *et al.* Lasofoxifene, a selective estrogen receptor modulator, prevents bone loss induced by aging and orchidectomy in the adult rat. *Endocrinology* 2000;141:1338–44
16. Alexandersen P, Riis BJ, Stakkestad JA, *et al.* Efficacy of levormeloxifene in the prevention of postmenopausal bone loss and on the lipid profile compared to low dose hormone replacement therapy. *J Clin Endocrinol Metab* 2001;86:755–60
17. Camerman N, Chan LY, Camerman A. Crystal and molecular structure of nafoxidine and stereochemical features of anticancer antiestrogens. *J Med Chem* 1980;23:941–5
18. Komm BS, Lyttle CR. Developing a SERM: stringent preclinical selection criteria leading to an acceptable candidate for clinical evaluation. *Ann NY Acad Sci* 2001;949:317–26
19. Rezandi M, Pedram A, Green GL, *et al.* Cell membrane and nuclear estrogen receptors originate from a single transcript: studies of ERα and ERβ expressed in Chinese hamster ovary cells. *Anat Embryol* 1999;199:379–90
20. Shugrue PJ, Merchenthaler I. Distribution of estrogen receptor α immunoreactivity in the central nervous system. *J Comp Neurol* 2001;43: 64–81
21. Kuipper GGJM, Shughrue PJ, Merchentaler I, *et al.* The estrogen receptor β subtype: a novel mediator of estrogen action in the neuroendocrine systems. *Front Neuroendocrinol* 1998;19:253–6
22. Gize EA, Venugopalan M, Glasebrook AL, *et al.* Characterization of raloxifene binding and transactivation properties of the estrogen receptor β. *J Bone Miner Res* 1997;12(Suppl 1):S428
23. Bowman SP, Leake A, Morris ID. Hypothalamic, pituitary and uterine cytosolic and nuclear oestrogen receptors and their relationship to the serum concentration of tamoxifen and its metabolite, 4-hydroxy-tamoxifen, in the ovariectomized rat. *J Endocrinol* 1982;94:167–75
24. Bryant HU, Bales KR, Paul SM, *et al.* Estrogen agonist effects of selective estrogen receptor modulators in ovariectomized rat brain. *Soc Neurosci Abstr* 1997;23:2377
25. Simard J, Labrie F. Keoxifene shows pure antiestrogenic activity in pituitary gonadotrophs. *Mol Cell Endocrinol* 1995;39:141–4
26. Clemens JA, Bennet DR, Black LH, *et al.* Effects of a new antiestrogen, keoxifene, on growth of carcinogen-induced mammary tumors and on LH and prolactin levels. *Life Sci* 1983;32:2869–75

27. Sanchez-Criado JE, Guelmes P, Bellido C, *et al.* Tamoxifen but not other selective estrogen receptor modulators antagonizes estrogen actions on luteinizing hormone secretion while inducing gonadotrophin-releasing hormone self-priming in the rat. *Neuroendocrinology* 2002;76:203–13
28. Pinilla L, Gonzalez LC, Tena-Sempere M, *et al.* Evidence for an estrogen-like action of raloxifene upon the hypothalamic-pituitary unit: raloxifene inhibits luteinizing hormone secretion and stimulates prolactin secretion in ovariectomized female rats. *Neurosci Lett* 2002;311:149–52
29. Genazzani AR, Bernardi F, Stomati M, *et al.* Effects of estradiol and raloxifene analog on brain, adrenal and serum allopregnenolone content in fertile ovariectomized female rats. *Neuroendocrinology* 2000;72:162–70
30. Engel JB, Felberbaum RE, Eilers W. Clomiphene-induced LH surges and cetrorelix. *Reprod Biomed Online* 2002;5:109–11
31. Boostanfar R, Jain JK, Mishell DR, *et al.* A prospective randomized trial comparing clomiphene citrate with tamoxifen citrate for ovulation induction. *Fertil Steril* 2001;75:1024–6
32. Genazzani AR, Bernardi F, Stomati M, *et al.* Raloxifene analog LY117018 effects on central and peripheral β-endorphin. *Gynecol Endocrinol* 1999; 13:249–58
33. Martinoli MG, Veilleux R, Pelletier G. Effects of triiodothyronine, dexamethasone and estradiol 17β on GH mRNA in rat pituitary cells in culture as revealed by *in situ* hybridization. *Acta Endocrinol* 1991;124:83–90
34. Woolley C, McEwen BS. Estradiol mediates fluctuation in hippocampal synapse density during the estrous cycle in the adult rat. *J Neurosci* 1992; 12:2549–54
35. Sohrabji F, Green LA, Miranda RC, *et al.* Reciprocal regulation of estrogen and NGF receptors by their ligands in PC12 cells. *J Neurobiol* 1994;25:974–88
36. Nilsen J, Mor G, Naftolin F. Raloxifene induces neurite outgrowth in estrogen receptor positive PC12 cells. *Menopause* 1998;5:211–16
37. Krishnan V, Wagle A, Singh JP, Yang NN, Bryant HU. Neuroprotective effects of 17β-estradiol are mediated by ERα and ERβ. Presented at the *Gordon Research Conference*, Hong Kong, June 2000:abstr
38. Hlatky MA, Boothroyd D, Vittinghoff E, *et al.* Quality of life and depressive symptoms in postmenopausal women after receiving hormone therapy. *J Am Med Assoc* 2002;287:591–7
39. Riecher-Rossler A, Hafner H. Schizophrenia and oestrogen – is there an association? *Eur Arch Psychiatry Clin Neurosci* 1993;242:323–8
40. Muir JL. Acetylcholine, aging and Alzheimer's disease. *Pharmacol Biochem Behav* 1997;56:155–63
41. Ohara T, Tanaka K, Fukaya H, *et al.* SDZ ENA 713 facilitates central cholinergic function and ameliorates spatial memory impairment in rats. *Behav Brain Res* 1997;83:229–33
42. Singh M, Meyer EM, Millard WJ, *et al.* Ovarian steroid deprivation results in a reversible learning impairment and compromised cholinergic function in female Sprague Dawley rats. *Brain Res* 1994;644:305–12
43. Wu X, Glinn MA, Ostrowski NL, *et al.* Raloxifene and estradiol benzoate both fully restore hippocampal choline acetyltransferase activity in ovariectomized rats. *Brain Res* 1999;847:98–104
44. Cyr M, Landry M, DiPaolo T. Modulation of estrogen receptor directed drugs of 5-hydroxytryptamine-2A receptors in rat brain. *Neuropsychopharmacology* 2000;23:69–78
45. Osterlund MK, Overstreet DH, Hurd YL. The Flinders sensitive line rats, a genetic model of depression, show abnormal serotonin receptor mRNA expression in the brain that is reversed by 17β-estradiol. *Mol Brain Res* 1999;74:158–66
46. Sumner BEH, Grant KE, Rosie R, *et al.* Effects of tamoxifen on serotonin transporter and 5-hydroxytryptamine 2A receptor binding sites and mRNA levels in the brain of ovariectomized rats with or without acute estradiol replacement. *Mol Brain Res* 1999;73:119–28
47. Zhou W, Koldzic-Zivanovic N, Clarke CH, *et al.* Selective estrogen receptor modulator effects in the rat brain. *Neuroendocrinology* 2002;75:24–33
48. Bethea CL, Mirkes SJ, Su A, *et al.* Effects of oral estrogen, raloxifene and arzoxifene on gene expression in serotonin neurons of macaques. *Psychoneuroendocrinology* 2002;27:431–45
49. Bethea CL, Mirkes SJ, Shively CA, *et al.* Steroid regulation of tryptophan hydroxylase protein in the dorsal raphe of macaques. *Biol Psychiatry* 2000;47:562–76
50. Van Hartesveldt C, Joyce JN. Effects of estrogen on the basal ganglia. *Neurosci Biobehav Rev* 1986; 10:1–14
51. Landry M, Levesque D, DiPaolo T. Estrogenic properties of raloxifene, but not tamoxifen, on D2 and D3 dopamine receptors in the rat forebrain. *Neuroendocrinology* 2002;76:214–22
52. Grandbois M, Morissette M, Callier S, *et al.* Ovarian steroids and raloxifene prevent MPTP-induced dopamine depletion in mice. *NeuroReport* 2000;11:343–6
53. Saunders-Pullman R, Gordon-Elliot J, Parides M, *et al.* The effect of estrogen replacement on early Parkinson's disease. *Neurology* 1999;52:1417–21
54. Bliss TV, Collingridge GL. A synaptic model of memory: long-term potentiation in the hippocampus. *Nature (London)* 1993;361:31–9
55. Dunnett SB, Bjorklund A. Prospects for new restorative and neuroprotective treatments in Parkinson's disease. *Nature (London)* 1999;399: A32–9

56. Cyr M, Thibault C, Morissette M, *et al.* Estrogen-like activity of tamoxifen and raloxifene on NMDA receptor binding and expression of its subunits in rat brain. *Neuropsychopharmacology* 2001;25:242-57
57. Cyr M, Ghribi O, Thibault C, *et al.* Ovarian steroids and selective estrogen receptor modulators activity on rat brain NMDA and AMPA receptors. *Brain Res Rev* 2001;37:153-61
58. Littleton-Kearney, Ostrowski NL, Cox DA, *et al.* Selective estrogen receptor modulators: tissue actions and potential for CNS protection. *CNS Drug Rev* 2002;8:309-30
59. Yaffe K, Sawaya G, Lieberberg, *et al.* Estrogen therapy in postmenopausal women: effects on cognitive function and dementia. *J Am Med Assoc* 1998;279:688-95
60. Hernandez ML, Fernandez-Ruiz JJ, De Miguel R, *et al.* Time-dependent effects of ovarian steroids on tyrosine hydroxylase activity in the limbic forebrain of female rats. *J Neural Transm Gen Sect* 1991;83:77-84
61. Paganini-Hill A, Clark LJ. Preliminary assessment of cognitive function in breast cancer patients treated with tamoxifen. *Breast Cancer Res Treat* 2000;64:165-76
62. Ernst T, Chang L, Cooray D, *et al.* The effects of tamoxifen and estrogen on brain metabolism in elderly women. *J Natl Cancer Inst* 2002;94:592-7
63. Nickelsen T, Lufkin EG, Riggs BL, *et al.* Raloxifene hydrochloride, a selective estrogen receptor modulator: safety assessment of effects on cognitive function and mood in postmenopausal women. *Psychoneuroendocrinology* 1999;24:115-28
64. Yaffe K, Krueger K, Sarkar S, *et al.* Cognitive function in postmenopausal women treated with raloxifene. *N Engl J Med* 2001;344:1207-13
65. Yaffe K, Krueger K, Blackwell T, *et al* Effect of raloxifene on the prevention of dementia and cognitive impairment in older women: results from the Multiple Outcomes of Raloxifene evaluation trial. Presented at the *Conference on Alzheimer's Disease*, Stockholm, 2002:abstr 274
66. Neele SJM, Rombouts SARB, Bierlaagh MA, *et al.* Raloxifene affects brain activation patterns in postmenopausal women during visual encoding. *J Clin Endocrinol Metab* 2001;86:1422-4
67. Shaywitz SE, Shawitz BA, Pugh KR, *et al.* Effect of estrogen on brain activation patterns in postmenopausal women during working memory tasks. *J Am Med Assoc* 1999;281:1197-202
68. Voss S, Quail D, Dawson A, *et al.* A randomized, double-blind trial comparing raloxifene HCl and continuous combined hormone replacement therapy in postmenopausal women: effects on compliance and quality of life. *Br J Obstet Gynaecol* 2002;109:874-85
69. Lacreuse A, Wilson ME, Herndon. Estradiol, but not raloxifene, improves aspects of spatial working memory in aged ovariectomized rhesus monkeys. *Neurobiol Aging* 2002;23:589-600
70. Rusa R, Alkayed NJ, Traystman RJ, *et al.* Estrogen replacement therapy is protective in experimental stroke. *Stroke* 1999:30:1665-70
71. Kimelberg HK, Feustel PJ, Jin Y, *et al.* Acute treatment with tamoxifen reduces ischemic damage following middle cerebral artery occlusion. *NeuroReport* 2000;11:2675-9
72. Osuka K, Fuestel PJ, Mongin AA, *et al.* Tamoxifen inhibits nitrotyrosine formation after reversible middle cerebral artery occlusion in the rat. *J Neurochem* 2001;76:1842-50
73. Simoncini T, Genazzani AR. Raloxifene acutely stimulates nitric oxide release from human endothelial cells via an activation of endothelial nitric oxide synthase. *J Clin Endocrinol Metab* 2000;85:2966-9
74. Rossberg MI, Murphy SJ, Traystman RJ, *et al.* LY353381.HCl, a selective estrogen receptor modulator, and experimental stroke. *Stroke* 2000;31:3041-6
75. Merchenthaler I, Funkhauser JM, Carver JM, *et al.* The effect of estrogens and antiestrogens in a rat model for hot flush. *Maturitas* 1998;30:307-16
76. Green PS, Yang SH, Simpkins JW. Neuroprotective effects of phenolic A ring oestrogens. *Novartis Foundation Symp* 2000;230:202-20
77. Siefer DB, Roa-Pena L, Keefe DL, *et al.* Increasing hypothalamic arcuate nucleus glial peroxidase activity in aging female rats is reduced by an antiestrogen and a gonadotropin-releasing hormone agonist. *Menopause* 1994;1:83-90

Index